CLINICAL INSTRUCTION AND EVALUATION

A Teaching Resource

Andrea B. O'Connor

NLN
P R E S S

CLINICAL INSTRUCTION AND EVALUATION

A Teaching Resource

Andrea B. O'Connor, EdD, JD, RN

Professor
Department of Nursing
Western Connecticut State University
Danbury, Connecticut

JONES AND BARTLETT PUBLISHERS
Sudbury, Massachusetts
BOSTON   TORONTO   LONDON   SINGAPORE

National League for Nursing

World Headquarters
Jones and Bartlett Publishers
40 Tall Pine Drive
Sudbury, MA 01776
978-443-5000
www.jbpub.com
info@jbpub.com

Jones and Bartlett Publishers Canada
2406 Nikanna Road
Mississauga, ON L5C 2W6
CANADA

Jones and Bartlett Publishers International
Barb House, Barb Mews
London W6 7PA
UK

Library of Congress Cataloging-in-Publication Data

O'Connor, Andrea B.
   Clinical instruction and evaluation: a teaching resource / Andrea B. O'Connor.
     p.cm.
   Includes bibliographical references and index.
   ISBN 0-7637-1687-1 (alk. paper)
   1. Nursing—Study and teaching. 2. Clinical medicine—Study and teaching. I. Title.

ORT73 .O26 2001
610.73'071'1—dc21

2001017383

Production Credits
Acquisitions Editor: Penny M. Glynn
Associate Editor: Christine Tridente
Production Editor: AnnMarie Lemoine
Editorial Assistant: Thomas Prindle
Manufacturing Buyer: Amy Duddridge
Cover Design: AnnMarie Lemoine
Design and Composition: Carlisle Communications, Ltd.
Printing and Binding: Malloy Lithographing

Printed in the United States of America
05   10 9 8 7 6 5 4

PREFACE

Effective clinical teaching is an essential component of nursing education programs. Unlike other professions (for example, architecture, law, medicine), in which formal education is designed with the expectation that the graduate of the program will enter an apprenticeship in order to develop functional proficiency and expertise, nursing programs are expected to produce competent practitioners upon graduation. This requires that programs invest faculty resources in educational experiences in clinical settings, where students learn to integrate theoretical content with practical skills in the care of patients.

Numerous qualified faculty are required to deliver the many hours of clinical learning experiences that are necessary to enable students to meet the expectations of the regulators who license them, the employers who hire them, and the patients who are recipients of their care upon graduation. Clinical learning experiences must be designed and supervised by qualified nursing faculty who collectively have knowledge and expertise in the various specialty areas that must be covered in a program preparing professional nurses. It is neither practical nor economically feasible to maintain a roster of full-time faculty reflecting such a diversity of clinical specialization. Therefore, most nursing education programs turn to clinically expert practitioners to teach on a part-time basis, with their assignments almost exclusively involving clinical instruction.

Although they are prepared at the graduate level in nursing, clinically expert nurses have had little or no preparation for the role of nursing educator. Academic institutions may provide course-specific orientation for part-time faculty, but cannot undertake the task of teaching them how to teach. Clinical nursing education should not be left to chance. Trial-and-error approaches to the work of clinical instruction and evaluation shortchange the student, the nursing education program, and, ultimately, the consumer of nursing services. Clinically expert nurses need guidance in putting their knowledge and skills to a new use: the education of nursing students.

Clinical instruction in nursing represents the most costly component of professional nursing education programs. Administrators need assurances that the faculty members entrusted with the important responsibility of teaching in the clinical setting are competent to do so. The relatively transient nature of part-time clinical instructors makes formal programs to orient them to the task an ineffective and costly approach. This book has been written to specifically address both the theoretical and practical know-how needed to succeed as a clinical nursing instructor and provide the highest quality of clinical education for nursing students.

This book addresses the unique tasks of clinical teaching and evaluation in nursing. It is a down-to-earth, practical guide to the nuts-and-bolts of clinical teaching and evaluation in nursing education programs. It has been developed so that each section can be used independently of the others. The reader may enter the guide at any section for content related to an immediate problem, or read those sections that seem most relevant to the clinical situation in which she is teaching. The guide illustrates content with examples drawn from actual situations encountered by clinical instructors, to demonstrate the application of theories of teaching, learning, and evaluation in clinical settings.

Much of the guide is based on my own experiences as a nursing instructor and as the director of the baccalaureate nursing program at Western Connecticut State University in Danbury, CT. Interviews with both experienced and neophyte faculty helped to validate issues and approaches in clinical nursing education and provide insight into areas in which I have had limited or no personal experience. I am especially indebted to my colleagues Dr. Barbara Piscopo, Chair, Department of Nursing, and Professor Eileen "Pat" Geraci, Coordinator, BSN Program, both of Western Connecticut State University, for sharing their experiences and insights with me. Literature sources, both books and articles, provided a rich resource of material concerning clinical teaching and evaluation in nursing, including theoretical perspectives and alternative approaches to specific problems in clinical instruction.

Teaching nursing in the clinical setting is challenging as well as exhausting. Like clinical nursing, teaching requires intellectual, technical, and interpersonal expertise in order to communicate the complex art of nursing to students and help them develop the competence to deliver skilled care. The opportunity to provide clinical instruction for nursing students is a distinct privilege that gives immense satisfaction and ample rewards to the clinically expert nurses who undertake this task.

A NOTE ON STYLE . . .

For ease in reading, nursing students and instructors are referred to with feminine pronouns throughout this book; to avoid confusion, patients are referred to with masculine pronouns. The term "patient" has been used, rather than the more inclusive term "client," because this is the term most nurses use to describe the people for whom they provide care.

CONTENTS

PREFACE   v

1 GOALS OF CLINICAL NURSING EDUCATION   1

Applying Theoretical Learning to Patient Care Situations   2

Developing Communication Skills   3

Demonstrating Skill in the Use of Therapeutic Nursing
    Interventions   5

Evidencing Caring Behaviors in Nursing Actions   6

Considering the Ethical Implications of Clinical Decisions and
    Nursing Actions   7

Gaining a Perspective on the Contextual Environment   9

Experiencing the Variety of Professional Nursing Roles   11

Summary   12

References   12

2 ENTERING THE INSTRUCTIONAL ROLE   13

The Academic Environment   14

    Becoming a Member of the Nursing Department Faculty   14

    Expectations of the Clinical Instructor   16

    Developing Collegial Relationships within the Nursing Department   21

The Clinical Setting   22

    Demands of Clinical Teaching   23

    Expectations of Clinical Staff   24

    Expectations of Students   26

    Orientation to the Clinical Setting   26

Summary   28

References   28

3   THEORETICAL APPROACHES TO TEACHING AND LEARNING IN CLINICAL
NURSING EDUCATION   29

How Learners Learn   30
    Psychological Theories   30
    Developmental Theories   33
    Social Theories   34
Behavioral Domains and Hierarchies of Learning   35
    Cognitive Domain   36
    Psychomotor Domain   36
    Affective Domain   40
Nature of the Adult Learner   44
    Assumptions of Andragogy   45
    Conditions for Learning   46
Benner's Framework for the Development of Clinical Expertise   48
Summary   50
References   51

4   GETTING STARTED   53

Program Faculty   53
Clinical Staff   56
The Clinical Group   58
Before the Clinical Experience Begins   59
The First Clinical Day   60
    Orientation   61
    Establishing Ground Rules   63
    Setting Expectations   66

5   TEACHING AND LEARNING STRATEGIES FOR THE COLLEGE LABORATORY
SETTING   69

The Laboratory Setting   71
Uses of the College Laboratory   73
Instructional Materials   73
Structuring the Laboratory Experience   77
The Process of Learning a Psychomotor Skill   78
Integrating the Cognitive Basis for Psychomotor Skills   81
Summary   82
References   83

6 ORGANIZING AND MANAGING INSTRUCTION IN THE CLINICAL PRACTICE
SETTING   85

Expectations, Hopes, and Fears   87
    Causing No Harm to the Patient   87
    Helping Patients   88
    Integrating Theory into Clinical Practice   89
    Learning Clinical Practice Skills   89
    Looking Good as a Nurse and as a Student   90
Selecting Clinical Learning Experiences   91
    Curricular Goals   91
    Learning Environment   92
    Instructor Expertise   93
    Learner Characteristics   95
    Other Considerations   96
    Alternative Approaches   97
Techniques to Help Students Prepare for Clinical Learning
    Experiences   97
    Teacher-Created Data Collection Forms   98
    Daily Nursing Care Plans   99
    The "Verbal Connection"   99
    Clinical Focus Guidelines   100
    Clinical Concept Mapping   100
The Clinical Preconference   103
Guiding Student Learning in the Clinical Setting   104
    Teaching-Learning Principles Underlying Instruction   105
    Modeling the Professional Nursing Role   109
Managing Off-Unit Experiences   112
Taking Advantage of Serendipitous Opportunities   114
The Clinical Postconference   114
Summary   116
References   117

7 TEACHING AND LEARNING STRATEGIES FOR THE CLINICAL PRACTICE
SETTING   119

Instructional Techniques for the Clinical Setting   121
    Demonstration   121
    War Stories   122

Questioning   122
Listening   124
Supervision of Student Performance of Technical Skills   125
Process of Skill Mastery   125
How to Let Go   128
When to Jump In   129
Ensuring That Patient Needs Are Met   130
Promoting the Integration of Theory and Practice   132
Case Studies   135
Seminars   135
Nursing Rounds   136
Written Assignments   137
Developing Critical Thinking Skills and Reflective Practice   139
What Is Critical Thinking?   140
The Role of Reflective Practice   141
Strategies for Promoting Critical Thinking and Reflective Practice   142
The Affective Domain: Fostering Caring in Clinical Practice   147
Summary   148
References   149

8

SPECIAL TECHNIQUES FOR SPECIAL SETTINGS   151

The Maternity Setting: Managing Instruction to Capture the
    Cyclical Nature of the Maternity Experience   151
The Pediatric Setting: The Problem of a Disappearing Clientele   153
The Mental Health Setting: It's Communication, But Is It
    Therapeutic?   155
Community Health Settings: Independent Practice in
    Unstructured Settings   157

9

THEORETICAL APPROACHES TO THE EVALUATION OF LEARNING IN THE
LABORATORY AND CLINICAL PRACTICE SETTINGS   163

Philosophies of Evaluation   164
Purposes of Evaluation   166
The Evaluation Process   167
Goals of Evaluation   168
Standards for Evaluation   169
Evaluation Methods   170
Analyzing Results   172

Reporting Results and Making Decisions 172
Using Results 173
Evaluating the Evaluation Process 173
Summary 175
References 175

10 EVALUATION STRATEGIES FOR THE LABORATORY AND CLINICAL PRACTICE SETTINGS 177

Identifying the Goals of Evaluation 178
Clarifying the Standards for Evaluation 181
Selecting and Applying Evaluation Methods 185
Observations 190
Written Work 192
Oral Presentations 192
Simulations 193
Self-Evaluations 194
Testimonials 194
Analyzing Results 195
Reporting Results 195
Due Process Issues 197
Confidentiality Issues 198
Making Decisions 198
Using Results 199
Evaluating the Evaluation Process 199
References 199

11 INTERPERSONAL ISSUES IN CLINICAL NURSING EDUCATION 201

The Instructional Role 202
The Clinical Instructor as Teacher 203
The Clinical Instructor as Supervisor 204
The Clinical Instructor as Evaluator 206
The Clinical Instructor as Nurse 206
Communicating Caring 207
Conveying Enthusiasm 209
Communication Strategies 210
Setting Goals 210
Communicating Values 211
Motivating Performance 212

Praising   212
Providing Corrective Feedback   212
Preventing Unsafe Practice   212
Describing Performance Deficits   214
Disciplining a Student   215
Failing a Student   215
Removing a Student from the Clinical Area   215

Responding to Student Stress   216
Helping Students to Cope with . . .   218
    . . . Death and Dying   219
    . . . Disfigurement, Deformities, Wounds, and Other Alterations
            in Body Integrity   220
    .. . . A Patient's Sexuality   221
    . . . Racist or Sexist Remarks by Patients   222
    . . . Staff or Physician Harassment   222

Strategies for Working with the . . .   223
    . . . Reluctant Learner   223
    . . . Reticent Learner   223
    . . . Monopolizer   224
    . . . Distractor   225
    . . . Student Who Lies   225
    . . . Student Who Plagiarizes   226
    . . . Student Who Exhibits Inappropriate Behavior   227
    . . . Student Who Is Defiant   228
    . . . Student Who Is Poorly Groomed   228
    . . . Student Who Is a Family Member or Friend   228
    . . . Older Student   228
    . . . Male Student   229
    . . . Student Who Is Repeating the Course   229
    . . . Student Who Is Licensed as an LPN or RN   229
    . . . Student for Whom English Is a Second Language   230

Maintaining Relationships with Staff   230
Controlling Emotions   231
Summary   232
References   232

12 ETHICAL AND LEGAL ISSUES IN NURSING EDUCATION 233

Ethical Issues in Nursing Education 234
    Ethical Systems and Analytical Tools 234
    Approaches to Guiding Students through Ethical Dilemmas
        in Practice 235
    Ethical Issues Related to the Instructional Role 239
LEGAL ISSUES IN NURSING EDUCATION 242
    Licensure Issues 243
    Due Process Issues 246
    The Student with a Disability 247
    Contractual Issues 248
Summary 249
References 249

APPENDICES **251**

A SAMPLE PROGRAM, LEVEL, AND RELATED COURSE OBJECTIVES FOR A
BACCALAUREATE NURSING PROGRAM 251

B SAMPLE COURSE OUTLINE FOR A NURSING COURSE WITH A CLINICAL
COMPONENT 257

C SAMPLE CLINICAL EVALUATION FORM 263

D SAMPLE ANECDOTAL NOTES 267

E SAMPLE AGENCY AFFILIATION AGREEMENT 269

F SAMPLE CLINICAL PREPARATION FORMS 273

G SAMPLE GUIDELINES FOR OFF-UNIT EXPERIENCES 279

LIST OF TABLES

3-1   DESCRIPTIONS AND CHARACTERISTIC BEHAVIORS OF THE
        HIERARCHICAL CATEGORIES IN THE COGNITIVE DOMAIN   37

3-2   DESCRIPTIONS AND CHARACTERISTIC BEHAVIORS OF THE
        HIERARCHICAL CATEGORIES IN THE PSYCHOMOTOR DOMAIN   39

3-3   DESCRIPTIONS AND CHARACTERISTIC BEHAVIORS OF THE
        HIERARCHICAL CATEGORIES IN THE AFFECTIVE DOMAIN   41

5-1   LEARNING STYLES   71

5-2   GRONLUND'S HIERARCHY OF THE PSYCHOMOTOR DOMAIN   78

5-3   GUINEE'S HIERARCHY OF THE PSYCHOMOTOR DOMAIN   79

6-1   ROLE MODEL BEHAVIORS IN THE CLINICAL SETTING   111

7-1   HIERARCHICAL STRUCTURE OF BEHAVIORS IN THE
        COGNITIVE DOMAIN   133

7-2   INDICATORS OF CRITICAL THINKING APPLIED TO
        NURSING CONTEXTS   141

7-3   QUESTIONS REFLECTING THE HIERARCHICAL STRUCTURE OF
        COGNITIVE KNOWLEDGE   145

10-1   THE EVALUATION PROCESS   179

10-2   LEVELS OF STUDENT PERFORMANCE IN CLINICAL PRACTICE   182

10-3   DEFINITION OF TERMS RELATED TO OVERRIDERS   184

10-4   GUIDELINES FOR PROVIDING ACADEMIC DUE PROCESS
FOR STUDENTS   196

12-1   PRINCIPLES UNDERLYING ETHICAL DILEMMAS   238

12-2   SELECTED PROVISIONS OF THE CONNECTICUT STATE
NURSE PRACTICE ACT   244

LIST OF FIGURES

3-1   LAWS OF CLOSURE AND CONTINUITY   31

5-1   CONCEPT MAPPING   82

5-2   VEE HEURISTIC   83

6-1   CLINICAL CONCEPT MAP DEVELOPMENT   101

LIST OF BOXES

4-1   DIRECTIONS FOR SCAVENGER HUNT   62

4-2   GROUND RULES FOR COLLEGE LABORATORY EXPERIENCES   67

4-3   EXPECTATIONS FOR CLINICAL EXPERIENCES   68

12-1   AMERICAN NURSES' ASSOCIATION CODE FOR NURSES   237

CHAPTER 1

GOALS OF CLINICAL NURSING EDUCATION

Applying Theoretical Learning to Patient Care Situations   2
Developing Communication Skills   3
Demonstrating Skill in the Use of Therapeutic Nursing Interventions   5
Evidencing Caring Behaviors in Nursing Actions   6
Considering the Ethical Implications of Clinical Decisions and Nursing Actions   7
Gaining a Perspective on the Contextual Environment   9
Experiencing the Variety of Professional Nursing Roles   11
Summary   12
References   12

The ultimate goal of nursing education is to prepare the student to think critically, communicate accurately, and perform indicated therapeutic nursing interventions in patient care situations; exhibit the caring behaviors inherent in nursing actions; apply an ethical perspective in clinical decision making; and function effectively as a team member within the organizational structures surrounding the delivery of patient care. The clinical laboratory is the place where much of this learning occurs.

The goals of clinical nursing education are to enable the student to

1. Apply theoretical learning to patient care situations through the use of critical thinking skills to recognize and resolve patient care problems and the use of the nursing process to design therapeutic nursing interventions and evaluate their effectiveness
2. Develop communication skills in working with patients, their families, and other health care providers
3. Demonstrate skill in the safe use of therapeutic nursing interventions in providing care to patients
4. Evidence caring behaviors in nursing actions
5. Consider the ethical implications of clinical decisions and nursing actions

6. Gain a perspective on the contextual environment of health care delivery
7. Experience the various roles of the professional nurse within the health care delivery system

APPLYING THEORETICAL LEARNING TO PATIENT CARE SITUATIONS

Clinical nursing education enables students to move from theoretical learning about nursing, based on textbook and classroom explanations of human responses to illness and its treatment, to practical learning in making the observations and performing the interventions necessary to manage those responses in real-life situations. Theory becomes reality as students begin to make connections between the generic "usual" case presented in the classroom and the specific "actual" case with which they are involved.

The clinical laboratory is the place where the theoretical begins to make sense, and a great deal of integration of theoretical with practical knowledge becomes possible as students search out explanations for the phenomena they are witnessing in the clinical situations to which they are exposed. Abandoning the safety of "book learning" for the real world of patient care is frightening. Students enter this aspect of their education with eager trepidation. The clinical instructor must be skilled in assessing the degree of anxiety presented by each student and able to channel unfocused functional anxiety to maximize learning and defuse dysfunctional anxiety to permit safe performance.

Students see how the theoretical "ideal" plays out in the clinical "real" as they embark on the critical thinking process of problem identification, sorting through theoretical as well as experiential knowledge to determine what is relevant in the present situation and applying this knowledge to the design of interventions. Exposure to an array of clinical situations is essential to fine-tune the student's observational skills, recall and application abilities, and problem solving skills, and such exposure is impossible in the relatively brief time allotted to clinical learning. Therefore, the clinical instructor must devise approaches to enhance critical thinking, for example, through conferencing, where students compare and contrast their individual experiences; journaling, where students reflect on the clinical experience and begin to make the intellectual connections that might have eluded them during the experience; structured questioning that presents "what if" situations, where the student is encouraged to explore alternative scenarios that might occur; and "war stories" that recount the instructor's experiences with similar situations.

The nursing process makes it easier to understand the intellectual connections that are necessary to apply theory in practice. When the nursing process is used as a guide to critical thinking that emphasizes the connections between making observations and assessments, analyzing these to formulate tentative diagnoses, selecting approaches to address the problems identified through the diagnostic process, implementing interventions, and evaluating the effectiveness of interventions as well as the accuracy of initial diagnoses, students can embrace it as a useful tool for clinical decision making. The clinical instructor can facilitate this use of the nursing process by articulating her own thinking through of clinical problems.

Written care plans, usually based on a nursing process format, require the student to make explicit the intellectual connections she has (or has not) made, and force the integration of theoretical learning in the case being addressed. Such assignments are a useful adjunct to clinical learning and checking the degree to which each student is successfully connecting theory to practice. However, when the nursing process is reduced to a framework for the written care plan rather than an active approach to thinking about clinical situations, students may devalue the critical thinking that is an inherent aspect of developing theory-applied, clinical knowledge.

DEVELOPING COMMUNICATION SKILLS

Transitioning from a predominantly social style of communication to the situationally determined communication styles required in nursing practice is an essential component of clinical learning. No amount of classroom or college laboratory practice can prepare the student for this communication challenge.

The development of therapeutic communication skills is the primary focus of theoretical learning about communication in nursing education programs. The student must be guided to recognize the full repertoire of communication strategies and to become skilled in selecting and using appropriate strategies in specific situations. In addition to therapeutic communications, nurses must be adept at interviewing, counseling, and teaching patients; documenting observations and interventions, both orally and in writing; and delegating up and down the chain of health care workers. Each of these strategies requires attentiveness to the objective of the interaction, the best means of structuring the interaction, and the applicable language to use.

Unlike social communications, professional communications are goal-directed. Students need help in identifying the objective of their communication strategies as well as the information necessary to achieve that objective. Initial interactions need to be as carefully planned and mentally rehearsed as administering an intramuscular injection or changing a dressing.

Students also need to be skilled in listening to and observing their communication partners, hearing and absorbing what is said, interpreting what is said, and then crafting a response. Too often students are so anxious to deliver a message that they fail to listen to the responses that would improve that message. Clinical instructors can assist the student to listen better by encouraging her to slow down to allow silence to provide the time and space needed for both partners to think before talking.

Nurses tend to use "common language" with patients and their families, readily translating medical jargon into terms that patients can understand. In using common language, nurses make adjustments based on the patient's age, educational level, culture, native language, and existing communication problems—such as hearing deficits or an inability to speak around an endotracheal tube—as well as the patient's level of anxiety or alertness. Nurses also make full use of nonverbal communication such as touch, facial expressions, and reassuring vocalizations. By observing the interactions of staff and the clinical instructor with patients, students learn the nuances of skilled communication with patients. When the clinical instructor points out an especially effective approach, or one that is less than successful, and articulates the critical elements of the interaction, students are better able to grasp the full dynamic of the episode.

Nurses use "nurse-talk" with one another, particularly co-workers. Nurse-talk is an abbreviated communication style loaded with acronyms and terms specific to the clinical environment. Such talk suits the rapidly changing clinical situation and the limited time that nurses have to brief one another. For students nurse-talk can be both baffling and intimidating. Unable to decipher the language and afraid to display ignorance by requesting a translation, students may muddle through a clinical experience with little understanding of what is going on. This problem is exacerbated if some students in the clinical group, who have had work experiences in an environment similar to the clinical area in which they are learning, use their mastery of nurse-talk to feign clinical expertise. The clinical instructor must serve as translator, accepting students' inability to negotiate nurse-talk at this stage of their professional development and interpreting the nurse-talk for them. Providing translation presents an excellent opportunity to reinforce theoretical content. For example, when a staff nurse refers to "the cabbage in Room 304," the clinical instructor can explain that "cabbage" refers to the acronym "CABG," which stands for "coronary artery bypass graft," and then provide a brief overview of indications for the procedure, what the procedure accomplishes, and practice pointers such as the need to monitor both the primary and donor operative sites. This also would be an opportune time to reinforce the concept that patients are people, not medical diagnoses or procedures.

"Delegation-talk" is another type of communication to be mastered by students. Delegation occurs "down" when an aspect of nursing care is to be provided by another; delegation occurs "up" when the nurse is requesting an intervention by a physician or supervisor. Delegation-talk uses explicit language to communicate to the delegatee what needs to be done and why, when it needs to be done, how it should be done, and expectations for response or report back to the delegator. Delegation-talk must clearly identify "who" is to perform the delegated task; "someone ought to . . ." is unlikely to accomplish the objective of delegation-talk. Students are uncomfortable delegating to individuals who are more knowledgeable and/or skilled than they are, which can interfere with communication. Shared responsibility for health care delivery demands delegation, and students must become skilled in and comfortable with the use of delegation-talk. Practicing with one another can help master this language.

They must also learn the "professional tongue." The professional tongue uses medical and nursing terminology to provide a precise description or explanation of a situation. It is used to communicate with those who are less familiar with the existing situation, as in completing written documentation on a patient's status, giving an end-of-shift report, discussing a patient's condition during "rounds," or in teaching other professionals. The development of the professional tongue can be enhanced by insisting on its use in student reports to staff members at the conclusion of the clinical day or in conference presentations.

While it is impossible for the clinical instructor to witness each episode of communication in order to provide students with practical pointers on fine-tuning communication skills, this aspect of clinical education must become part of their curriculum. Process recordings are a useful device for helping students to focus on their communication skills and need not be confined to therapeutic interactions.

DEMONSTRATING SKILL IN THE USE OF THERAPEUTIC NURSING INTERVENTIONS

The clinical area is the place where students learn their technical skills. Opportunities to learn and practice specific skills in the controlled college laboratory setting, while valuable, are not a substitute for using these skills with patients. Hands-on care propels the student toward the goal of becoming a nurse, progress that is measured by an ever-lengthening list of technical skills that have been performed—if not mastered—in the clinical area.

Doing transcends thinking or communicating, especially in early clinical experiences. Doing enables the student to feel useful and is generally accompanied by a sense of accomplishment. Access to the patient is facilitated when the student has a purpose for entering the patient's domain, and so the need to provide physical care or render a treatment makes approaching the patient less intimidating. A patient assignment that does not involve the use of technical skills feels like a waste of time and energy to most students, who tend not to seek out or respond to other patient needs such as teaching or counseling.

For the clinical instructor who knows that technical skills are only a small component of the professional nursing role, this focus on doing can be distressing. Komorita et al. (1991) report that "nurses have a tendency to consider comfort and trusting relationship items [reflecting caring] as most important while patients perceive behaviors associated with physical care most important" (p. 23). Students enter nursing education programs sharing many perceptions with patients; these perceptions change as students incorporate the values of the profession into their view of nursing.

Despite its centrality for students, the goal of developing the technical skills of practice is a source of intense anxiety. Students are afraid to make an error and harm—or even kill—the patient. They worry that the patient will find them inept, will feel like a guinea pig, or will insist that the student be replaced by a "real nurse." The urge to "care" competes with the real need to learn through practice; the two motives feel incompatible.

Developing skills to deliver therapeutic nursing interventions involves more than technical expertise. It requires the simultaneous performance of caring behaviors, technical skills, and the intellectual manipulations of critical thinking, which can only be achieved when technique—the "how to" of the skill component—is so well mastered that it no longer requires conscious mental attention for successful performance. It is at this point that the nursing student—or, more likely, graduate nurse—is able to focus on the "whole picture" and respond to the patient who is receiving the intervention. The clinical instructor can advance skill development by attending to the details the student is unable to see when performing a technical task, especially for the first time. For example, the instructor can explain the procedure to the patient, provide comfort—such as holding the patient's hand—and observe the patient's response to the intervention. In this way the instructor can complement the student's activities to model the "whole" performance. Assuming a complementary role also helps the instructor to refrain from taking over for the student in the midst of a procedure.

For the clinical instructor safety is a primary concern when students are learning technical skills in the clinical setting. Like the students, the instructor is concerned that errors will occur and patients will be harmed, a concern that is multiplied by the number of students being supervised in the clinical area. Knowing that she cannot be with every student at all times, the clinical instructor must allocate time fairly to provide all students with relatively equivalent opportunities to learn the technical skills required. Keeping track of levels of experience and competence achieved by each student in each skill, coupled with the instructor's overriding concern with safety, can create the impression that students are correct: technical skill mastery *is* what clinical learning is all about. The instructor's skillful use of questioning and verbal rehearsals of care activities can create opportunities for teaching the "why" behind the "how," as well as alerting students to the clinical issues associated with interventions.

EVIDENCING CARING BEHAVIORS IN NURSING ACTIONS

It is a rare student who fails to express the desire to "care for others" as a primary reason for becoming a nurse. Students usually cannot articulate what they mean by "caring," but we can assume that it involves relief of suffering, providing comfort, and a general "connectedness" with the patient.

Almon (1999) suggests that caring expressed by "doing for" needs to be replaced with caring that is enabling and empowering—a caring "about" the person of the patient who is struggling to cope with illness and its treatment or to incorporate a necessary change into his lifestyle. But "doing for" is highly valued by students for many reasons and it is difficult to shift their emphasis toward a conception of caring as providing the patient with the support necessary to achieve and maintain wellness.

Students are unable to see the "big picture." They do not view the patient as a functioning whole, as a member of a family system or a society. They do not consider the situation from which the patient enters the health care system and to which he will return. This tunnel vision is not due to lack of data on these larger issues; indeed, the student may have collected all the relevant data herself. The student's focus is on the immediate situation, and is more self-absorbed than other-directed as the student struggles with the tasks and issues presented by the clinical assignment. Students are likely to monitor IV drip rates without checking to see that the IV site and tubing are intact; they are likely to watch a cardiac monitor display of an arrhythmia without checking the patient's response to the arrhythmia.

Students are able to recognize caring when they see it, therefore, role modeling the caring component of nursing care delivery is an essential part of the clinical instructor's role. Complimenting students when the instructor has observed caring actions signals to students their capacity to develop this aspect of their profession and reinforces caring behaviors.

Students are also able to recognize the failure to care in other staff members and are often verbal about this. Channeling their outrage into a discussion of why the observed episode was "uncaring," what might have contributed to staff behavior, and what actions might have been taken to transform the interaction into a caring one helps students to understand caring as reflected in actions, as well as in general attitudes of concern and compassion.

CONSIDERING THE ETHICAL IMPLICATIONS OF CLINICAL DECISIONS AND NURSING ACTIONS

Ethical considerations in nursing care delivery are intimately entwined with caring. Ethical action involves "doing what is right" in situations that involve alternative possibilities for action. In responding to a situation ethically, the nurse does not substitute her judgment for that of the patient, but, rather, considers which clinical decisions and nursing actions best reflect the patient's expressed wishes and underlying values. While ethical considerations encompass such major issues as the right to self-determination, the right to privacy, and the right to be treated with dignity, ethics also entails the consideration of clinical decisions and nursing actions reflecting the "best good" in the situation from the patient's perspective.

Despite their general tendency toward caring in their interactions with patients, nursing students are often self- rather than other-centered. In an effort to perform competently, the student focuses on the performance more than on the recipient of the care being performed. Actual or perceived expectations of the instructor also divert the student's attention away from the patient and toward the tasks to be completed.

Translating a code of ethics presented in the classroom into action in individual patient situations is beyond the ability of most nursing students. The student's clinical knowledge base is still developing. The student has not yet encountered a sufficient number of practice situations to enable her to recognize the ethical issues in day-to-day practice, identify acceptable alternatives for action, and set priorities that exemplify patient-centered care. The student can't perceive the subtleties of a given situation that suggest the need for a discretionary response. The student is unaware of the parameters within which discretion can be exercised.

The nursing student is unable to fully evaluate the patient's situation, with all its distinctiveness, as a basis for considering alternatives that would represent an ethical response. For example, the nursing student is unlikely to consider deferring morning care until later in the day if the patient has had a difficult night, or to take time to allow the patient to elaborate on concerns when a routine blood pressure reading is scheduled, or to encourage the patient to participate in physical therapy despite complaints of assorted aches and pains.

The clinical instructor can use conference time to review each student's plan of care for the day, pointing out specific situations that might call for a change in the routine approach for a given patient. Focused questioning of what constitutes the "best good" for this patient at this time can help the student to consider the ethical implications of the clinical situation and the alternative approaches available to achieve an optimal outcome.

Ethical behavior also entails taking responsibility for one's actions. Students often bring a classroom morality to the clinical setting. That morality includes guessing when unsure of an answer, avoiding asking for assistance, ignoring problem situations in the hope that no one will notice, and, in many settings, cheating. Such behaviors are obviously incompatible with safe patient care, and the clinical instructor must establish standards of clinical morality at the outset of the clinical experience. This involves encouraging questions, consultation with others, looking up answers, verifying activities before performing them, and admitting to errors. Students need to learn that it is okay to make mistakes while learning, but wrong to cover them up. Consistency in managing student errors, while maintaining patient safety, is essential in promoting clinical morality.

GAINING A PERSPECTIVE ON THE CONTEXTUAL ENVIRONMENT

Clinical nursing education takes students through a series of experiences with patients of all ages receiving health care for a full array of conditions in a variety of settings. Experiences focus on health maintenance and health promotion, acute illness, and chronic conditions that occur in institutional and community settings. Each of these experiences has a unique contextual environment. Although they are affected by the characteristics of the environments in which learning occurs, students often are unaware of their effects on patient care.

Each clinical setting varies in the pace of activities that occur there. Pace is reflected in the urgency of time constraints, as well as in the rapidity of changes in patient condition. Even the most slow-paced environment, as in the skilled nursing facility, contains time pressures for beginning nursing students. As skilled performance of routine care activities evolves, this environment may begin to feel sluggish. As students progress to more acute situations, they must learn to keep pace with rapidly evolving environments. Priorities for care activities must shift in accordance with changes in patient condition and the student must become attuned and responsive to these changes. The orientation to the clinical setting provided by the clinical instructor should include pace and time constraints as factors impacting on patient care.

Related to pace is the amount of noise in the clinical environment. Background sounds can soothe or energize, and their effects are felt not only by patients, but also by health care workers. Acute care environments are notoriously noisy, and this noise can increase student anxiety and even interfere with their ability to think through clinical situations. Students need to be told to control noise whenever possible, as in turning down a TV set when attempting to interview a patient, or learning to alter their natural response to contextual noise by ignoring the noise when it interferes with performance. The clinical instructor also needs to be aware of the effect of contextual noise on her own behaviors, especially when several students are competing for attention and asking questions simultaneously. A "time-out" to reorganize the situation, or move it to a quieter venue, may be the answer when the instructor becomes frazzled due to noise overload.

Institutional environments also contain many workers, who affect the atmosphere of the setting, and often compete with one another for access to the patient. The clinical instructor's assistance in identifying the roles and functions of all the workers in the health care facility helps students to cope with this variable. Students often feel subordinate to all other workers, and need the instructor's support in asserting their rightful position as care providers and patient advocates.

The amount of technical equipment and the degree to which health care providers rely on technology in monitoring patients' conditions varies with each setting. Each machine encountered by the student presents a challenge apart from the person connected to it. Greater reliance on technology tends to result in a degree of depersonalization. This tendency toward depersonalization is further exacerbated by the student's tendency toward self-absorption and focus on tasks, now represented by the technology. Care is provided to the machine rather than to the patient. The clinical instructor can help to overcome the depersonalization that occurs with increased technology, while at the same time teaching students how to utilize equipment, by focusing on how the equipment is being used in the specific patient situation, and what observations of the patient are necessary to support the technology. Because the type of equipment used for specific purposes varies from institution to institution, the instructor also needs to familiarize students with the underlying mechanism of the technology so that they can readily transfer this knowledge to new situations. Knowing the how and why of equipment operation enables the student to master technology and stay connected to the patient.

The clinical instructor needs to alert students to the governing rules and operational realities of a given clinical setting. Documentation procedures vary from setting to setting. Priority tasks to which other activities are subordinate may characterize a clinical area, as on a surgical unit where preoperative preparation of patients scheduled for surgery is the dominant morning activity. Staff practices may be diametrically opposed to those taught to students, as in managing used linen, which they routinely toss on the floor. In the institutional setting, supervision and consultation are readily available; community settings—in particular, the home care environment—lack these backup supports. Recognition of the great variety of rules and realities in clinical situations helps students to ask rather than assume when they move from setting to setting.

In today's health care system economics affects the care environment. Waste of materials—inevitable when students are learning—may be viewed as a minor catastrophe by staff. Small economies may be practiced, such as changing linens on alternate days if they are not soiled. Charges for supplies must be accurately allocated. Early discharge of patients, often unexpected, disrupts the rhythm of the day and compresses the time available for teaching. Staffing may be adjusted because students are scheduled to be on the unit, despite contractual stipulations that students will not substitute as staff. In the past, health care institutions have been willing to absorb the costs associated with serving as a clinical setting for nursing education. More recently, these same institutions have attempted to charge a fee to the educational institution for the use of the facility. Few colleges can afford this, leading to competition for clinical settings, which may influence scheduling of student activities on specific units. Sensitizing students to economic realities while maintaining an environment that is supportive of learning and that maintains standards of care is a vital yet difficult task for the clinical instructor.

The various clinical settings that students traverse in the course of their education have contextual differences that they must recognize and respond to if they are to learn and operate successfully in each setting. Providing an orientation to the contextual variables that are likely to be encountered enables students to better "read" the environments in which they are learning, and make the necessary adjustments to support success.

EXPERIENCING THE VARIETY OF PROFESSIONAL NURSING ROLES

In most clinical learning situations, students are charged with providing full care to one or more patients, except for treatments they have not yet learned. The experience of providing full patient care helps students sort out what to delegate, and what to do themselves, and to anticipate outcomes and cues that signal deviation from a normal or expected clinical course. The clinical instructor can assist the student in developing such insights. Yet the reality of the clinical practice setting is that the professional nurse rarely, if ever, provides full care to patients. The nurse accomplishes patient care goals by delegating and by managing a multiworker/multitask approach to patient care. Mundt (1997) argues that, as integrated health care networks evolve, "The major focus of the clinical learning will be nursing management through the continuum of care, collaboration, team building, and the study of patient outcomes within the organizational context of [the] network" (p. 310). Students can't master the critical role of coordinating care unless they have a structured clinical experience that allows them to practice delegating and the necessary oversight that accompanies it.

During their early clinical experiences students execute a care plan created by others. Students need help to recognize that this is not a delegated role, but rather a collaborative role, because many nurses will use the plan in their work with patients. As students work with existing care plans, they should be encouraged to critique the plans based on their own observations of patient responses to the care being provided. The notion that the care plan is a dynamic instrument for moving the patient toward desired outcomes helps students to better grasp the concept of continuity in care, and can be used to help them trace patient progress.

Leadership involves articulating a goal that can be embraced by others and motivating performance toward goal achievement. While leadership is often conceptualized as the management of nursing care delivery, in reality the management role is more one of resource allocation and coordination. Nursing leadership can be demonstrated in direct patient care, as when the nurse works with a patient to identify goals and the means to achieve them, and then motivates the patient to achieve those goals.

Change agency, research, and advocacy are nursing roles that are similarly inherent in students' clinical experiences. Highlighting these roles, for example, in postconference activities, increases students' awareness of the multi-faceted profession they are about to enter.

SUMMARY

The overall goal of clinical nursing education is to prepare students for future practice through current learning experiences. Because of the rapid changes likely to occur in health care, understanding is more important than doing and rationale more important than technique. The clinical instructor must maintain a focus on the essential knowledge to be mastered through clinical learning, while orchestrating students' care activities in a way that ensures patient safety, provides opportunities for students to perform successfully in the clinical area, and communicates the fullness of the professional nursing role.

REFERENCES

Almon, M.E. (1999). Thoughts on nursing; Where it has been and where it is going. *Nursing and Health Care Perspectives*, 20, 20–25.

Komorita, N.I., Doehring, K.M., & Hirchert, P.W. (1991). Perceptions of caring by nurse educators. *Journal of Nursing Education*, 30, 23–29.

Mundt, M.H. (1997). A model for clinical learning experiences in integrated health care networks. *Journal of Nursing Education*, 36, 309–316.

CHAPTER 2

ENTERING THE INSTRUCTIONAL ROLE

The Academic Environment   14
    Becoming a Member of the Nursing Department Faculty   14
    Expectations of the Clinical Instructor   16
    Developing Collegial Relationships within the Nursing
    Department   21
The Clinical Setting   22
    Demands of Clinical Teaching   23
    Expectations of Clinical Staff   24
    Expectations of Students   26
    Orientation to the Clinical Setting   26
Summary   28
References   28

In describing the transition from nurse clinician to nurse educator, Esper (1995) remarks, "The position of nurse educator seems to have it all: prestige, a great schedule, and an opportunity to make a mark on the future direction of nursing" (p. 89). All of this is true. But entering the educator role also involves developing new skills (teaching and evaluation), adjusting to an often unfamiliar clinical setting, becoming acquainted with the academic environment, and functioning as a liaison between the clinical and academic settings. Clinical expertise may be one basis for selecting nursing faculty, but that alone is not sufficient for being an educator.

Whether hired as a full-time faculty member, with both classroom and clinical teaching responsibilities, or as a part-time faculty member with only a clinical teaching assignment, the new faculty member can ease the transition to educator by gathering the information needed to succeed as a clinical instructor. Despite the recognized need for orientation and mentoring programs for new faculty, few such programs are in place. Instead, the new faculty member must reach out for the help she needs.

The clinical instructor has a foot in each of two very different organizations: the academic institution of which she is now a member and the clinical setting in which she is now a guest. Familiarity with both settings eases the transition to the educator role.

THE ACADEMIC ENVIRONMENT

The academic environment has distinct characteristics, unlike any work environments that the nurse has experienced. While nursing faculty, more than faculty in other academic departments, operate as a team in delivering the curriculum, much of the work is done by individuals in isolation from one another. While this gives the faculty member free rein in teaching activities, it is often difficult to locate a fellow faculty member for a quick consultation on an emerging problem, especially in the clinical area. Compared to the fast-paced clinical environment, especially within hospitals, the academic environment is sluggish. There is a predictable ebb and flow of activity, with chaos at the start of every semester, a calm middle, and a frenzied end, but there are limited crises and most are readily managed. Decisions are made at a leisurely pace, and there is no rush to communicate decisions to those affected by them. The new faculty member is likely to experience this first hand in the hiring process, which spans several weeks if not months. Finally, despite its central mission of creating and communicating knowledge, there is a decidedly low tolerance for change and innovation. Change that does occur is incremental, and usually in response to external forces, such as accrediting agencies.

Becoming a Member of the Nursing Department Faculty

Full-time faculty members are hired following a formal "search"—the academic process for inviting applications for available positions—interviewing qualified candidates, and making recommendations for hire to administration. The search is conducted by faculty members within the academic department,[1] so the applicant has the opportunity to meet at least some of the people with whom she will be working. Part-time faculty (also called "adjunct faculty") are hired by one or two members of the department, usually the department chair and/or the coordinator of the level at which the faculty member will be teaching. While administrative approval is required for these appointments, there is less scrutiny of the applicant and fewer opportunities for the applicant to interact with other faculty members prior to accepting the position.

---

[1]The term "department" is used to describe the nursing unit within the college or university. The nursing unit may be a larger unit, such as a division, school, or college.

Full-time faculty members can be hired on a "tenure track" or as temporary faculty. The distinction is important for several reasons. Tenure track faculty appointments are continued from year to year without the need for an additional search. The faculty member is granted a continuing appointment every one to two years[2] based on a favorable recommendation by faculty peers who have evaluated the faculty member's performance in the prior term. In the sixth year of appointment, the faculty member applies for tenure, which—if awarded—essentially guarantees employment for as long as the faculty member wishes to remain at the institution.[3] Because of this guarantee of lifetime employment, tenure decisions are made with great care. If the faculty member fails to be awarded tenure, a terminal one-year appointment is granted, after which the faculty member must leave the institution. Temporary full-time faculty are given one-year appointments that must be renewed the following year. The length of time a person can remain in a temporary position is dictated by institutional policy. However, if the temporary full-time faculty is eventually granted a tenure-track position, the tenure "clock" (reflecting the six-year probationary period) often starts with the initial temporary appointment. Because the tenure decision is based on a cumulative record of achievement, a temporary faculty member who believes she may be interested in a tenure-track position will need to build a track record early, including formal evaluations by students and faculty peers, to meet the criteria for tenure.

Part-time faculty members usually are not eligible for tenure, although a solid performance often is rewarded with an offer to continue in the position. Student and faculty-peer evaluations may or may not be done to support such an offer. Part-time appointments are made for one semester. A maximum workload[4] for the part-time faculty member is usually set by policy; exceeding this maximum places the faculty member in a category similar to a temporary full-time faculty member.

Compensation for both full-time and part-time faculty is based on rank. These ranks are Instructor, Assistant Professor, Associate Professor, and Professor, and are based on education and years of teaching experience. A range of salaries exists in each rank, so there is some room for negotiation upon hire. After initial hire, however, the faculty member's salary only increases with across-the-board raises, unless there is a promotion, in which case the faculty member most often is paid the beginning rate for the new rank. Compensation includes a full package of benefits for full-time faculty; part-time faculty usually are ineligible for most benefits, although perks such as free tuition at the institution may be available.

---

[2]The length of continuing appointments, as well as procedures and criteria for review, reflect institutional policy, usually based on a collective bargaining agreement, most often with the American Association of University Professors (AAUP).

[3]While there are criteria and procedures for removing tenured faculty, it is a very rare occurrence.

[4]Workload, or some other, similar term, is the unit used to determine full-time versus part-time status as well as pay rates for part-time faculty.

Temporary full-time and part-time faculty are offered a contract that out-lines the term of the appointment, rank, rate of pay, and teaching responsi-bilities. Return of the signed contract signals the faculty member's acceptance of the appointment.

Workload unit discriminates between full-time and part-time faculty, but does not fully reflect the actual workload of the faculty member. Workload units may be based on or derived from the academic credit assigned to a course, or the workload unit may be the assigned course, regardless of the number of academic credits it carries. Thus, a 3-credit course involving 3 hours of classroom teaching over a 15-week semester may carry 3 workload units for the faculty member teaching the course (that is, 1 workload unit for each 1 credit of classroom teaching), or 1 workload unit if the course represents a unit. Workload units for college and clinical laboratories are determined by in-stitutional policy, and usually are based on the actual number of hours in-volved in one week in the laboratory. Students earn 1 academic credit for each 3 hours in a laboratory experience that spans the full 15-week semester.

Although the full-time workload per semester usually is computed based on teaching responsibilities, the faculty member also must meet other obli-gations. Preparation for classroom teaching is not compensated separately and can represent upward of 3 hours for each hour of classroom instruction. Creating and correcting tests and grading other assignments is configured as part of the preparatory time. Similarly, preparation for the college or clinical laboratory, which may require many hours per week as faculty search for the best experiences for students, often is not a part of the workload computation. Correcting and grading written assignments in conjunction with laboratory ex-periences is also part of preparatory time. Conferences with students—to an-swer questions, review clinical progress, and communicate the results of eval-uation—are a necessary component of teaching, but not part of the workload computation. Faculty members may be required to schedule a minimum number of office hours per week during which they are available to students; many faculty members exceed this minimum. Additional office hours usually are scheduled during the time students are registering for next semester's courses, which may require meeting with a faculty advisor for approval of the planned course schedule. Finally, time must be made available for meetings, including general faculty meetings, department meetings, and committee meetings, at which faculty participate in the overall governance of the institu-tion and the department.

Part-time faculty are not similarly burdened. While their preparatory time is not counted in workload unit computation, and part-time faculty must arrange time for conferences with students in their clinical groups, they are usually not required to advise during registration or attend meetings.

Expectations of the Clinical Instructor

The clinical instructor is expected to conduct the clinical component of the as-signed course so that students are able to correlate classroom content with the practical realities of the clinical setting. The clinical instructor facilitates the students' achievement of course objectives, and prepares the students to move forward in the program. The clinical instructor must provide a minimum of an interim and final evaluation of individual student performance that con- tributes to the student's success or failure in the clinical course. Such evalua- tion includes conferencing with each student to communicate progress, and may include conferencing with the lead faculty member for the course. Where a student's performance is borderline or failing, more frequent evaluation and conferencing may be necessary. The clinical instructor is expected to follow the policies and procedures of the department and the clinical facility, as well as any rules and regulations enunciated by government bodies, such as the state board of nursing. Finally, the clinical instructor is expected to maintain a positive image of the nursing program and the educational institution in which it is housed. To deliver on such expectations, the clinical instructor needs a good deal of information.

Correlating Classroom and Clinical Content to Achieve Objectives.   Each clinical experience in a nursing program is either a component of or connected to a classroom course, which itself is a component of the larger curriculum. A curriculum is a program of study that is intended to progressively build knowl- edge and skills to achieve identified outcomes. The sequencing of content and associated clinical experiences usually is guided by one or more organi- zational schemes. These organizational schemes are one component of the conceptual framework of the program, which also describes the conceptual- ization of nursing that has been adopted by the faculty.

The organizational scheme for sequencing courses within the curriculum usually is reflected in behavioral objectives for each year (sometimes termed "level") in the program, culminating in a set of program objectives or out- comes, which are presumably achieved by each student upon graduation. Each course taken at a program level has its own objectives which, in con- junction with those of other courses taken at the same level, contribute to ob- jectives for the level. The sequencing, organization, and forward movement of the curriculum depend on each faculty member delivering on the promise of the objectives, and faculty at the next program level should be able to rely on students having achieved the objectives set for the previous level. (Appendix A contains sample program, level, and related course objectives for a baccalaureate nursing program.)

Objectives, whether program, level, or course, tend to be global. Although the objectives usually indicate the type of patient (adult, child), setting (acute, chronic, community), and general category of health problem (med- ical, surgical, psychiatric), they are not specific enough to show the instructor whether the student has been exposed to principles in the care of the dia- betic patient. That information is contained in the course outline which clari- fies the classroom content. (Appendix B contains a sample course outline for a course with a clinical component.) Missing entirely from either the objec- tives or the course outlines is information concerning technical skills that have been introduced to, practiced by, and mastered by the student. This information requires further digging, usually through consultation with faculty who have taught the clinical component of the preceding courses or, more efficiently, by querying the students.

To succeed in correlating clinical experiences with classroom content (to the extent that this is even possible), the clinical instructor must know what is being taught in the classes, and when it is being taught. To succeed in ensuring that students achieve course objectives, the clinical instructor must know what students have already learned as well as the nature of their associated clinical experiences, and the learning and experiences that will build upon this course later in the program. The clinical instructor should request the following documents and resources to guide clinical teaching:

1. Program objectives, and the level objectives that contribute to their achievement
2. Conceptual framework of the program
3. Course outlines for all nursing courses preceding or offered concurrently with the course in which she is teaching, along with the outline for that course
4. Course materials given to students, including the schedule of clinical experiences
5. A copy of any text being used for the course[5]

To succeed in guiding students' clinical learning, the instructor must be able to understand the conceptualization of nursing being used by the students to organize their nursing knowledge. This conceptualization is articulated in the program's framework. It may reflect an existing theory of nursing such as Orem's self-care deficit theory or Roy's adaptation model, or it may be an amalgam of several theoretical perspectives. This aspect of the conceptual framework addresses what nursing is, its goals for patients, and how nurses work with patients to accomplish these goals. Each conceptual framework uses its own language to describe nursing concepts, and the clinical instructor must understand what terms mean within the larger framework to work effectively with students.

Evaluating Student Performance.   Evaluating students' clinical performance is a major challenge for all faculty, and particularly difficult for the new clinical instructor, who often lacks experience in formal evaluation procedures. Of vital importance in evaluation is fairness in the application of a published standard of performance. Problems arise when students can justifiably assert that they were treated differently than other students in the group or that they were unaware of the criteria to be used in evaluating performance.

---

[5]Such texts are called "desk copies," and usually are provided by the publisher to faculty at no charge. Inquire in the department to determine how to order a "desk copy" of texts being used in the course.

The availability of a standardized clinical evaluation form used by all clinical instructors in the course (or even better, the program) is an excellent beginning point for undertaking student evaluation. (Appendix C contains a sample clinical evaluation form.) To use the form effectively, the clinical instructor must inquire about its interpretation. Which grading options are in use (e.g., pass/fail; letter or numeric grades)? Which standards are associated with each option (e.g., performs independently or with minimum assistance; consistently demonstrates unsafe practice)? If the form is based on course objectives or other behavior-related scheme, which grade or how many passing ratings must be achieved to pass the clinical component of the course (e.g., if a pass/fail system is used, must the student pass each objective; is a passing rating required in some "critical" objectives but not others)? A review of completed forms is useful in determining how the form is used. The clinical instructor also needs to know the consequences of a failing clinical grade. In most nursing programs, a failed clinical experience results in failure of the entire course.

Each student should receive a copy of the clinical evaluation form at the beginning of the clinical experience, and the instructor should review the form with the students, providing specific examples of behaviors that would result in a passing or failing rating. For example, the instructor might inform students that being late more than once during the semester or failure to call the unit when the student is unable to attend clinical on a given day will result in a failing rating on the objective related to professional responsibility. The instructor also needs to provide examples of unsafe performance, emphasizing that making errors is a part of learning, but failing to recognize, report, and correct those errors can have dire consequences for patient safety and will result in a clinical failure. Ultimately, it is the instructor's interpretation of what constitutes a satisfactory performance that will yield the final rating. Communicating this interpretation alerts everyone to the instructor's standards.

The drawback of a checklist evaluation form is that it can only briefly summarize performance spanning several weeks of clinical experience. Some documentation of the events that contribute to clinical evaluation is necessary, and is best done through anecdotal records kept by the instructor and periodically shared with students. (Sample anecdotal notes appear in Appendix D.) These records note the circumstances of the observed incident (e.g., the type of patient, clinical problem, necessary assessment or intervention) and the behavior of the student during the incident. Records should be kept for every student, not just those having difficulty in the clinical setting, and should include both positive and negative examples of behavior. Anecdotal records provide objective, contemporaneous data that will contribute to the final evaluation. The problems associated with recall are minimized. The instructor is alerted to an uneven pattern of evaluation, if this has occurred inadvertently. Providing objective descriptions of performance deficits is useful in counseling students to improve their performance.

The clinical instructor must be familiar with evaluation policies and procedures. Such policies and procedures include ways to ensure a student's right to due process protection in the event of a grade dispute, options for borderline or failing students to receive remediation, and options for borderline or failing students to withdraw from the course. These may be found in the institution's student handbook or in a departmental policy manual. It is essential to seek out and consult these references before problems arise.

Following Established Policies and Procedures.   Many policies related to students and to faculty exist in any nursing program, but they are not always clear. It becomes the instructor's task to find the information she needs. A calendar indicating school holidays and breaks is essential, as well as a breakdown of student schedules away from the clinical unit. A clear understanding of start and stop times and the time allotted for meal breaks ensures that all clinical groups in a course are in the clinical area for roughly the same amount of time.[6] Provisions for making up a clinical absence need to be clear, as well as the maximum number of clinical days that can be missed in a semester and the consequences of extended absences.

All programs have requirements pertaining to health concerns. Each student is usually required to have a physical examination at the start of the program, and to maintain immunizations required by the college and/or the clinical setting. The usual immunizations include measles, rubella, and hepatitis B (or appropriately documented declination). Frequently, an annual tuberculin test is required. Department staff are responsible for verifying health information, but the instructor should double check to be certain all students in the clinical group are in compliance. Most programs require students to be annually certified in cardiopulmonary resuscitation (CPR); as with health information, this documentation is maintained by the department. Additional health-related issues include mandatory annual OSHA reviews prior to entering the clinical area, as well as policies related to students becoming ill while in the clinical area and managing potential hepatitis B/HIV exposures, as with needlesticks or contact with contaminated materials.

Upon hire, faculty are required to provide evidence of education by submitting official transcripts of all collegiate work to the appropriate college office. In most nursing programs, a masters degree in nursing or a related field is required for all instructors, both part-time and full-time. Evidence of current licensure as a registered professional nurse in the state in which the program is located as well as in the state in which the clinical experience will occur must be on file and updated annually. Annual CPR recertification is required for all

---

[6]The concept of "academic freedom," which has been interpreted by some as "do your own thing," does not apply to the scheduling of clinical experiences, which are negotiated in advance. While faculty and students need not simply "do their time" in the clinical area, and can modify the experience on a particularly slow day, it is best to adhere to the posted days and hours as closely as possible.

clinical faculty, as is evidence of complying with the health requirements mandated by the agency, usually the same as those required for students in the program.

State regulations governing nursing programs may impact clinical instruction. For example, regulations may stipulate a specific faculty:student ratio in the clinical area, such as 1:8 or 1:10, and that the faculty be available within the setting at all times students are there. Clinical instructors assigned to community settings need to determine how required availability is maintained, as through a beeper system, and who is responsible for providing and paying for the equipment.

Maintaining a Positive Image for the Program.   Even if the clinical experience is the faculty member's only assignment in the nursing program, she is considered a representative and ambassador for the program. The instructor's own clinical expertise, skill in managing the learning experiences of students, and willingness to contribute to the well-being of the clinical unit and its staff contribute to the agency's evaluation of the experience, and hence the program. There is keen competition for clinical placements for nursing students. The instructor's ability to cement relationships at the clinical level makes negotiation for subsequent placements less difficult.

The clinical instructor may be asked questions about the nursing program, and should have some general sense of the available offerings. For example, she should be aware of whether there is a degree-completion program for RNs, a graduate program, or continuing education offerings and who should be contacted for information about these programs.

Developing Collegial Relationships within the Nursing Department

Because faculty usually operate in isolation from one another in their teaching activities and have schedules that differ dramatically from those of their co-workers, they need to structure opportunities for the collegial sharing that provides support, encouragement, and informal learning. Each department develops its own approach to enhancing collegiality; morale declines if this aspect of work life is neglected.

Clinical instructors are rarely scheduled to be at the college, and so are likely to be left out of the majority of socializing activities. By arranging to come in to the college on a day when most faculty are there, the clinical instructor can interface with full-time faculty and develop a better perspective on the program. This is a good time to connect with the lead instructor in the course with which the clinical instructor is involved, to get a sense of how classes are going and whether students' comments reflect relevant clinical learning experiences. Some new instructors attend several (or even all) classes to get a feel for the level of content being presented and to assist in the task of correlating classroom content with clinical experiences. This should only be done with the permission of the classroom faculty. Although not required to attend, part-time faculty usually are welcome at department faculty meetings and even committee meetings. Participating in these meetings gives the part-time faculty member a sense of belonging to the faculty as a whole, and provides some insights into the issues that affect program functioning.

In the clinical setting the instructor can seek out other program faculty members during mealtimes. Just knowing who else from the program is teaching in the same facility at the same time can be reassuring and supportive.

Developing a friendship with an established faculty member can help the neophyte to "read" the history and politics of the department, which goes a long way in explaining interactions among faculty and enables the new faculty member to fit in.

THE CLINICAL SETTING

While nursing programs often are affiliated with a primary facility in which clinical experiences occur, most of them try to provide students with a range of experiences in a variety of health care facilities. Competition for clinical placements also sends programs on a search for suitable placements that may be far afield of the geographical location of the program. Clinical affiliations are selected by the department chair, program coordinator, and, often, the clinical faculty who will be teaching at the facility. The final arrangements with the facility are confirmed in a contractual agreement that outlines the roles and obligations of both the college and the clinical facility in relation to the clinical affiliation. It is wise for the new clinical instructor to request a copy of the agreement pertaining to the facility in which she will be teaching students. A sample of such an agreement appears in Appendix E.

Nursing program personnel seek clinical placements in accredited agencies whose philosophy of care is congruent with the program's philosophy; that maintain high standards of patient care and of nursing practice; provide the types of clinical experiences that permit achievement of course objectives and that fit with the overall curriculum design; and accept the student placements without raising too many barriers, such as charging a fee for the use of the facility or demanding unrealistically low ratios of students to faculty. It is essential that students be permitted to have a full range of experiences (e.g., no restrictions on giving medications, observing procedures) during learning activities in the facility. Ideally, the presence of students on the unit is not considered in staffing patterns.

Of concern, too, is that the facility is within reasonable commuting distance from the college (or the students, if the student population is primarily commuters), that there's parking, and storage for students' coats and books. If students are at the facility for a full shift, a cafeteria or food service should be available to them. Conference space, for pre- and post-conferences as well as individual conferences with students, is an important amenity, especially space adjacent to the clinical area. A bonus is a medical library that can be used by students.

In the best of possible clinical worlds, the staff is eager to have students in the clinical area for the sheer joy and satisfaction of facilitating their entry into the profession and the intellectual stimulation their presence provides. It is the clinical instructor who makes or breaks the staff's reception of students into the clinical area.

Demands of Clinical Teaching

The role of the clinical instructor is multifaceted and complex, requiring the instructor to juggle many responsibilities and respond to competing demands. Oermann's study of work-related stress in clinical nursing faculty suggests that they have many stresses.

> The extent of knowledge and skills to be developed by students in the clinical setting, limited time for teaching, acuity of patients, and number of students for whom the clinical teacher is responsible may contribute to creating a stressful work environment for faculty. Maintaining positive relations with staff, becoming familiar with agency policies and norms, and balancing learning experiences with patient needs and welfare are important responsibilities of the faculty to ensure a positive learning environment for students. (1998, p. 302)

Boughn (1992) adds,

> There is extensive preparation required for clinical teaching. The clinical instructor must possess an in-depth working knowledge of the patients assigned to their students. They must keep current on a wide variety of health care problems, treatments, procedures, and policies. (p. 217)

While all students in the clinical group are pursuing the same objectives, and have the same frame of reference in terms of classroom content, they are not alike in terms of learning needs. One student may be able to prioritize care activities and approach the clinical day in an organized fashion; another may be struggling to determine what should be done first. Some students may be overdependent on the instructor, seeking guidance and affirmation before providing any aspect of care; others may be intent on avoiding the instructor. Crises inevitably arise during the course of the clinical experience to which the student and instructor must respond, which pulls the instructor away from other students. Supervision of an activity with one student may take more time than originally planned, as when a student contaminates many dressing kits, leaving limited time to supervise another student.

Although the students and their learning needs are at the center of the clinical instructor's attention, others—most notably, patients and staff—also compete for that attention and cannot be ignored. The clinical instructor's primary role is educator, but she is a professional colleague to staff and a nurse to patients. Her warmth and responsiveness to staff will create a positive learning environment for students. The instructor's concern for patients and communication with them will make them more receptive to accepting students as care providers. At the same time, the instructor cannot become overinvolved with patients by taking over for a student or absenting herself from the instructional role in order to provide direct patient care.

Even if the clinical instructor is teaching in a facility in which she was once or is now employed, she remains a guest in the facility, and must remain aware of that status. For example, an instructor who also maintains an employment relationship with the facility must guard against inevitable role confusion, as may occur when the staff needs her while she is trying to teach. Being a guest involves knowing and conforming to the operating policies and practices of the facility and the clinical unit. The clinical instructor must learn to "go with the flow," and avoid criticizing staff or established routines. While the clinical instructor may need to explain discrepancies between staff practices and the standards to which students are held, this needs to be done in terms of differences in approach, avoiding value judgments. Students need to know there is more than one "right" way to do things, and that different nurses approach patient care in different ways. Mastering one technique, and knowing the rationale for it, enables the student to make adjustments in future practice. When warranted, the instructor should compliment staff on the care they are providing, or their innovative approach to a patient problem. Citing a staff member as an outstanding role model helps students to recognize excellence and gives staff a real boost.

The clinical instructor should be cautious about initiating change on the clinical unit because it may be interpreted as criticism. Students can be the vehicle for introducing change through their genuine questions about existing practices.

The clinical instructor needs to remain responsive to staff socially, even in the face of student demands for attention. Having a cup of coffee with staff keeps the instructor from appearing aloof and "above it all." Bringing in a can of coffee and an occasional goodie for the coffee break also is appreciated, especially if students have been invited too.

Expectations of Clinical Staff

At the beginning of the experience clinical staff need a general idea of the course content and objectives, as well as the level of students—beginners or near graduation. As the experience progresses, they need a brief overview of activities that are planned for that clinical day, along with any changes in the usual time students will be on the unit. Staff need to know which patients have been selected for student assignments, and in which activities students will engage. It's vital that they know about students' responsibility for administering medication and with what dose of medication this responsibility begins and ends. Will students be doing formal documentation on care activities or simply providing reports to the primary nurse or charge nurse? Ideally, student assignments are made the day before the clinical and communicated to staff at that time; however, early discharge of a patient or a student absence will require a change in plans, which must be communicated.

While staff do not expect to be involved in making student-patient assignments, they do appreciate being consulted about patients who might best enable students to meet objectives, and those that should be avoided if possible. This collaboration engages staff in the educational effort, and enables them to better understand the learning needs of the student group.

Staff expect that care activities will be completed in accordance with operating routines. This includes timely administration and accurate documentation of medications and recording of vital signs. They expect that changes in a patient's condition will be reported promptly to the appropriate staff member rather than held until the end of the clinical day.

Staff expect that students will have questions regarding the location of supplies and equipment as well as patient preferences, but they also expect that the instructor will have provided a thorough orientation for students to reduce the number of such questions. Computerization of patient records, including reports of test results and documentation about administering medication and other treatments, creates special problems for the clinical instructor. Usually, the instructor, but not the students, is given access to the computer. When students need to consult the patient record, they access it through the instructor, who may be working with another student, or through a staff member, who is unlikely to appreciate this interruption. This issue should be addressed before the clinical experience begins, so that the instructor can direct the student to appropriate sources for assistance.

Positive relationships with staff can be fostered by encouraging students to ask them about the best way to care for specific patients. For example, over a period of time, nursing assistants in a skilled nursing facility develop better approaches with patients for whom they regularly provide care. It is both practical and flattering for students to ask to learn these techniques. Students should be encouraged to offer assistance to staff when appropriate, as with helping in repositioning a patient or emptying a bedpan.

Staff expect that the instructor will intervene if things go wrong in a student's care of a patient. They are aware that they walk a fine line in this regard, and are careful not to interfere with the teaching-learning process while remaining acutely aware of patient safety and welfare concerns. Open lines of communication are essential if the clinical instructor is to feel comfortable in asking for staff assistance and staff comfortable with offering such assistance when a patient's condition changes or the demands of care become overwhelming for the student.

Staff hold the clinical instructor ultimately responsible for the care provided by students to patients on the unit. The instructor needs to provide staff with a means of contacting her after the clinical experience has ended in the event problems arise related to the care that the student provided.

Expectations of Students

Reeve (1994) summarizes the results of studies describing characteristics of the effective clinical instructor:

> The instructor should have a professional manner and the ability to function as a role model, the ability to provide appropriate evaluation and feedback, to be a resource person and be able to assist students to meet objectives without taking over, to have good interpersonal relationships and communication skills, to display respect for the student, and to have appropriate teaching practices. (p. 15)

Students expect that the clinical instructor will help them apply theoretical knowledge to the patient care situations with which they are involved. They expect to be guided in making observations, reaching conclusions, selecting and performing interventions, and evaluating outcomes. They want to be as independent as possible in their practice with patients, but, at the same time, have the instructor available. Students expect that the instructor will answer questions pertaining to patient care, or guide them to resources that can provide the answers. An important aspect of role modeling is to enable students to recognize that no nurse knows everything, and that it is important to seek the answers to questions as they arise rather than muddle through with a guess or a hunch.

Students expect the clinical instructor to be comfortable in the clinical environment and be able to provide the care that the students are expected to provide, including the performance of various skilled activities.

Davis et al. (1992) identify the ability to remain calm as an important characteristic of the instructional role. Students expect that the clinical instructor will be able to manage crises and conflicts without falling apart or flying into a rage. They expect the clinical instructor to operate "above the fray," not getting involved in staff politics or student battles. Students hope that the clinical instructor will act as an advocate for them with staff when necessary.

Students expect to be treated with the dignity and caring afforded the patients in their care. They are very aware of their relatively low status within the clinical area, and seek the instructor's support and respect in their efforts to learn while doing. They anticipate that they will need to be corrected as they learn, but expect that this will be a learning experience rather than a humiliating confrontation.

Orientation to the Clinical Setting

Clinical instructors new to a facility are required to participate in an orientation similar (or identical) to that provided for new employees. Often, the staff education department is responsible for arranging the details of the orientation of clinical instructors, and also serves as liaison with the instructors and the nursing programs they represent. It is essential that the new instructor attend the orientation activities as scheduled. Making personal contact with the staff education liaison provides the instructor with an additional resource within the clinical setting.

While much of the information provided in the facility's standardized orientation will be irrelevant to the instructional role, an awareness of the institutional philosophy and mission, organizational structure, and key personnel is useful as a frame of reference for assessing the clinical learning environment. For example, an institution with a strong educational and research mission is likely to have systems in place that support and facilitate clinical learning experiences. Fire, safety, and biohazard reviews provide some details on policies and procedures in use in the facility, and should prompt the instructor to note questions for the nurse manager of the clinical unit, such as, what is the students' role if a fire occurs? Operation of a computerized patient information system, systems for charging supplies, documentation practices, medication administration policies and procedures, including the management of controlled substances, are areas of vital importance to the clinical instructor. Hopefully, the facility will provide written materials containing this information; if not, the instructor will need to know where to locate such information on the unit.

In the initial meeting with the nurse manager, the clinical instructor should seek information that will guide the selection of appropriate assignments for students. For example, the instructor will need to know the usual clinical problems encountered on the unit, the range of ages of patients, average patient acuity and length of stay, average census, and availability of off-unit observational experiences, as in diagnostic laboratories. If possible, previous experiences with students from this or other programs should be explored with the nurse manager. Such a discussion might involve practices by previous instructors that were particularly useful in managing clinical instruction or that posed problems for the staff. Preferences for student-staff interactions should be determined, including whether each patient for whom students provide care will also have a primary nurse; the anticipated role of the primary nurse in relation to care activities and student learning; and procedures for getting a report on patients at the beginning of the clinical day and reporting off at the end of the experience. Unit routines should be noted, such as the standard times to administer medication and times at which meals are served. To minimize reliance on staff for information, the nurse manager can be asked to identify key personnel to whom specific types of questions might be addressed.

A tour of the unit is essential. The clinical instructor must become familiar with the general layout of patient rooms and central supply and equipment areas. The location of frequently used supplies and equipment, including emergency equipment, must be determined. The supplies and equipment should be examined and manipulated if possible, so that the instructor is confident in using these in patient care. The instructor should ask to access sample patient records to identify the information they contain. This enables the instructor to direct the student to the appropriate location of patient-specific information.

Ideally, the clinical instructor should arrange to work on the unit in the staff nurse role for several days to become completely acclimated to the environment and its routines. If this is impossible, the instructor should ask to "shadow" one or more staff for a day or two to observe the nuances of the environment of care.

SUMMARY

Piscopo (1994) describes the clinical faculty role as "boundary spanning." The clinical instructor is active in both the academic and clinical environments and must adjust to the special nature of each. She must bring the standards and agenda (as reflected in the curriculum and objectives) of the educational program to the clinical setting and manage the clinical experience to achieve those standards and agenda. At the same time, she must cope with the realities of the clinical setting, which may render the educational agenda irrelevant or impossible to achieve. The clinical instructor is a guest in the clinical environment in which she spends most of her time, and a stranger in the academic environment in which she is employed. No wonder clinical nursing faculty report as stressors

> coping with job expectations associated with their clinical teaching roles; feeling physically and emotionally drained at the end of a clinical teaching day; job demands that interfere with activities of personal importance; heavy workload; pressure to maintain clinical competence or a clinical practice without time to do so; feeling unable to satisfy the demands of work-related constituencies (e.g., students, clinical agency personnel, patients); and teaching inadequately prepared students (Oermann, 1998, p. 302).

REFERENCES

Boughn, S. (1992). An immodest proposal: Pay equity for nursing faculty who do clinical teaching. *Journal of Nursing Education*, 31, 215–220.

Davis, D.C, Dearman, C., Schwab, C., & Kitchens, E. (1992). Competencies of novice nurse educators. *Journal of Nursing Education*, 31, 159–164.

Esper, P.S. (1995). Facing transition—Nurse clinician to nurse educator. *Journal of Nursing Education*, 34, 89–91.

Oermann, M.H. (1998). Work-related stress of clinical nursing faculty. *Journal of Nursing Education*, 37, 302–304.

Piscopo, B. (1994). Organizational climate, communication, and role strain in clinical nursing faculty. *Journal of Professional Nursing*, 10, 112–119.

Reeve, M.M. (1994). Development of an instrument to measure effectiveness of clinical instructors. *Journal of Nursing Education*, 33, 15–20.

CHAPTER 3

THEORETICAL APPROACHES TO TEACHING AND LEARNING IN CLINICAL NURSING EDUCATION

How Learners Learn   30
   Psychological Theories   30
   Developmental Theories   33
   Social Theories   34
Behavioral Domains and Hierarchies of Learning   35
   Cognitive Domain   36
   Psychomotor Domain   36
   Affective Domain   40
Nature of the Adult Learner   44
   Assumptions of Andragogy   45
   Conditions for Learning   46
Benner's Framework for the Development of Clinical Expertise   48
Summary   50
References   51

How is it that students learn such a complex applied field as nursing? How do they come to recognize the connections between their knowledge of the anatomy and physiology of cardiovascular function and the signs and symptoms exhibited by a patient, as well as what needs to be done in the situation? The capacity of the human brain to retain and recall many diverse facts, and then apply these thoughtfully in the immediate situation is the matter of educational theory. Learning theories seek to understand how learning occurs. Their practical application is in manipulating approaches to teaching that will enhance learning.

How Learners Learn

Numerous theories have been proposed to explain how learning occurs. These theories are categorized on the basis of their dominant perspective.

Psychological Theories[1]

Behavioral psychology assumes that learning proceeds on a trial-and-error basis, and that learning occurs when correct responses are reinforced or incorrect responses punished. It is the outcome of the learning that is the focus of concern rather than the intellectual processes that resulted in that outcome. In this theoretical approach, the learning process occurs in a "black box," and only the outcome of learning is available for study. An extension of the behaviorist approach (also called S-R [stimulus-response] associationism) involves stimulus substitution, where a second stimulus, usually unassociated with the primary stimulus-evoking behavior, is substituted for the first to yield a response. The Pavlovian response typifies stimulus substitution, where a dog salivates when presented with a steak, a bell rings simultaneously with the presentation of the steak, and the dog eventually "learns" to associate the bell with the steak and salivates when the bell rings, in the absence of the steak. In the context of nursing education, behaviorism can be exemplified using the process of learning the required sequence of actions in performing CPR. The initial stimulus, an unconscious person, evokes a response: attempting to rouse the individual. A second stimulus, the failure of the person to respond, evokes yet another response: checking for breathing, and so forth. Stimulus substitution is exemplified in the response to an announced "code"; the nurse need not witness the unconscious individual to know what is happening and to respond.

Nursing education has been profoundly affected by behaviorism, best evidenced by its focus on objectives, or goals, to be mastered throughout the educational process. The ability to demonstrate the behavior identified in an objective is assumed to reflect learning, and there has been little concern with how that learning occurred.

A second psychological theory is derived from Gestalt psychology. Its focus is on the learner's thought processes, or cognition. Learning involves the development of insights (or the modification of old insights) in an effort to organize and interpret components of the stimulus situation. *Insight* is a key principle of this theory, and reflects the learner's ability to recognize patterns and relationships that are present in the stimulus situation that give meaning to the whole. The laws of *relativism*—a second principle of this theory—help the person to organize and understand her perceptions. The principle of rela-

---

[1]This section draws upon O'Connor, A.B. (1986). *Nursing staff development and continuing education.* Boston: Little, Brown, pp. 39–44.

tivism proposes that components of the whole are seen in relation to one another, and it is on the basis of these relationships, rather than the components themselves, that meaning is derived.

Several laws of relativism guide perceptions. The law of *similarity* prompts the learner to organize the components in a situation on the basis of their similarity to one another. Learning requires recognition of the salient aspects of components that make them similar—or dissimilar—to one another. For example, IV tubing and gastric tubing are similar in those aspects that characterize "tubes," and dissimilar in those aspects concerning placement and use. The law of *proximity* groups components on the basis of their proximity to one another. A nurse does not expect to find sterile supplies in a utility room. The law of *closure* causes the learner to fill in empty spaces in a picture, using the assumptions underlying the laws of *continuity*. Thus, Figure 3–1 shows a circle (law of closure), and the line completing the circle is assumed to continue on a steady path rather than moving off into space (law of continuity). The law of *membership* involves making sense of the unknown through attentiveness to context, assuming that each unknown component in a situation carries the characteristics of or is somehow related to other components. This is the

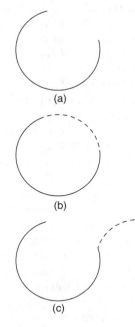

(a)

(b)

(c)

Figure 3–1 The law of closure suggests that the viewer will assume Figure (a) to be part of a completed circle (b). The law of continuity suggests that the line that will complete Figure (a) will continue on a steady path, resulting in circle (b), rather than move in a new direction (c).

phenomenon that underlies stereotyping. It is important for the educator to recognize that the utility of the laws of relativism diminishes as more assumptions—not based on what is actually present in the situation—must be made by the learner. Helping learners to make the fine-tuned discriminations necessary in nursing contexts requires pointing out the salient features of each situation that contribute to total understanding.

In the nursing context, Gestalt psychology prompts nurses to look at the "whole picture," rather than discrete aspects of the situation. Thus, a blood pressure reading is interpreted within the context of other patient signs and symptoms, such as pulse rate, color, subjective response, and so forth, to help evaluate the patient's condition.

A third theory, cognitive-field psychology, looks at the psychological context within which learning occurs and proposes that that context (field) affects knowing (cognition) in profound ways. In this theory, cognitive learning is similar to the learning described by Gestalt psychology, involving the development of insights and depending on relationships within—but also outside—the stimulus situation. Learning occurs through *differentiation*, which enables the learner to perceive subtle differences among similar objects, as in recognizing intramuscular, subcutaneous, and suture needles within the broad category of needles; *generalization*, which enables the learner to perceive similarities among disparate objects, as in recognizing the function of postoperative drains, regardless of type or location; and *restructuralization*, which enables the learner to regroup concepts to derive a better understanding of the stimulus situation, as in recognizing restlessness and irritability as possible signs of pain.

Unique to the cognitive-field theory of learning are principles that take into consideration the psychological environment of the learner as she perceives the personal, physical, and social world. The first principle views *perception as relativistic*, in that it is influenced not only by other components of the stimulus situation, but also by past, present, and imagined future events; by abstract as well as concrete concepts; and by the real as well as the imagined. Thus, each learner "perceives" in unique ways. This helps to explain why all students don't "see" the situation in the same way, or as the clinical instructor sees it. The second principle envisions *human behavior as purposive* and learning as goal-directed. The degree of goal-directedness of an individual learner is determined by the degree to which the learner is attracted to or repulsed by the goal. It is important to note that behavior that moves the learner *away* from an undesired goal is purposive. This is encountered when a student is in a nursing program because someone else thinks she would be a fine nurse, but hasn't embraced this goal for herself. A third principle defines *learning as a psychological event* that can occur in the absence of observed behavioral change, in opposition to behaviorist psychology. Fourth, learning is *situational*. It occurs in a context, and is affected by that context, which will form part of the relativistic perceptual world of the learner in future situations. The final principle, *contemporaneity*, suggests that events that occur simultaneously with learning also become part of the relativistic perceptual world of the learner, and are evoked in similar future circumstances.

In nursing education, the cognitive-field theory offers an explanation of the problems inherent in transferring theory to practice. Classroom learning occurs in a context very dissimilar to that of the clinical environment, a context that lacks the richness of stimuli presented by patient problems. Obviously, performing CPR on a mannequin in the controlled setting of the college laboratory is vastly different from performing CPR in the clinical setting. But note also the conversations among nurses that occur after a "code" in the clinical area, where talk of previous experiences with codes reveals the contextual environment within which the current event has been perceived and understood.

While the psychological theories of learning offer perspectives on how learners respond to and understand the world, their focus is on cognition (what is known rather than what is experienced) and the changes that occur in the internal psychological environment of the learner. Other learning theories discuss the interplay of the individual and the external environment, and consider more than just the psychological and cognitive aspects of the learner.

Developmental Theories

Many theories of learning propose that readiness to learn is determined by biological, psychological, and social development as well as social pressure to learn. In line with general theories of growth and development, developmental theories of learning assert that learning is orderly and sequential in nature, with each level building upon or evolving from a previous level, in a pattern that is followed by all learners, although at different rates.

Piaget's (1962) theory of cognitive development in children, for example, proposes that the initial sensorimotor stage, in which the infant explores the environment, is a prelude to the preoperational stage, in which the child begins to use symbols, such as words and pictures, that represent aspects of the environment. In the concrete operational stage, the child is able to manipulate concrete objects in the environment, such as sorting blocks by color or shape. The ability to manipulate abstract concepts does not emerge until the formal operational stage. Piaget's theory applies to childhood learning, and does not attempt to explain the further intellectual development of adults.

Havighurst (1953) proposed that learning occurs to achieve developmental tasks related to occupational roles, family roles, and civic responsibility. This perspective exemplifies the belief of developmental theorists that social pressure contributes to learning. Havighurst's theory is limited by its basis in a singular sociocultural condition (heterosexual marriage with children) which does not reflect modern society. Nurse educators, however, need to be alert to the numerous social pressures that students have in the course of their education. Many are parents; even more must work to support themselves and their families. Entering the nursing field may be viewed by these students as a means to better meet these obligations in the future, but the time and energy they have available to study today may impact their success in school.

Kohlberg's (1981) theory of moral reasoning and the feminist perspective on his theory offered by Gilligan (1982) attempt to trace the development of the sense of right and wrong. Both theories loosely follow Piaget's sequence of cognitive development. Moral reasoning proceeds from a self-centered perspective (fear of consequences to self, e.g., punishment or possibility of reward motivates obedience to rules) to an other-centered perspective, where choosing the right or avoiding the wrong is based on the desires or values of an admired other or established authority. The final stage of development, which may not be reached by all, involves an internalized system of morality that forms the basis for actions.

In nursing, Benner (1982) has applied the Dreyfus model of skill acquisition to the sequential development of nursing expertise. This model suggests that expertise is acquired through the application of knowledge in interaction with the environment, and progresses as the learner becomes more attuned to the subtleties of the situations she encounters. The sequence of practice development proposed by Benner moves from novice to advanced beginner to competent to proficient to expert.

Developmental theories of learning help to explain the concept of "readiness" to learn, by revealing the prerequisite intellectual understandings and skills necessary to engage in more advanced learning. These theories also recognize the differences in the pace of learning evidenced by individual students who would seem, by their placement in the program, to be at the same level.

Social Theories

Social theories of learning propose that knowledge is socially constructed, in interaction with others, and interpreted through the lens of what is known and what is culturally acceptable. Friere (1970) proposed that learning emerges from the social situation in which people find themselves, which prompts them to seek the knowledge and skills that will enable them to extricate themselves from that situation and rise above it. In Friere's view, learning is a collective process among individuals who, together, seek solutions to the everyday problems of life. Knowles's (1980) theory of adult learning also proposes that the need to learn is prompted by the demands of the immediate situation, and that the shared knowledge and perspectives of a group of learners is the source of new learning. In this approach, the educator is a facilitator rather than a provider of learning, and the responsibility for learning rests with the group.

A collection of theories being applied in nursing education—humanistic-educative, phenomenological, feminist pedagogy, critical social theory—shift the emphasis in the educational process to the learner, and how she is affected by learning. The humanistic-educative model views learning as the process of developing the learner's highest potential. The phenomenological approach seeks to understand the lived experiences of both students and patients, and focuses on the whole picture in contrast to a technical skills orientation. Feminist pedagogy seeks to incorporate a feminist perspective on human experiences, as a response to a male-dominated system of knowledge and its transmission that may exclude alternative perspectives. Like the phenomenological approach, feminist pedagogy is rooted in and sensitive to the experiences of women, as students, as educators, and as patients. Critical social theory attempts to counterbalance what is termed the "received view," the conventionally accepted explanation of a phenomenon, with a view that is derived from the social experience as it is exists in reality (Kirschling et al., 1995; Norton, 1998). Each of these theories focuses on the person of the learner and the social context within which learning occurs and knowledge will be applied.

In a movement that has been called the "curriculum revolution" (Bevis, 1988), nursing educators have proposed that nursing education abandon its behaviorist roots, which emphasize outcomes of learning as evidenced by learner behaviors, to embrace a humanistic-educative approach that focuses on transactions between teachers and students and among students, which is where learning occurs. In contrast to the behaviorist model, in which the teacher appears to be continually evaluating the student's performance in accordance with objectives, the humanistic model fosters the development of the student-teacher relationship, in which each shares in the learning that is prompted by the immediate situation.

BEHAVIORAL DOMAINS AND HIERARCHIES OF LEARNING

Despite a movement toward a humanistic model of teaching and learning, nursing education is still deeply embedded in the behaviorist model. There is an emphasis on outcomes of learning as reflected in the achievement of a collection of behavioral objectives that permeate courses and the larger curriculum. This emphasis is in keeping with prevalent trends in education, as well as with the structure of guidelines for nursing program accreditation. Behavioral objectives describe observable changes in learner behavior that reflect progress toward or achievement of goals established for the course or curriculum. Behavioral objectives reflect three aspects of learning: cognitive (intellect), psychomotor (performance), and affective (emotion). Within each of these domains, knowledge is acquired, a skill is mastered, or a value is adopted in accordance with a hierarchical structure specific to the domain. A behavioral objective identifies the observable student behavior that reflects achievement of a specific hierarchical level of a specific domain. Only one behavior—and one domain and level within that domain—is included in any given behavioral objective. One criticism of behavioral objectives (among many) is that they are reductionist in nature, and fail to capture the complexity of applied knowledge necessary to succeed in clinical nursing education.

Although they are used in all aspects of nursing education, behavioral objectives may be *least* relevant in the clinical setting, where the domains of knowledge interact simultaneously and are interdependent. Accurately calculating the dosage requirement for an intramuscular injection (cognitive domain) and drawing up the appropriate amount of medication in a syringe (psychomotor domain) might be disentangled from one another in expressing a behavioral objective related to administering medication (although one would want both behaviors to be demonstrated); but what about the process of locating a site for injection, which involves knowing appropriate sites for this type of injection (cognitive domain), palpating for anatomical landmarks to select the area for the injection (psychomotor domain), and choosing the site least likely to cause discomfort (affective domain)? This "experiential" domain, which represents the integration of knowledge from the three recognized domains, is a neglected area in the literature describing learning in applied fields (Menix, 1996). Rather than develop this domain, educators focus behavioral objectives on the dominant behavior to be observed, or on the cognitive, under the assumption that the associated psychomotor and affective components of the behavior are subordinate to the cognitive and will follow.

Cognitive Domain

The cognitive domain concerns intellectual operations based on acquired knowledge of facts and theories. Table 3–1 describes major categories within the cognitive domain as a guide to the level of learning each represents, as well as descriptions of characteristic behaviors reflecting each level in this domain.

Behavioral objectives concerned with knowledge and comprehension are inappropriate in the clinical setting, where the focus should be on application, analysis, synthesis, and evaluation. The clinical instructor's skilled questioning of students should reflect this focus. A student's recitation of the normal range of pulse rate is irrelevant clinically unless that knowledge is applied in evaluating a patient's pulse rate and analyzed in relation to other aspects of the clinical situation.

The cognitive domain is the most well developed of the three behavioral domains, and most commonly encountered in nursing education. This tends to place an emphasis (intended or not) on "knowing that," often at the expense of "knowing how" and incorporating values into actions, one of the criticisms of the behaviorist approach to education.

Psychomotor Domain

The psychomotor domain concerns skills involving neuromuscular activities and physical manipulations. Table 3–2 describes major categories within one scheme of the psychomotor domain as a guide to the level of learning each

TABLE 3–1 DESCRIPTIONS AND CHARACTERISTIC BEHAVIORS OF THE
HIERARCHICAL CATEGORIES IN THE COGNITIVE DOMAIN

1. **Knowledge.** Knowledge is defined as the remembering of previously learned material. This involves the recall of a wide range of material, from specific facts to complete theories, but all that is required is the bringing to mind of the appropriate information. Knowledge represents the lowest level of learning outcomes in the cognitive domain.

   Characteristic behaviors

   Knowledge of specifics

    Knowledge of terminology

    Knowledge of specific facts

   Knowledge of ways and means of dealing with specifics

    Knowledge of conventions

    Knowledge of trends and sequences

    Knowledge of classifications and categories

    Knowledge of criteria

    Knowledge of methods

   Knowledge of universals and abstractions in the field

    Knowledge of principles and generalizations

    Knowledge of theories and structures

2. **Comprehension.** Comprehension is defined as the ability to grasp the meaning of material. This may be shown by translating material from one form to another (words to numbers), by interpreting material (explaining or summarizing), and by estimating future trends (predicting consequences or effects). These learning outcomes go one step beyond the simple remembering of material, and represent the lowest level of understanding.

   Characteristic behaviors

   Translation

   Interpretation

   Extrapolation

3. **Application.** Application refers to the ability to use learned material in new and concrete situations. This includes the application of such things as rules, methods, concepts, principles, laws, and theories. Learning outcomes in this area require a higher level of understanding than those under comprehension.

4. **Analysis.** Analysis refers to the ability to break down material into its component parts so that its organizational structure may be understood. This includes the identification of the parts, analysis of the relationships between parts, and recognition of the organizational principles involved.

TABLE 3–1 CONTINUED

Learning outcomes here represent a higher intellectual level than comprehension and application because they require an understanding of both the content and the structural form of the material.

Characteristic behaviors

Analysis of elements

Analysis of relationships

Analysis of organizational principles

5. **Synthesis.**   Synthesis refers to the ability to put parts together to form a new whole. This involves the production of a unique communication (theme or speech), a plan of operations (research proposal), or a set of abstract relations (scheme for classifying information). Learning outcomes in this area stress creative behaviors, with major emphasis on the formulation of new patterns of structures.

Characteristic behaviors

Production of a unique communication

Production of a plan or proposed set of operations

Derivation of a set of abstract relations

6. **Evaluation.**   Evaluation is concerned with the ability to judge the value of material (statement, novel, poem, research report) for a given purpose. The judgments are to be based on definite criteria. These may be internal criteria (organization) or external criteria (relevance to the purpose) and the student may determine the criteria or be given them. Learning outcomes in this area are highest in the cognitive hierarchy because they contain elements of all of the other categories, plus conscious value judgments based on clearly defined criteria.

Characteristic behaviors

Judgments in terms of internal criteria

Judgments in terms of external criteria

Note. Adapted from Gronlund, N.E. (1991). *How to write and use instructional objectives* (4th ed.), p. 32. New York, NY: Macmillan; Kibler, R.J., Barker, L.L., & Miles, D.T. (1970). *Behavioral objectives and instruction*, pp. 44–55. Boston: Allyn and Bacon.

represents, as well as descriptions of characteristic behaviors reflecting each level in this domain.

Initial instruction in psychomotor skills often occurs in the controlled environment of the college laboratory. In this setting, students have the opportunity to manipulate and become familiar with supplies and equipment. Trial and error approaches to practicing a skill enable students to develop the body sense (through kinesthetic feedback) that signals developing fluidity and control in carrying out the skill. (Nursing faculty often are divided about the

TABLE 3–2 Descriptions and Characteristic Behaviors of the Hierarchical Categories in the Psychomotor Domain

1. **Perception.** The first level is concerned with the use of the sense organs to obtain cues that guide motor activity.
   Characteristic behaviors
   Awareness of a stimulus
   Selection of task-relevant cues
   Translation of cue perception to action in a performance

2. **Set.** Set refers to readiness to take a particular type of action. Perception of cues serves as an important prerequisite for this level.
   Characteristic behaviors
   Mental readiness to act
   Physical readiness to act
   Willingness to act

3. **Guided Response.** Guided response is concerned with the early stages in learning a complex skill. Adequacy of performance is judged by an instructor or by a suitable set of criteria.
   Characteristic behaviors
   Imitation of instructor's demonstration
   Continuous referral to model performance
   Trial and error

4. **Mechanism.** Mechanism is concerned with performance acts where the learned responses have become habitual and the movements can be performed with some confidence and proficiency. Learning outcomes at this level are concerned with performance skills of various types, but the movement patterns are less complex than at the next higher level.

5. **Complex Overt Response.** Complex Overt Response is concerned with the skillful performance of motor acts that involve complex movement patterns. Proficiency is indicated by a quick, smooth, accurate performance, requiring a minimum of energy. Learning outcomes at this level include highly coordinated motor activities.
   Characteristic behaviors
   Performance without hesitation
   Movements exhibit ease and good muscle control
   Coordinated, fluid, timely, and automatic performance

6. **Adaptation.** Adaptation is concerned with skills that are so well developed that the individual can modify movement patterns to fit special requirements or to meet a problem situation.

TABLE 3–2 Continued

7. **Origination.**   Origination refers to the creating of new movement patterns to fit a particular situation or specific problem. Learning outcomes at this level emphasize creativity based upon highly developed skills.

Note. Adapted from Gronlund, N.E. (1991). *How to write and use instructional objectives* (4th ed.), p. 36. New York, NY: Macmillan.

usefulness of the college laboratory for skill instruction. Because such learning must eventually be transferred to the clinical setting, some prefer to do the initial instruction in that setting. Issues related to patient comfort and safety, waste of supplies, and dysfunctional anxiety levels of students are arguments supporting the use of the college laboratory for initial skill instruction.)

The mastery of psychomotor skills requires practice. Feedback that compliments performances that approach mastery is useful in helping the student to further develop the body sense that accompanies skilled performance. Careful observation of a student's performance can yield clues to behaviors that may be interfering with skill mastery. For example, standing too far away from patients in performing skills, contributes to the students' muscular fatigue. Simply encouraging the student to move closer, to raise the bed, to take down the side rail may be all that is needed to move the student's level of performance further toward mastery.

In the initial stages of learning skills, students become very tightly focused on the mechanics of the procedure. They are unable to attend to other cues in the environment, and often are unable to think or talk at the same time they are performing. Suggesting that the student talk through the steps of a procedure while doing it may be useful in relieving the tension that accompanies such an intense focus on mechanics, without interfering with the necessary concentration on what is being done.

Coordinating cognitive content with psychomotor learning is essential if students are to understand the rationale underlying their actions. Rationale eventually replaces step-by-step adherence to a procedure, and permits the development of the higher level of learning that permits adaptation of a technique in a situation that does not permit strict adherence to procedural guidelines. This is particularly important in community-based practice, where the setting is less controlled. Once students are liberated from intense reliance on procedure, they become free to invent solutions to problems encountered in practice, the highest level of learning in this domain.

Affective Domain

The affective domain concerns emotional responses to phenomena. It incorporates awareness of feelings generated in response to phenomena as well as value judgments about those phenomena. Table 3–3 describes major

TABLE 3–3   Descriptions and Characteristic Behaviors of the Hierarchical Categories in the Affective Domain

1. **Receiving.**   Receiving refers to the student's willingness to attend to particular phenomena or stimuli (classroom activities, textbook, music, etc.). From a teaching standpoint, it is concerned with getting, holding, and directing the student's attention. Learning outcomes in this area range from the simple awareness that a thing exists to selective attention on the part of the learner. Receiving represents the lowest level of learning outcomes in the affective domain.

   Characteristic behaviors

   Awareness

   Willingness to receive

   Controlled or selected attention

2. **Responding.**   Responding refers to active participation on the part of the student. At this level he or she not only attends to a particular phenomenon but also reacts to it in some way. Learning outcomes in this area emphasize acquiescence in responding (reads assigned material), willingness to respond (voluntarily reads beyond assignment), or satisfaction in responding (reads for pleasure or enjoyment). The higher levels of this category include those instructional objectives that are commonly classified under "interests"; that is, those that stress the seeking out and enjoyment of particular activities.

   Characteristic behaviors

   Acquiescence in responding

   Willingness to respond

   Satisfaction in response

3. **Valuing.**   Valuing is concerned with the worth or value a student attaches to a particular object, phenomenon, or behavior. This ranges in degree from the more simple acceptance of a value (desires to improve group skills) to the more complex level of commitment (assumes responsibility for the effective functioning of the group). Valuing is based on the internalization of a set of specified values, but clues to these values are expressed in the student's overt behavior. Learning outcomes in this area are concerned with behavior that is consistent and stable enough to make the value clearly identifiable. Instructional objectives that are commonly classified under "attitudes" and "appreciation" fall into this category.

   Characteristic behaviors

   Acceptance of a value

   Preference for a value

   Commitment

TABLE 3–3 CONTINUED

4. **Organization.**   Organization is concerned with bringing together different values, resolving conflicts between them, and beginning the building of an internally consistent value system. Thus the emphasis is on comparing, relating, and synthesizing values. Learning outcomes are concerned with the conceptualization of a value (recognizes the responsibility of each individual for improving human relations) or with the organization of a value system (develops a vocational plan that satisfies his or her need for both economic security and social service). Instructional objectives relating to the development of a philosophy of life fall into this category.

   Characteristic behaviors

   Conceptualization of a value

   Organization of a value system

5. **Characterization by a Value or Value Complex.**   At this level of the affective domain, the individual has a value system that has controlled his or her behavior for a sufficiently long time for him or her to have developed a characteristic "lifestyle." Thus the behavior is pervasive, consistent, and predictable. Learning outcomes at this level cover a broad range of activities, but the major emphasis is on the fact that the behavior is typical or characteristic of the student. Instructional objectives that are concerned with the student's general patterns of adjustment (personal, social, emotional) are appropriate here.

   Characteristic behaviors

   Generalized set

   Characterization

Note. Adapted from Gronlund, N.E. (1991). *How to write and use instructional objectives* (4th ed.), p. 34. New York, NY: Macmillan; Kibler, R.J., Barker, L.L., & Miles, D.T. (1970). *Behavioral objectives and instruction*, pp. 55–66. Boston: Allyn and Bacon.

categories within one scheme of the affective domain as a guide to the level of learning each represents, as well as descriptions of characteristic behaviors reflecting each level in this domain.

The affective domain is a complex, ill-defined, and difficult to measure aspect of learning. But many of the values in nursing, such as empathy and caring in response to patients, derive from the affective domain. Descriptors of the categories within the domain don't give a full picture of the multidimensional nature of this domain, which encompasses attitudes, appreciation, and valuing. An attitude is a disposition toward or against a phenomenon that leads to an inclination to behave in ways reflecting the attitude. Appreciation involves enjoyment of and experiencing pleasure in relation to a phenomenon. Valuing involves the evaluation of a phenomenon as having worth, utility, and importance.

The clinical setting stimulates affective learning by presenting multiple phenomena that trigger the emotional responses of students. Because attitudes, preferences, and values tend to be highly individualized, students may be hesitant to discuss feelings prompted by clinical situations. In reality, though, most students experience similar responses to similar situations. It is important for the clinical instructor to create a climate of trust in which students feel free to express their emotional responses, begin to reflect on their meaning, and formulate ways of behaving in the circumstances that generated the response. Sometimes, it is the student's behavior that reveals an underlying emotional response that the student is unaware of or unable to articulate. By describing the observed behavior to the student, the instructor may be able to bring the stimulating attitude into the student's awareness. A personal experience might illustrate this. As a student I was assigned to care for an obese African American man who had syphilis. My West Indian instructor remarked on the difference in the care I provided for this patient as opposed to my other patients. There was a distancing in my care activities that suggested I was prejudiced, presumably because the patient was Black. While I knew that race was not an issue here, my instructor's comments caused me to recognize my behavior and search for its origin. I found that I was, indeed, prejudiced, but toward the patient's obesity. This opportunity to reflect on a situation about which I was previously unaware enabled me to recognize feelings of prejudice when they occurred in future patient encounters, and to respond more appropriately.

Instructors can promote affective learning through the use of experiential/perceptual techniques and values clarification during the clinical postconference. Experiential/perceptual approaches encourage students to imagine themselves in a stimulus situation and then discuss their responses to the situation. The approach can be used to enhance empathic capacity, permit confrontation with potentially anxiety-producing situations, and stimulate discussion of values in relation to the situation. After using relaxation techniques to settle the group, the instructor presents a situation in the form of a poem, meditation, or brief scenario, inviting the students to enter the situation and experience it on an emotional level. Students then are asked to share their experiences with the group. Materials related to aging, dying, suffering, and hopelessness, for example, can stimulate enhanced awareness of what being in these states might be like for patients as well as attitudes toward and caring responses in these situations. Experiential/perceptual techniques permit a focus on a conceptual issue rather than a problem in the immediate clinical situation, and so involve the whole clinical group. Within the hierarchical framework outlined for the affective domain, experiential/perceptual techniques promote learning at the lower levels of receiving and responding.

Values clarification is used to help students explore their own feelings about fundamental issues in nursing. The goals of values clarification are to promote awareness of self and the values one holds, validate one's own values and those of others as legitimate, and interact socially in discussing alternative viewpoints on issues raised. It is the exposure to and acceptance of others' values (without necessarily adopting those values) that helps to clarify each student's own values. The process moves students' affective learning into the levels of valuing and organizing. A values clarification exercise can use as the stimulus an existing clinical situation or one commonly encountered in practice. Students are encouraged to identify their values in relation to the situation (called "choosing"). To encourage full participation, this is best done individually, by having students write down their responses. Next, students share their values with the group (called "prizing") and their reasons for thinking this way. Social interaction around values issues is encouraged through such techniques as values voting, where students indicate support for or against a statement; construction of a values continuum, where alternative responses are bounded by two extremes; completion of unfinished sentences concerning the issue; and problem-solving exercises. It is vital that values clarification exercises take place in a trusting, supportive, and nonjudgmental atmosphere, where students feel free to express—and own—their values without fear of ridicule or condemnation. Such an atmosphere promotes awareness that others hold values different from one's own. The cognitive dissonance that such an enhanced awareness creates prompts students to further explore their own value stances and increases tolerance of alternative value systems.

NATURE OF THE ADULT LEARNER

Adult learning theory proposes that adults differ from children in their approaches to learning. Adult learning theory has been labeled "andragogy" as distinct from "pedagogy." Children tend to be dependent learners, relying heavily on direction from the teacher. Adults, who have already achieved independence in other aspects of their lives, prefer to design their education around identified needs, using resources provided by the teacher as well as those they find for themselves. Children have limited life experiences on which to draw, limiting the numbers and quality of insights developed in relation to stimulus situations in the learning environment. Adults, on the other hand, learn best by relating new information to what is already known. For children, learning is part of the general process of growth and development; for adults, learning is more situationally based, in response to current developmental needs, such as preparing for a career. Situational issues also impact learning, as when family and job responsibilities interfere with learning. Children often are viewed as receptacles for the information deposited by their teachers, building a storehouse of content that can be accessed when needed; adults tend to seek education to meet specific present-day needs, and are frustrated when learning cannot be immediately applied. Finally, the education of children tends to be subject-centered, with the organization of learning based on the logical development of a topic. Adult education strategies tend to be more problem-centered, with a focus on specific problems to be solved (Knowles, 1980).

More often than not, nursing education programs are organized using the principles of pedagogy rather than andragogy. Nursing students tend to be in transition toward adulthood, and have come to the nursing program well attuned to the structure and direction provided by the pedagogical approach. Even among the significant numbers of nontraditional learners[2] entering nursing programs, the pedagogical approach is familiar, and therefore comfortable.

The clinical setting provides an excellent opportunity to use an andragogical approach to teaching and learning. By applying the assumptions of andragogy concerning the learner's self-concept, life experience, learning readiness, time perspective, and learning orientation and establishing the conditions for learning described later in this section, the clinical instructor can transform the traditional learning experience. The clinical instructor's role is one of facilitator of learning rather than provider of instruction. In organizing the clinical day and making assignments, the instructor is setting the scene for learning to occur. Students are encouraged to use the instructor as a resource person as they negotiate the problems associated with the day's assignment. As students become more attuned to this approach, they can begin to take charge of their own learning, a skill that will be needed in their professional lives.

Assumptions of Andragogy

Self-concept of independence rather than dependence.   In the clinical setting, each student's independence in learning can be fostered, because each student will be engaged in somewhat different activities to meet objectives for the course. Students can be encouraged to collaborate with the instructor in identifying appropriate activities that will enhance learning. For example, a student may identify a need to perform a procedure or to care for a patient in a specific age category.

Wealth of life experiences.   The instructor can draw on life experiences to enhance learning and promote the intellectual connections that facilitate the application of theory to practice. Collectively, the clinical group has many experiences to share that can help to illustrate a concept, even in the absence of a pertinent clinical example on the unit. The sharing of "war stories" by students, instructor, and staff is one way of building knowledge based on the rich experiences of others. It is important to recognize that life experiences can also interfere with learning. The student who is in the midst of grieving the loss of a close relative may have difficulty in caring for a patient who is dying from a similar condition.

---

[2]Nontraditional learners are variously defined, but tend to be 26 years of age or older and have had previous work and/or educational experience.

Learning readiness based on developmental needs.   Students are eager to engage in clinical learning because this seems most relevant to their goal of becoming professional nurses. By encouraging wide exploration of the clinical scene and the knowledge it contains, the instructor can take advantage of students' natural readiness to learn. The instructor also needs to be aware of lifestyle issues that may be interfering with learning, and respond appropriately. For example, students are rarely (if ever) permitted to carry pagers or cell phones while on the clinical unit, but some means of communication must be provided for students who also are parents in the event personnel at the child's school need to contact the parent.

Time perspective present- rather than future-oriented.   The clinical instructor should take advantage of clinical learning opportunities as these present themselves rather than steadfastly attending to stated objectives. It is seldom possible to correlate classroom content in a given week with the clinical experiences of students in that same week. By viewing the clinical experience as a whole that will, over time, enable each student to achieve desired objectives, the instructor becomes free to design the learning environment to maximize available opportunities. This approach permits both student and instructor to take advantage of the serendipitous learning that can take place in the clinical setting, rather than deferring it until the theoretical content has been presented in class. The immediate need for knowledge to solve an existing clinical problem moves the student into the learning situation and is likely to ensure that what is learned is retained.

Problem-centered rather than subject-centered learning orientation.   A problem-centered approach is ideal for the clinical setting, which presents a series of problems to be solved. Assisting students to accurately identify problems based on assessment data and theoretical knowledge, and then working with them to develop solutions to those problems that address the multiple facets of the situation, promotes students' ability to think critically and holistically rather than apply a textbook recipe to the problems encountered in patient care.

Conditions for Learning
In addition to assumptions about adult learners, Knowles (1980) proposed ideal conditions under which adults learn best.

Learners feel the need to learn.   Problem-centered approaches enable learners to identify learning experiences that address specific problems being encountered by the learner. If the learner is unable to recognize deficits, raising questions concerning the problem situation may stimulate increased self-awareness of the need to learn.

The learning environment is characterized by physical comfort, trust, respect, helpfulness, freedom of expression, and acceptance of differences. Andragogy can work only in a climate of trust and respect. Instructor and student explore possibilities together in a search for knowledge that will resolve clinical problems. The instructor's willingness to say, "I don't know the answer to your question. Let's find out," demonstrates that no one can be expected to have all the answers; it is the continual search for knowledge that marks the professional. A learning environment that permits freedom of expression and is receptive and accepting of differences among learners encourages the sharing of viewpoints and reactions. This is critical to the development of a value system in relation to clinical phenomena, the basis of ethical knowledge in nursing.

Learners espouse the goals of learning as their own goals. The learner's goals and the instructional goals must be congruent for the learner to engage in the learning situation. Part of the instructor's role is to point out the salience of learning activities in relation to development of clinical nursing expertise.

Learners share responsibility for planning and implementing the learning experience. Learners need to be given options in terms of learning activities and in terms of how they will approach the learning situation. Collaborating with the learner as she develops and implements an approach to a clinical situation ensures attention to significant priorities while giving the learner increased control of the situation.

Learners participate actively in the learning process, which uses a variety of strategies and techniques to permit the learner to use a personal learning style. While learners who have been exposed to a variety of teaching strategies have learned to vary their learning style to best accommodate the instruction, all learners have a preferred learning style. Students need to be given the opportunity to select whether to review a procedure in a manual, watch a film strip or video, observe someone else performing the procedure, or jump into the situation immediately. When multiple options for learning exist, students are able to make the most of the opportunities available by selecting those that best match their preferred learning style. This is particularly important in the college laboratory setting, where students initially practice skills.

The learning process relates to and makes use of the learner's experiences. Drawing on students' past experiences empowers them in the current situation and provides a pool of information for the entire clinical group. Students with significant clinical experience as nursing assistants or licensed practical nurses can be recruited as peer instructors. Teaching others in the clinical group how to perform a task refines the experienced student's skills; having a peer as an instructor makes it easier for students to ask questions.

Learners sense progress toward goals. The best motivator for continued learning is achievement. Corrective feedback needs to be balanced with a generous amount of positive feedback. Pointing out what was done correctly, and then showing how to improve the performance gives the student the sense that there is hope for eventually learning the skill. It is particularly important to comment on the more intangible aspects of clinical performance, such as effective communication or decisions and actions reflecting caring, so that students become aware that these behaviors are as commendable as technical skill performance.

BENNER'S FRAMEWORK FOR THE DEVELOPMENT OF CLINICAL EXPERTISE

Of all the explanations of how learners learn, Benner's perspective on how nurses develop clinical expertise (Benner, 1982; Benner, Tanner, & Chesla, 1996) has the most relevance for clinical instruction in nursing. Benner's work uses hermeneutical phenomenology, an approach to the interpretation of human concerns and behaviors as they exist in the contexts in which they occur, in this instance, nurses' development of clinical knowledge and judgment. Hermeneutical phenomenology analyzes narratives (stories) provided by those in the situation of interest in response to questions that ask what an experience has been like for the reporter. Benner's work has involved nurses at all stages of their careers. Based on their stories, Benner described the sequence—novice, advanced beginner, competent, proficient, expert—in which nurses develop expertise in practice. Three major themes that emerged from Benner's work clarify the differences in these stages of development.

The first of these themes is that skilled nursing does not rely on theoretical knowledge alone. Practical or clinical knowledge, embedded in the clinical situations nurses encounter, is necessary to explicate, understand, and apply the theory. From this perspective, the goal of nursing education to enable students to apply theory to practice is incompletely stated; its corollary, to apply practice to the understanding of theory, is an equally valid goal for education, a goal that only can be achieved in the clinical setting.

The second theme is that the ability to grasp a clinical situation is dependent on the ability to single out the relevant from the irrelevant elements of the situation. Benner labels this ability "perceptual awareness." Perceptual awareness does not involve detached rule-guided reasoning; the nurse "sees" what is most salient in the situation in identifying a clinical problem. Perceptual awareness is most manifested in the nurse's intuitive grasp of the clinical situation. Intuition in this context involves knowledge derived from the clinical situation in interaction with knowledge derived from other situations experienced by the nurse to yield an understanding that seems to defy explanation. Intuition is not guessing or feeling; it is deep knowing, and a necessary element of expert practice.

The third theme is that clinical expertise requires emotional, caring, morally responsible involvement with patients, and that there is no theoretical approach to teaching this involvement. Involvement requires the "being of the nurse" to engage with the "being of the patient" in situations that frequently involve the most intimate and private aspects of life: care of the body, birthing, suffering, dying. This involvement of the personhood of the nurse with those she cares for leads to the development of "involved intuitive responses" to clinical situations: knowing not only what is most salient in the situation, but also what should be done in the situation.

Novice. This initial stage of development describes the nursing student. Learning must begin somewhere; theoretical learning in nursing begins with descriptions of context-free features of clinical conditions that can be understood without the benefit of experience, and providing rules for action based on these features. In clinical learning, the novice's focus is on rule-based activities and the application of theoretical knowledge. The task of the novice is to import classroom learning to the clinical situation to begin to see how theory "plays out" in reality. The novice should be able to recognize which rules are relevant in a situation, what to look for, and possible actions to be taken. Benner et al. (1996) suggest encouraging students to prepare for the clinical experience by applying "clinical forethought" based on theory: "I should be looking for *a, b, c*; the patient is likely to need *m, n, o*; *r, s*, and/or *t* might happen, and my response should be *x, y, z*."

The clinical instructor can assist the novice in seeing the interplay of clinical content with theoretical content in the creation of clinical knowledge by pointing out the relevant aspects of the situation. Comparing and contrasting among clinical situations is also important for the novice, who needs guidance in recognizing nuances in patients' conditions. Consider the sign, "diaphoresis," which accompanies many conditions. There are qualitative differences between the diaphoresis that accompanies a myocardial infarction, a febrile state, and anxiety. The textbook description can never capture these nuances; they must be learned through observation in the clinical arena.

The novice also needs to learn about individualizing care, that is, modifying the rule-driven list of tasks to meet patient needs as perceived and expressed by the patient. It is only through beginning involvement with the patient that the novice can begin to recognize the importance and meaning of individualizing care.

Finally, the novice should be encouraged to reflect critically on the practice that has occurred in the clinical experience, by reviewing and recalling aspects of the experience to better understand what was going on, what was experienced, what was learned, what was missed, and what might be done better. Such critical reflection allows the student to perceive much that was "missed" in the midst of the experience, and begin to make sense of the multiple stimuli present in the clinical environment. Journaling is an excellent mechanism for fostering critical reflection. The instructor's periodic review of students' journals can provide important feedback to students who may be uncertain of their clinical thinking and performance. The journals also can provide insights for the instructor as to what is going on with students.

Advanced beginner. This stage describes the newly graduated nurse, although there should be glimpses of advanced beginner practice prior to graduation. This stage occurs only after the learner has had ample experience in real situations. The advanced beginner is able to recognize elements that are germane to a situation when they reoccur. The advanced beginner is aware of the richness of the clinical situation, and may be overwhelmed by the abundance of observed elements in the situation. Despite the ability to recognize theoretical signs and symptoms in the real situation, the advanced beginner still has difficulty "translating this theoretical learning into the practical implications for particular patients with multiple problems" (Benner et al., 1996, p. 54).

The focus of advanced beginner practice is on tasks to be completed and routines to be followed. There is limited connection to patient needs. Task-completion rather than patient management is the goal of the advanced beginner. Theoretical understanding has been enriched by practical experience, but there is still a heavy reliance on theory as a guide to practice.

Competent.   The competent nurse deals with the relevant elements identified in a situation by organizing them in a hierarchical manner. There is less dependence on abstract rules, and more dependence on organizing the situation with rules derived from the experience to identify what is important and what is not. There is increased involvement with the person of the patient, and, concomitantly, an increased sense of personal responsibility for the decisions made on the patient's behalf.

Proficient.   The proficient nurse operates more intuitively than does the competent nurse. Rules are replaced with situational discriminations and associated responses. The proficient nurse engages less in detached reflection about what is going on, but must still consciously decide what to do about it.

Expert.   The expert nurse's intuitive grasp of the situation, based on long experience, guides the nurse's actions in response to the situation as well as her understanding of what is going on. Knowing what to do is based as much on knowledge of the individual patient as on knowledge of the patient's condition.

In an article describing a student's experience in learning to think, Ironside (1999) reports the student's excitement about learning to "think like a nurse," fostered when the clinical instructor engaged her in a problem-solving dialogue that revealed the instructor's thought processes. The student distinguishes between "critical thinking," which she equates with answering questions, and "nurse thinking," which resides in the situation and requires consideration of its multiple facets and possibilities. Perhaps clinical learning in nursing can best be fostered by revealing "nurse thinking" to students as they engage in the reality of practice.

SUMMARY

In an editorial titled "Lessons on Learning," Tanner (1998) summarized Ewell's insights on learning based on accumulated research focusing on the act of learning rather than the act of teaching:

- The learner is not a receptacle for knowledge but rather creates his or her learning actively and uniquely.
- Learning is about making meaning for each individual learner by establishing and reworking patterns, relationships, and connections.
- Every student learns all the time, both with us and despite us.
- Direct experience decisively shapes individual understanding.
- Learning occurs best in the context of a compelling "presenting problem."
- Beyond stimulation, learning requires reflection.
- Learning occurs best in a cultural context that provides both enjoyable interaction and substantial personal support. (pp. 195–196)

REFERENCES

Benner, P. (1982). From novice to expert. *American Journal of Nursing, 82,* 402–407.

Benner, P., Tanner, C.A., & Chesla, C.A. (1996). *Expertise in nursing practice; Caring, clinical judgment, and ethics.* New York: Springer.

Bevis, E.O. (1988). New directions for a new age. In National League for Nursing, *Curriculum revolution: Mandate for change.* New York: NLN.

Friere, P. (1970). *Pedagogy of the oppressed.* New York: The Seabury Press.

Gilligan, C. (1982). *In a different voice: Psychological theory and women's development.* Cambridge, MA: Harvard University Press.

Gronlund, N.E. (1991). *How to write and use instructional objectives* (4th ed.). New York, NY: Macmillan.

Havighurst, R.J. (1953). *Human development and education.* New York: Longmans, Green.

Ironside, P.M. (1999). Thinking in nursing education. *Nursing and Health Care Perspectives, 20,* 238–247.

Kibler, R.J., Barker, L.L., & Miles, D.T. (1970). *Behavioral objectives and instruction.* Boston: Allyn and Bacon.

Kirschling, J.M., Fields, J., Imle, M., Mowery, M., Tanner, C.A., Perrin, N., & Stewart, B.J. (1995). Evaluating teaching effectiveness. *Journal of Nursing Education, 34,* 401–410.

Knowles, M.S. (1980). *The modern practice of adult education* (rev. ed.). Chicago: Association Press.

Kohlberg, L. (1981). *The philosophy of moral development.* San Francisco: Harper & Row.

Menix, K.D. (1996). Domains of learning: Interdependent components of achievable learning outcomes. *Journal of Continuing Education in Nursing, 27,* 200–208.

Norton, B. (1998). From teaching to learning: Theoretical foundations. (pp. 211–245). In Billings, D.M. & Halstead, J.A., *Teaching in nursing: A guide for faculty.* Philadelphia: Saunders.

O'Connor, A.B. (1986). *Nursing staff development and continuing education.* (pp. 39–44). Boston: Little, Brown.

Piaget, J. (1962). *Play, dreams, and imitation in childhood.* New York: W.W. Norton & Company.

Tanner, C.A. (1998). Editorial: Lessons on learning. *Journal of Nursing Education, 37,* 195–196.

CHAPTER 4

GETTING STARTED

Program Faculty   53
Clinical Staff   56
The Clinical Group   58
Before the Clinical Experience Begins   59
The First Clinical Day   60
    Orientation   61
    Establishing Ground Rules   63
    Setting Expectations   66

As a colleague maintains, "Nursing is a team sport." So, too, is nursing education, particularly the education that occurs in the clinical setting. Success as a clinical nursing instructor requires careful attention to nurturing team members, promoting collegiality among them, and fostering the teamwork that will lead to a satisfying experience for everyone involved. Team members include the nursing program faculty and support staff, clinical staff and liaison support personnel, and the students comprising the clinical group. Getting started as a clinical instructor requires a thorough understanding of the expectations, desires, and potential contributions of each of these team subgroups.

PROGRAM FACULTY

The clinical component of each nursing course is intended to enhance and supplement the classroom component by demonstrating the connections between theoretical knowledge of health problems and their treatment and the application of this knowledge in health care delivery. Nursing assessments of patients' responses to illness and its treatment, and the selection and implementation of appropriate interventions to meet patients' needs, are the primary focus of clinical learning. Each clinical experience in the nursing education program builds upon the previous experience, so that students are enabled to develop confidence in their emerging competence in interactions with patients and in their delivery of skilled nursing care. As they progress through the program, students also become aware of the different ways patients manifest and respond to illness and its treatment and gain increasing sensitivity to patients as unique individuals.

The logical beginning point for the clinical instructor is to get information about the course with which the clinical experience is associated, the objectives for the clinical experience, and the placement of the course within the sequence of educational experiences, both theoretical and clinical. Written course materials and a copy of the course texts give essential background information. Conversations with the lead instructor in the course will flesh out these documents to provide a clearer understanding of the flow of the course as well as the expectations for students at various points during the semester. The important goal of connecting theoretical learning with clinical observations and experiences cannot be achieved without some familiarity with what is transpiring in the classroom. Some sense of the "typical" student's level of competence at this point in the program is useful to the instructor in beginning to develop reasonable expectations for student performance.

As contributors to a team effort, nursing educators strive to deliver on a common curriculum and agreed-upon objectives. They seek to provide learning experiences that are essentially comparable for all students, recognizing that the unique circumstances of each clinical setting cannot be replicated for all student groups, or even among students in one clinical group. Academic freedom, a fundamental value in academe, gives instructors wide-ranging liberties in the ways they choose to deliver on a curriculum and its objectives. The tension that exists between program goals as expressed in the curriculum, with deep roots in the standards of professional nursing practice, and the principles underlying academic freedom can create a dilemma for the neophyte instructor. Should the unprepared student be sent off the unit to gather the information necessary to complete an assignment, or assigned to shadow the primary nurse who must now pick up that assignment, or "buddy up" with a fellow student? If the patient population is low, should students be sent to a clinic providing care for similar patients, to an observational experience in a diagnostic laboratory, to the library? Must each student provide total care for assigned patients, or can students work together when care demands are heavy or complex? Can the focus of the clinical experience be different for each student on a given day, with some students fine-tuning assessment skills while others engage in direct-care activities? Can students be sent off the unit to attend a unique event, such as clinical rounds on a patient they have cared for, or must all activities be centered on the assigned unit? By brainstorming with other clinical faculty about such potential situations, the clinical instructor can gain a feeling for the "norms" surrounding the management of clinical learning experiences, and the degree of academic freedom tolerated in the educational program and/or clinical setting.

Written assignments and presentations that are a required component of the course and arise from the clinical learning experience should be identified early in the semester. Differences in the ways in which various clinical instructors manage these assignments, which usually contribute to the final course grade, can be a source of frustration for students. Therefore, the clinical instructor needs to be thoroughly familiar with the guidelines for assignments, including grading criteria, before the assignment is presented to students in the clinical group. Coordination and communication are crucial to ensuring that these assignments contribute to learning rather than competitive anxiety for students. The instructor needs to be familiar with the criteria to be used in evaluating clinical performance, and the schedule for midsemester and final evaluations. A clear understanding of what constitutes an acceptable level of performance at this stage of the program is essential to ensure equitable grading.

The instructor also needs pragmatic information about the actual dates on which clinical experiences will occur (including a schedule of school holidays, time allocated for on-campus testing, as of skills), start and stop times for the clinical experience, and off-unit experiences that need to be built into the clinical schedule (such as observational experiences in the operating room or attendance at a professional conference). A list of the students assigned to the clinical group also is essential. Policy issues, including management of student absences, student injury or illness while engaged in the clinical learning experience, and errors in patient care, need to be thoroughly reviewed and understood. The instructor needs to know whom to contact to help resolve these kinds of issues.

The clinical instructor should develop channels of communication with the lead instructor of the course as well as the program coordinator and/or department chair. Periodic conversations with the lead instructor to see if students are successfully connecting theory with clinical learning in the classroom, as evidenced by questions, comments, and responses on exams, enables the clinical instructor to gain a sense of how well the clinical experience is "tracking" classroom instruction. Conversations with other clinical instructors involved in the same course also provide a reference point for evaluating one's own management of the clinical learning experience. Knowledge of the chain of command to be followed in processing student issues or in seeking resolution of an issue arising in the course of clinical instruction enables the instructor to act promptly and appropriately when necessary. Full-time faculty members appreciate questions concerning procedural steps to be taken in the event a problem arises, since this suggests that they will be informed of such issues promptly.

The clinical instructor can feel isolated from the rest of the program faculty, especially if there is little need to be on campus, as when the teaching assignment involves only clinical instruction. It is the instructor who must forge the relationships and develop the communication channels to ensure full participation on the faculty "team" in delivering high quality nursing education.

CLINICAL STAFF

Clinical instructors usually are responsible for supervising 8 to 10 students in a clinical setting. By definition, students are learners in this situation, and do not yet have the knowledge and competence to perform independently. Consequently, the clinical instructor assumes responsibility not only for student learning in this setting, but also for the safe care of the patients for whom students are assigned to care. The logistics of such responsibility are overwhelming, and the task cannot be accomplished without the full support of staff. Developing rapport with staff is vital to gaining this support. When staff and the clinical instructor work as a team in educating students, learning is enhanced and staff satisfaction grows. Staff participation in the educational experience frees the instructor to interact with and guide the learning of all students rather than requiring that she remain focused on monitoring the less skilled and potentially unsafe students.

Trust is the most essential component in building a successful team relationship with clinical staff. Clinical staff need to trust that the instructor has the necessary knowledge base and clinical skills to function competently in the clinical area. They need to feel confident in the care that the instructor will be providing for patients, both directly and through the students she is supervising. Such trust also involves the instructor's recognition of her own limitations, and her willingness to reveal such limitations by asking pertinent questions and seeking guidance from staff when unusual situations arise. Clinical staff also need to trust that the instructor will follow established policies and procedures in the delivery of care, particularly in relation to medication administration and documentation practices.

Clinical staff need to trust that the instructor will keep them informed of events as they occur during the clinical experience, even if this entails reporting for the student. The instructor can never communicate too much, especially concerning student problems and the steps being taken to resolve them. When staff trust that they will be informed promptly of a change in a patient's condition, or a response to a treatment, or a student's inability to complete a task before leaving the unit, they will not feel the need to double-check on students' work or seek constant reassurances that necessary treatments are being provided.

Clinical staff need to trust that the instructor will remain open to criticisms and suggestions about the course of the clinical experience and the performance of individual students. The instructor can invite such feedback by asking staff if there is anything about which the instructor should be aware, or simply asking how the day went after students have left the clinical area. When problems are identified, the instructor should deal with these and then report back to staff that the problem has been addressed. This indicates that the instructor values and is attentive to the staff's input into the educational experience of students.

Developing a trusting relationship with clinical staff must begin well before students arrive on the clinical unit. The instructor must spend time on the unit to learn the unit's physical setup, to learn about the patients, to assimilate unit routines, and to master the policies and procedures regarding patient care. Working on the unit is the best way to learn its operations and to demonstrate the clinical competence that contributes to the development of trust and acceptance. As the instructor becomes familiar with the unit, its patients, and its routines, she also will begin to develop relationships with clinical and support staff and physicians who are regularly present on the unit. This familiarity with personnel enables the instructor to pave the way for student activities on the unit, and for their own interactions with staff and physicians.

A second component of team-building with clinical staff is respect. Clinical staff need to feel supported in their roles as nurses. This is best expressed through sharing in staff efforts to provide quality patient care. A willingness to pitch in and help when help is needed reciprocates for the efforts staff make in helping students. Encouraging students to help within the limits of their abilities—to answer call lights, empty bedpans, assist in making beds or ambulating a patient—contributes to the sense of a team effort, and helps to ensure that instructor and students are not "dumping" on staff those tasks that are not a part of the formal assignment. Demonstrating respect for staff also involves consulting them with questions concerning patient care, and not second-guessing their approaches to providing such care. Alternative approaches can be discussed in a conference away from the unit, as a means of broadening students' appreciation for the variety of ways in which nurses solve patient problems.

A third component of team-building is communication. Staff need to know what the students will be doing on a given clinical day. They need to be clear about the objectives of the experience and the types of activities students will be engaged in, as well as the aspects of care the students will not be providing. Staff need to know the students' names and some sense of their abilities; it is prudent to let the primary nurse know that a student needs extra observation or follow-up, or assistance with some aspect of care. If students will be leaving the unit earlier than usual, staff need to know this early in the day to plan for patients' needs.

Staff also need to know whom to contact at the college if problems arise in the clinical setting that cannot be resolved with the instructor. By providing the names and telephone numbers of the department chairperson, secretary, and the program coordinator, the instructor is acknowledging that problems can—and should—be brought to a higher level if necessary. Similarly, the instructor should provide key staff with her own phone numbers and schedule in the event she needs to be contacted after the clinical experience is over to verify that a medication or treatment was completed, or to report an incident. Providing for such communication is one more way of demonstrating respect for staff and the work they do as well as showing that the instructor shares their concerns that care be provided competently and completely.

The time spent in gaining the support and enthusiasm of staff as essential partners in the educational effort is well worth the investment. The clinical day is apt to flow more smoothly, students are more likely to be exposed to a fuller range of positive learning experiences, and the goals of the instructional role will appear more achievable in such a climate of teamwork.

THE CLINICAL GROUP

The group of students joining the instructor in the clinical setting has already developed a history and a personality of its own. These students have shared laboratories in such courses as anatomy and physiology and microbiology, and developed ways of working together. They have shared classroom experiences, and struggled together to master theory. Many clinical groups remain essentially intact as they proceed to successive clinical experiences, and group members share perceptions—both positive and negative—of what the typical clinical experience is like. Students are heavily invested in informal communication channels that report on each clinical setting and clinical instructor others have experienced. The clinical instructor needs to harness this group spirit and take hold of the leadership of the group without destroying or undoing the positive aspects of group membership. This is best done by establishing and communicating a goal that is larger than the day-to-day activities of learning and a process by which that goal can be achieved that makes learning exciting and possible.

For students, the overriding goal of learning activities is achieving confidence in their ability to become competent caregivers and to succeed in their aspirations to become professional nurses. The instructor's enthusiasm and passion for nursing is the means by which this overriding goal can be established for and openly embraced by the clinical group. From the very first contact with students in the clinical group, the clinical instructor needs to convey an energy and excitement about nursing that makes students want to be a part of this important endeavor. By demonstrating how much she values her own practice, the instructor communicates a work ethic that embraces high standards, an openness to new experiences and continued learning, and a willingness to push hard in order to achieve excellence in the practice of nursing.

Learning becomes exciting and goal achievement possible when students are valued participants in the learning effort. Establishing a relaxed, collegial environment for learning decreases student anxiety and frees energy and attention for learning. Give students the freedom to learn by doing, without hovering over them or peeking behind the curtain surrounding student and patient. Use other students and staff for teaching. Set high standards coupled with an expectation that students can and will meet them ("You can do this!"). A positive tone empowers students. Engage in collaborative problem solving with students as they struggle with the day's assignment. This encourages them to take risks and challenge themselves to higher levels of achievement.

Provide constructive criticism that includes comments on positive as well as negative behaviors and is phrased to build students' confidence in their potential to succeed. When students can trust that the instructor will not reprimand them in public, they lose the fear of being humiliated in front of staff, peers, and patients and become more accepting of corrective feedback. Work with students as they engage in care activities. Seeing the instructor in action develops students' confidence in the instructor's ability—and willingness—to be involved in the real work of nursing. At the same time, the instructor's ease and air of confidence in the clinical environment assures students that they will not be abandoned if things go wrong or they become overwhelmed by an assignment.

BEFORE THE CLINICAL EXPERIENCE BEGINS

If it is at all possible, assemble the clinical group before the first day of the experience. Even a few minutes spent together after class or during a break will help to establish a group identity that includes the instructor. Meeting the clinical instructor on the students' own turf (the campus setting) reinforces both the instructor's affiliation with the program and the group's goal of learning.

The initial meeting should be used for introductions and for providing necessary information related to the clinical setting. Establish a time and place where students will meet the instructor before proceeding to the clinical unit. Give students written directions to the facility from the college, including a map if the facility is not located in a familiar area, as well as information on parking. If the clinical day will span mealtime, indicate whether or not there is a cafeteria at the facility, or if storage is available for students bringing a meal from home. Safety issues, including a reminder to leave valuables at home, should be addressed. Indicate what type of dress should be worn (uniform, lab coat, street clothes) and emphasize the need to wear the program name tag as identification. Let students know what, if any, equipment (stethoscope, scissors, etc.) should be brought on the first clinical day. Do not assume that students will bring a small notebook and pen; tell them to do so. If you are unable to meet with the student group prior to the first clinical day, at the very least post the necessary information on a bulletin board, or ask that it be distributed to students in the group by the course instructor.

If there is sufficient time, meet with each student to identify individual expectations and goals for this experience. This is a good time to review with the student the skills they have been able to develop in previous clinical experiences, and those they would like to develop in this setting. Encourage students to share any anxieties they may have concerning this clinical experience. For example, some students are afraid of caring for very young children or for the mentally ill. Others may have difficulty relating to the elderly, particularly if they have experienced a recent loss of a family member or a grandparent has developed a chronic condition, such as Alzheimer's disease. If the student has been or is currently employed in a health care setting, elicit information about the position and the responsibilities the student has undertaken in the past. Knowledge of such a background is useful in structuring clinical assignments that build on, rather than repeat previous experiences. For the student who has a well developed set of clinical skills (for example, the licensed practical nurse who is pursuing professional nursing education), the challenge of the clinical experience may be in developing critical thinking in the analysis of assessment data, clinical judgment in selecting nursing interventions, delegation skills, and so forth. Some students are reluctant to reveal their status as LPNs for fear they will be held to a higher standard of performance than are other students. This reluctance deprives them of the potential for an enhanced experience that acknowledges the presence of skills not yet mastered by others in the clinical group and fosters the development of intellectual skills necessary for professional practice.

Consider reviewing each student's college record to get a sense of academic achievement and aptitude, performance in previous clinical experiences, and any personal problems that have been communicated to faculty. Make note of any persistent problems that have occurred, such as frequent absences or errors. In conducting such a review of student records, try to "bracket" the information as background rather than a final picture of each student's potential clinical performance. Students who are struggling academically often perform at an excellent level in the concrete clinical setting, where theory takes on new meaning and begins to make sense. Honor roll students may have a great deal of difficulty with manipulative skills, and may never be able to function safely in this regard. Just as a nurse reviews a patient's record to gain a sense of his health condition, its treatment, and the patient's response to these, but relies heavily on her own observations and assessments to determine the patient's current status, so the nurse educator reviews the student's previous performance as a framework for anticipating and analyzing current performance. Much learning can occur in the intervening month or months between clinical experiences, as the student reflects on past events, and such learning has an impact on performance in the next experience.

THE FIRST CLINICAL DAY

Unless students have been in the clinical facility during a prior clinical rotation, it is rare for patient care assignments to begin at the start of the first clinical day. Instead, this day usually is devoted—in whole or in part—to an orientation of students to the clinical facility, the unit on which most experiences will occur, and the expectations of the clinical instructor.

Orientation

Many facilities will provide a basic orientation for students that includes an overview of the institution's history, mission, and patient services. A review of safety precautions (fire procedures, accident prevention, infection control and biohazard exposure systems, and the like) pertaining to the facility is generally included, as well as a review of patient rights. Specific aspects of the facility's philosophy of care, such as encouraging patients to wear street clothes rather than pajamas during the day hours or allowing family members to provide direct care to certain patients, usually are shared with students. A tour of the facility may or may not be included in the general orientation. Having participated in an orientation to the facility, the instructor should be prepared to fill in gaps as necessary or ask questions that students might be afraid to ask.

Orientation to the clinical unit on which students will have experiences should begin with a tour of the unit and an introduction to key staff members. While it is possible that the nurse manager will undertake this orientation, the instructor needs to be prepared to step in as necessary. Identify those staff members who will be particularly helpful in answering questions. If possible, use an empty patient room to demonstrate the operation of the bed controls, the call bell-intercom system, oxygen outlets, and other equipment. Outline shift routines, protocols for medication administration, charting and other documentation requirements and systems, and any other operating procedures that students need to know about. Provide a handout that reviews this information because students may be overwhelmed by the orientation and unable to sort out the essential from the "nice to know." Reviewing the patient's record is useful in helping students to obtain needed information in preparing for clinical assignments.

Special concerns related to specific patient populations should be addressed during the orientation. For example, a skilled nursing facility may require a minimum of two people to transfer or ambulate residents. The potential for inappropriate behavior among mentally ill patients should be anticipated, with guidelines for dealing with such behavior. In the pediatric setting, involvement of parents must be considered. Students also need guidance in managing their own emotional and/or visceral responses to clinical events in ways that do not offend or alarm patients or their families. For example, when feeling faint while observing a procedure, the student should quietly excuse herself from the room rather than hoping the feeling will pass before she passes out. Acknowledging that even experienced nurses have such responses begins to address unspoken student fears.

The first day of clinical often allows enough time for unit rounds, to acquaint students with the type of patients usually treated on the unit. This approach humanizes the orientation and helps to defuse anxiety. A scavenger hunt that requires pairs of students to seek out equipment and supplies reinforces the orientation to the physical plant of the unit. A list of items that might be included in a scavenger hunt appears in Box 4–1.

Box 4–1   Directions for Scavenger Hunt

Working in groups of 2 or 3, locate each of the items listed below, and describe its exact location (e.g., room, cabinet, drawer).

Biohazard waste containers

Gowns/gloves/masks for isolation

Emergency cart

Oxygen closet is next to _____

Periwash, razors

Kleenex, bedpan covers, toilet tissue

Urine hat

Combs, toothbrushes, toothpaste

Denture swabs

Sphygmomanometers

Hopper

Chux, sheets, bibs, disposable washcloths

Sheepskin and cushions, head protectors

Washcloths, towels; Are there bath blankets available?

Laundry chute

Bathtub

Electric thermometers

Two locations of fire alarms

Soiled work room

Clean work room

Kardexes/documentation book

Scavenger hunt devised for beginning students in a long-term care facility.

As part of the unit orientation, discuss the schedule students will follow during the clinical experience, including when and where the group will meet on the next clinical day. Will there be a preconference? Will it occur before or following report? Where will it be held? Will there be a postconference? When and where will it be held? Will meals be scheduled at a common time or staggered among group members? Discuss equipment, such as stethoscopes, that should be brought to the clinical experience. Indicate where coats and personal belongings can be stored, again with a caution concerning valuables.

Orientation also should include some brief introduction of the instructor. Students seek wisdom from their teachers, and the instructor's clinical expertise is the source of this wisdom for students in the clinical area. A discussion of the instructor's background of nursing education and work experiences, communicated with enthusiasm, can energize students. Students hope their clinical instructors will serve as role models; providing relevant information about membership in specialty organizations, research projects, or advanced education expands students' views of professional nursing activities. Be selective in the personal information shared with students; basic "demographic" information, such as marital status and numbers of children, is safe ground, while personal crises and dilemmas are not.

Orientation is necessarily information-laden. Attempt to schedule physical activities, such as the unit tour, between blocks of content. If possible, provide information in related locations, as in the nursing station when reviewing the location and organization of patient records. Expect, however, that most of what is covered in the orientation will be forgotten by the next clinical experience, and be tolerant of questions in the first few weeks of the experience.

Establishing Ground Rules

The initial meeting with students in the clinical setting sets the tone for the experience and provides the structure within which clinical learning will occur. Providing structure does not violate the principles of adult learning, which emphasize mutual sharing among learners and instructor. Providing structure clarifies for everyone involved in the experience the behavioral expectations surrounding clinical learning activities. These expectations are best presented as professional role behaviors observed by all nurses in their practice, and include accountability, responsibility, and professional decorum.

Accountability. As a team effort, nursing requires that everyone involved in the health care endeavor be accountable to the team as well as to the patients for whom care is provided. Accountability involves integrity and dependability.

Stress the need for honesty in every aspect of patient care with which the student is involved. Failure to report errors or omissions should be a cause for clinical failure. The evolving picture of the patient's condition demands accurate reporting of observations. Colleagues must be able to trust the data provided by others, and that treatments reported as completed have been. Acknowledge to students that uneven performance, omissions, errors, and other inadequacies are inherent in the clinical learning experience, but that covering up such problems will not be tolerated. Performance deficits serve as a base from which learning can proceed, but such learning can only occur if the student acknowledges the problem and seeks assistance in rectifying it.

Review with students the starting time of the clinical experience, and insist that they arrive on time—or early—for every clinical session. Students should plan for traffic and/or parking problems, as well as for shifting family responsibilities, such as child care, to others if the need arises. Emphasize acceptable reasons for absences from the clinical area (usually illness or death in the family) and the effect of absences (e.g., required makeup sessions if these are available, alternate assignments, required withdrawal from the course if a certain number of absences is exceeded). Required notifications in the event of an absence from the clinical area should include a call to the instructor as well as to the unit. Develop a plan for managing school cancellations due to weather, and review with students the college's procedures for notifications of such closures (e.g., computer announcements, radio/TV announcements, dedicated telephone number). Set up a telephone tree so that students can be alerted to closures or late starts.

Responsibility.   Students must take full responsibility for their assignments by being prepared, actively participating in all aspects of the clinical experience, completing assigned work in a timely fashion, and maintaining safety.

Preparation for the clinical experience varies with the nature of the clinical setting as well as the level of the student. When the patient population is relatively stable, the instructor can make assignments the day before the clinical, so that students can prepare for clinical ahead of time. Alternatively, students may be expected to arrive in advance of the start of the clinical day in order to review the assignment. A report from the previous shift or the primary nurse supplements, but is not a substitute for the student's own preparation. Student preparation should include an understanding of the patient's medical diagnoses and plan of care as well as related nursing diagnoses and interventions, both those derived from the existing plan of care and those that might be anticipated for this patient. A review of unfamiliar procedures and medications is warranted. Students must also have a sense of the patient's status in relation to goals outlined in the care plan as a guide to planning activities and setting priorities. Students should be encouraged to introduce themselves to assigned patients in advance of the clinical.

Students should anticipate responsibility for information concerning the patient's treatment plan even if they will not be involved in all aspects of care delivery. For example, students need to know about the medications the patient is receiving, especially their anticipated effects and potential side effects, despite not administering these medications, and should be expected to observe for drug effects.

Beginning students may need guidance in organizing the information gathered in preparation for the clinical. The instructor might devise a form as a framework for recording essential information, while encouraging students to develop their own system for preparing for the clinical day. Samples of such forms are shown in Appendix F.

Encourage students to participate in all available activities on the clinical unit. Actively engaging in learning helps students to master the information and techniques needed to practice nursing effectively. Because the clinical experience cannot be programmed to provide only experiences at the students' level of development, expect that students will be exposed to unplanned situations and facilitate their appropriate involvement. At the same time, students need to recognize the limits of their ability, and to ask questions and seek assistance as needed. Except in rare circumstances, as when a student's performance is being evaluated, providing help to a fellow student should be encouraged. Active participation in conferences is another important part of learning.

Timely completion of work includes timely administration of treatments and medications and timely reporting of a change in the patient's condition. Assist beginning students in planning their activities to allow "windows" of time to complete scheduled treatments, as a beginning step in learning to prioritize activities. Expect more advanced students to prioritize activities appropriately. Students often are unable to understand the significance of observed changes in a patient's condition, but are able to recognize such changes, particularly if they are alerted to the potential for changes, either through their own preparation for clinical or the guidance of the instructor. Such observations should be reported promptly, even though the student is uncertain of their importance, rather than held for the end-of-experience report.

Alertness to safety issues is another aspect of responsibility. Rather than leave a wheelchair in the middle of the corridor, the student should move it to an appropriate area. Spills should be cleaned promptly, or reported to the appropriate person. Asking for help in positioning or ambulating a patient— and providing such help to a fellow student or staff member—ensures that the move will be accomplished without injury to staff or patient. Asking questions and seeking guidance rather than guessing prevents unintended mishaps, as does double (or triple) checking medication orders, calculations, and doses. Students do not want to endanger patients, but need approaches to ensure that accidents are avoided.

Professional Decorum.   When students behave like the professionals they aspire to be, they attract the confidence of both patients and staff, and also enjoy a heightened self-esteem. Establishing and maintaining standards of professional decorum is difficult when staff members do not follow the same standards. Imagining oneself as a critically ill or dying patient being cared for by such a staff member may help the student to grasp the importance of professionalism in enhancing patient comfort and confidence.

Insist that students follow the dress code established by the program as part of the expectations for the clinical area. Uniforms should be clean, ironed, and of appropriate length and fit. Shoes should be appropriate for the unit and allow the student to be silently mobile. Emphasize that the uniform is not intended to be a fashion statement, but a sign of professionalism. Extremes in makeup and hair style should be avoided, as should long nails and colored nail polish. Jewelry often becomes an issue with students, particularly the newly engaged, who can't bear to remove the diamond ring. A caution about loosening the stone while making a bed, transmitting infections to others, or scratching the patient is usually sufficient. Earrings are another source of contention, particularly among students with multiple piercings. Dangling earrings are inappropriate; simple studs or small hoops are best. Jewelry in other body areas (eyebrows, lip, tongue) should be banned in the clinical area. Perfumes should be avoided, as these can be nauseating to certain patients. Students need to be cautioned about personal cleanliness, including control of body odor and halitosis. Persistent problems should be addressed privately with the student, but should not be ignored. Frame issues related to dress and grooming within the context of safety (as with the transmission of infection), patient sensitivities, and professionalism rather than as personal preferences.

Items that might interfere with the student's activities—such as cell phones and pagers—should be left at home, or secured in an appropriate place on the unit. Provision for essential communications, as with school-aged children, should be planned ahead of time so that clinical activities are the focus of the student's attention.

Comportment is another aspect of professional decorum worthy of comment. Students may need to be reminded of their surroundings, and cautioned to keep voices at a reasonable level. Giggling, horseplay, and practical jokes are inappropriate in the clinical area.

Collegiality with staff and other health care workers is another area to explore with students. Emphasize that patients are in the clinical facility because of their need for nursing, and that the nursing student is a partner with others in providing that care. Students must treat all workers with respect, but expect to be treated similarly. Students tend to be in awe of physicians, whose intrusions and demands need to be considered in the context of patient needs. Students should not hesitate to remain with the patient if this is appropriate, ask questions, and provide information when other health workers enter the patient's unit.

A final area of professional decorum is maintaining confidentiality regarding patients. Students need guidance about note taking when preparing for clinical, preparation of written reports and care plans concerning assigned patients, and conversations in public areas, such as the cafeteria, elevators, and restroom. Use of a patient's first name (if not unusual) or initials is appropriate for written materials, although the student should be cautioned to keep such papers from public view. Any discussion of patients should be avoided in public places. Students are eager to share their experiences with other students when they return to the college; such discussions need to be framed in a general way, without reference to the facility or unit at which the experience occurred. One never knows when a relative or friend of a patient is among those listening to the student's account.

Consider providing students with a written set of ground rules to clarify these guidelines and expectations for behavior while in the clinical setting. A sample of such written ground rules appears in Boxes 4–2 and 4–3.

Setting Expectations

Set expectations high, and students will strive to achieve them. By communicating trust in the students' ability and desire to perform at an excellent level,

Box 4–2 Ground Rules for College Laboratory Experiences

1. Attendance at all laboratory sessions is required. If you are unable to attend a laboratory session, you must notify the instructor in advance by leaving a message under the instructor's office door, in the instructor's mailbox in the nursing office, or on the instructor's voice mail. Missed laboratory sessions will require makeup work.

2. Be on time—or early—for every laboratory session. Laboratory experiences will begin promptly at 9:00 a.m. A late arrival will be treated as an absence. Plan ahead to avoid travel and/or parking problems.

3. Participate fully in all laboratory experiences. Actively engaging in learning will help you to master the information and techniques you will need in order to practice nursing effectively.

4. Ask questions (there are no "dumb" questions). Recognize the limits of your ability. Seek assistance when you need it.

5. Be completely honest in all the work you do.

6. Remember that you are a guest in the facilities you will be visiting. Dress and behave appropriately.

7. Be "street smart." Leave valuables at home or locked in your car trunk when you are making community visits.

Failure to conform to ground rules may result in a laboratory failure and failure in the course, regardless of academic performance.

Written expectations for students attending a college laboratory.

and identifying the instructor's role in making that happen, the clinical instructor establishes a goal for learning that underlies every activity in the clinical area.

Reveal your modus operandi (if you have one), so students know what to expect. For example, if you plan to challenge students by pushing them to the limits of their ability, let them know, along with the assurance that you will step in when needed if they feel overwhelmed. If you require students to seek you out before performing specific procedures, let them know this (and reinforce this requirement at the appropriate time).

Identify written assignments required in conjunction with the clinical experience, due dates, and criteria for their evaluation. A brief explanation of the assignments—to alert students to them—is all that is necessary initially; a more detailed description and discussion of the assignment can be provided at a later time.

Clarify clinical evaluation procedures. If you intend to keep anecdotal notes about incidents of student performance, let them know what these entail and

Box 4–3   Expectations for Clinical Experiences

1. Attendance in clinical areas is mandatory. Students must be in the clinical area at the specified time. Students must assume responsibility for arranging with the clinical instructor for makeup opportunities if clinical experiences are missed. It is also the student's responsibility to contact the clinical instructor and the clinical facility the morning of the absence. Facility phone numbers and contact persons are listed in your clinical packet.

2. A student may be asked to leave the clinical area if, in the judgment of the clinical instructor, his/her health status could adversely affect clients, or if the student is unprepared for the clinical assignment.

3. Students should dress in appropriate street clothing for this experience. Suggested attire includes pants, khakis, or a long skirt. Short skirts, jeans, and revealing clothing are not acceptable. Wear comfortable shoes (no sneakers). Please have your school name tag on every week.

4. Violation of the above dress code will result in the student being asked to leave the clinical area.

Written expectations for students attending a clinical experience in a mental health facility.

when and where they can review the notes. Distribute the clinical evaluation form being used in the course and review the types of behaviors that constitute excellent performance, satisfactory performance, or warrant a clinical failure. Explain the terms used on the evaluation form (usually worded in behavioral objective form). For example, the objective, "Evaluates the effectiveness of the nursing care plan, proposing revisions when necessary," can be explained in terms of determining the patient's response to an intervention and suggesting changes if the intervention is not moving the patient toward identified goals, rather than following the care plan regardless of its effectiveness.

Despite a desire to defuse anxiety by assuring students that there are "no dumb questions," that they won't be humiliated by the instructor, and that mistakes are an expected part of learning, students will remain unconvinced of the instructor's humanistic approach until they witness it among their peers or experience it themselves. The best way to begin the clinical experience is with an open, friendly, good-humored approach that lets students know that they will learn, despite their doubts and fears, and that learning can be a relaxing and enjoyable experience.

Chapter 5

Teaching and Learning Strategies for the College Laboratory Setting

The Laboratory Setting   71
Uses of the College Laboratory   73
Instructional Materials   73
Structuring the Laboratory Experience   74
The Process of Learning a Psychomotor Skill   78
Integrating the Cognitive Basis for Psychomotor Skills   81
Summary   82
References   83

The college laboratory is the place where students are introduced to the technical skills they will be using throughout their careers as professional nurses. The potential uses of the college laboratory are limited only by the instructor's imagination and creativity. Well designed laboratory exercises can enable students to practice a full range of nursing activities, including communication techniques, problem-solving strategies, and documentation practices, in addition to the usual array of technical skills. The practical, hands-on, concrete approach to learning in the laboratory is appealing to students, and provides a foundation for the eventual transfer of skills to the clinical setting. Research on the utility of the college laboratory in nursing education suggests that preclinical testing of skills is "an effective strategy for reducing anxiety related to initial transfer of skill learning from a laboratory to a clinical setting and enhancing self-confidence" (Bell, 1991, p. 222).

Skill learning is facilitated by the student's ability to focus on a single task, the absence of any fear of making a mistake and injuring or hurting the patient, as well as minimal competing stimuli in the learning environment. Laboratory sessions usually are focused on a single set of skills, and the student can "tune out" other aspects of the presenting situation.

Not all nursing educators agree on the utility of the college laboratory. Some educators believe that a thorough understanding of the conceptual basis of a skill (the "why") is the essential element, with manual dexterity developed over time in the clinical setting. Others believe that the mastery of technical skills requires a process that is somewhat different than the acquisition of cognitive content, and see the laboratory as a place where students can begin to mesh the "why" with the "how."

Educators postulate that there are three behavioral domains: the cognitive domain concerns intellectual skills; the psychomotor domain concerns neuromuscular and manipulative skills; and the affective domain concerns attitudes and values. There is significant interplay and overlap among the three domains, as reflected in the cognitive basis of psychomotor skill development, but each of the domains is somewhat unique, suggesting the need for different approaches to teaching. Learning psychomotor skills requires the development of a kinesthetic sensitivity (body sense), a mind-body "connect" in which the student acquires a physical sense of performing the activity correctly. This takes time and practice, which may not be available in the clinical setting.

A significant body of research has demonstrated that students approach learning using one of four different modes of learning: abstract conceptualization (thinking), reflective observation (watching), concrete experience (feeling), and active experimentation (doing). Abstract conceptualizers process words efficiently, and prefer to learn via the written or spoken word. Reflective observers learn best visually; they respond to demonstrations, diagrams, and visual media. Concrete experiencers prefer to try things out for themselves, but wish to do so in a controlled setting. Active experimenters learn best in the real world; although they would prefer to learn in the clinical setting, lifelike simulations and role playing exercises may provide sufficient stimuli for learners in this mode. Learning involves a four-stage cycle, moving from concrete experience to reflective observation to abstract conceptualization to active experimentation, with every learner gaining experience in each mode. While all learners are able to use any of the four modes, varying the approach to learning as needed, individual learners tend to prefer one of each of the polar opposites represented by the two continua of concrete experience—abstract conceptualization and active experimentation—reflective observation (Richardson, 1998, pp. 23–24). These preferences, called learning styles, carry with them the characteristic approaches to learning summarized in Table 5–1. The college laboratory provides an opportunity for students to use each of these learning modes and thus develop flexibility in their approaches to learning.

The college laboratory should be a place where learners are actively engaged in learning. It should not be used as an extension of the classroom. The role of the instructor in the laboratory setting involves

- facilitating: setting up the conditions under which learning will occur;
- guiding: setting goals and general principles for achieving them;

TABLE 5–1 LEARNING STYLES

Accommodative

Preference is for the concrete experience and active experimentation modes of learning

Orientation is to task accomplishment through feeling and doing

Less concerned with theoretical basis for actions

Tend to take risks and to solve problems through trial-and-error approaches

Assimilative

Preference is for the abstract conceptualization and reflective observation modes of learning

Excel at organizing diverse items into an integrated whole

Very concerned with abstract concepts

Less concerned with people and with application of ideas

Divergent

Preference is for the concrete experience and reflective observation modes of learning

Tend to be imaginative and good at generating ideas

Tend to be people-oriented

Tend to be emotional

Convergent

Preference is for the abstract conceptualization and active experimentation modes of learning

Like to deal with things rather than people

Source: Based on Kolb, D. (1976). *Learning style inventory: Technical manual*. Boston: McBer.

- stimulating: motivating performance;
- supporting: providing individual attention as needed; and
- supervising: overseeing the learning process to avoid error fixation (Infante, 1985).

Teaching in the laboratory setting challenges the creativity of the instructor to sustain students' interest, promote learning, and use time effectively.

THE LABORATORY SETTING

Most college laboratories are designed to simulate the hospital setting, with hospital beds and bedside furniture, curtain partitions, and equipment and supplies similar to those used in the clinical setting. The breadth and depth of equipment and supplies usually reflects the faculty's commitment to the college laboratory as a component of nursing education. The instructor is well advised to spend some time in the college laboratory to familiarize herself with what is available and where items are located.

Ideally, a laboratory will have sinks with running water, to reinforce the essential practice of hand washing before and after performing nursing procedures involving patient contact. Cabinets and drawers are generally labeled with their contents; some are likely to be locked, and the instructor will need to have access to the keys on days she is teaching in the lab. Expensive and sophisticated equipment, such as IV monitors, are unlikely to be available, but basic equipment to conduct a physical examination (stethoscopes, manometers, otoscopes, etc.) often are supplied for student use. Bed linens, hospital gowns, and isolation gear usually are available, as are standard bedside items, such as bedpan, urinal, wash basin, and emesis basin.

Mannequins of varying complexity (most permit practice in catheterizations and administering enemas; some have a tracheostomy and a colostomy) and anatomical models (arms for practice in starting IVs, torsos for practicing injection site location, for example) usually are available.

Disposable supplies, such as dressings, wound care kits, IV bags and tubing, needles and syringes, enema kits, and the like, often are available, although some programs require students to purchase their own prepackaged supplies for the lab, in which case the instructor will need to know what is available in the laboratory. Samples of more sophisticated supplies, such as central lines, may be provided for demonstration purposes. Most supplies are reused in the course of the semester and replenished at the start of the school year.

Knowing what is and isn't available enables the instructor to work with what is on hand and improvise the rest. By planning ahead, supplies needed for the upcoming lab session can be gathered together and set aside for use by the student group, and necessary adaptations in the teaching plan made to accommodate unavailable items.

In many programs, a laboratory assistant is charged with maintaining order in the lab, reorganizing cabinets and drawers, and restocking supplies as needed. The assistant is also available to provide assistance to students using the laboratory for individual practice. In other programs, each instructor is responsible for keeping the laboratory in order and for monitoring supplies.

Time in the college laboratory usually is scheduled to coincide with the hours students will be in the clinical setting. If the instructor plans to use the laboratory as a substitute for a clinical experience, she must check that the laboratory will be free at the time she is planning to use it. It also is important to know whether—and when—the laboratory is open to students for individual practice.

Because the college laboratory is a shared resource, the neophyte instructor must learn the mores surrounding its use and abide by any unwritten rules concerning the lab schedule, the use of supplies, and maintenance.

USES OF THE COLLEGE LABORATORY

The college laboratory may be a planned component of various nursing courses, a location for students to practice skills on their own, a site for competency testing to clear students for the clinical area, or any combination of these.

When laboratory time is incorporated into a course, the clinical instructor will need to determine which skills are designated to be taught in the course for which she is responsible. If students are expected to perform skills using a specified technique, the instructor will need to know what technique is preferred and whether guidelines or skills checklists exist for her reference, because these criteria will likely be the basis for future performance evaluations.

Knowledge of the skills students in her group should have mastered in previous courses is essential so that the instructor's expectations are realistic for the level of student she is teaching and so that she doesn't waste instructional time repeating prior content. If a student is unable to perform a skill that was previously taught, this knowledge enables the instructor to suggest to the student that she practice the skill during an open laboratory session.

Competency testing in conjunction with a given course is usually a group effort, involving all instructors teaching in the course. The neophyte instructor can contribute to the endeavor by suggesting scenarios, preparing the laboratory environment, and participating in testing students.

INSTRUCTIONAL MATERIALS

Skills instruction is enhanced through the use of available written and mediated materials. Nursing programs vary in the types and variety of such materials and the means by which they can be accessed by instructors and students.

Students generally are required to purchase textbooks in conjunction with their nursing courses, many of which contain sections devoted to basic and advanced nursing skills. Often a laboratory workbook or skills book is available as a separate resource that the student uses throughout the program. Handouts prepared by the lead instructor or provided by individual instructors may supplement these materials. It is important to review these materials carefully to identify any inaccuracies as well as variations in technique so that these can be pointed out to students. Students need to know that several approaches can be used in performing any skill, as long as critical elements are included and basic principles are adhered to.

Mediated materials that depict various nursing skills, such as filmstrips, single-concept film loops or cartridges, videos, and computer-assisted or computer-interactive programs, are commercially available. These materials should be reviewed by the instructor for accuracy and technique prior to being viewed by students.

Just as they are expected to prepare for the clinical experience, students should be expected to prepare for college laboratory sessions by reviewing the skills that will be the focus of the day's activities and, if possible, viewing any mediated materials that are available to students. Such preparation permits more efficient use of laboratory time that would be otherwise spent in explaining each step of the procedure or watching a film or video. If the college laboratory is accessible to students and the equipment is available, mediated materials can be housed in the lab for viewing at the students' convenience. However, if only one copy of mediated materials is available and students have limited access to its use the instructor should be prepared to use a portion of the laboratory time in showing the film or video so that all students are exposed to the same information.

A major advantage of the college laboratory is in giving students the opportunity to manipulate the materials they will be using in the clinical area without fear of wastage. A simple example involves adjusting the flow rate while administering an enema. Observation of the flow of fluid from the tubing when the enema solution is held at various heights gives students a better sense of the best rate of flow. The instructor who recognizes that most of the procedures students are learning are quite novel to them will take the opportunity to point out such small but important aspects of the skill.

The college laboratory also allows students to compare and contrast similar items, enabling them to develop the ability to discriminate among the available sizes and varieties within a category of items, such as needles for injection. The creative instructor might prepare a display of the needles used for parenteral drug administration, with an indication of the rationale for choosing one size over another in different situations. Both students and faculty members appreciate contributions such as these.

STRUCTURING THE LABORATORY EXPERIENCE

A typical laboratory session will involve instruction and practice in a group of related activities. For example, donning protective isolation gear, donning sterile gloves and establishing a sterile field, changing dressings, and wound irrigation may be scheduled for a single session. One skill is taught at a time. A general introduction to the skill usually is provided, pointing out the theory and principles involved with the activity. Following this orientation, the instructor shows the film or video depicting the skill if students have not been able to view it beforehand, and then takes questions. Then the instructor demonstrates the skill for students using a student volunteer or mannequin. Although students have viewed the mediated material, seeing the instructor performing the skill often reveals aspects of technique that are less noticeable on the film. The instructor generally talks through the procedure, pointing out the rationale for various aspects of the activity. It is helpful first to perform the skill without comment, so students can observe a fluid performance, and then repeat the demonstration with an explanatory narrative. After the instructor's demonstration, students practice the skill, either on their own or in pairs. The instructor observes their performance, offering suggestions and corrections and answering questions. When all students feel comfortable with the skill, or when each student has correctly repeated the instructor's demonstration, the instructor moves to the next skill to be covered that day.

A variation on this approach is to ask a student volunteer to perform the skill while the instructor provides the commentary along with any corrections in technique that are needed. Once the student has successfully performed the skill, she can be deputized as an assistant instructor, providing guidance for her peers as they practice the skill. Alternatively, the instructor can invite students to indicate their readiness to repeat the demonstration of the skill. Each student who successfully demonstrates the skill is deputized to both teach and evaluate other students. Spot checks of student technique by the instructor ensure that peer teachers are maintaining standards. These peer teaching techniques serve several purposes. First, the process of teaching enhances content mastery because the peer instructor is challenged to answer questions she may not have considered. Second, learners are more likely to ask questions of a peer than a less familiar instructor. Third, one-to-one or small group instruction is enhanced because an instructor can, indeed, be in two or three places at one time. Fourth, the approach makes use of the knowledge and skills that exist in the student group. Fifth, peer instruction is time efficient (Nabokov, 1978).

Another alternative is to have students pair up and practice the skill together, with each assuming first the role of the nurse and then the role of the patient. Being in the patient role enables the student to gain some sense of what the procedure feels like from the receiving end. This student also can provide corrective cues to her partner as she performs the skill. The second perspective on the skill helps to reinforce learning.

Yet another approach is to follow skill demonstration with an exercise in mental imagery, in which students are encouraged to imagine performing the skill in the clinical setting. The instructor reads from a prepared script that describes the setting and the steps in the skill, giving students sufficient time to visualize the entire process. Students then practice the skill in the lab. Alternatively, the mental imagery exercise can follow student practice. The combination of mental and physical practice has been found to be effective in motor skill learning (Doheny, 1993). Encouraging students to use mental practice before bedtime and before actually performing the skill in the clinical setting can help to reinforce the steps in the procedure and reduce anxiety when the skill is applied clinically.

Students need more than one opportunity to practice skills, and so the instructor should build some time for skill review into lab sessions. Stations can be set up within the lab, each with a brief written scenario that directs the student to perform a skill. These scenarios can include small details that make them more realistic. For example,

Mr. Brown's intravenous of 500 cc D5W was hung at 8:00 A.M. and is to be infused over 5 hours. It is now 10:00 A.M. Is the IV on time?
Tell me the steps you would take to check the IV.
The physician has changed the IV order to have the remaining D5W infuse over 6 hours. Adjust the drip rate (drop factor is 60 gtts/cc).

Cleanse Mrs. Smith's wound with normal saline.
Document the size and condition of the wound.
Redress the wound with a dry sterile dressing.

Students also can be encouraged to playact while performing the skills, explaining their actions to the mannequin or student-partner as they would with a patient. Many students find that talking through the procedure aloud as they perform it helps them to recall the sequence of performance.

Similar scenarios can be created for competency testing. Students are required to complete all stations, or might draw a given number of skills from a fishbowl and then perform these while being observed and rated by instructors.

Psychomotor skills are not the only skills that can be taught in the college laboratory session. Practice with interviewing and therapeutic communication techniques can be accomplished as well. Students form groups of three. One takes the role of nurse, the second the role of patient, and the third acts as an observer. The instructor provides a stimulus question (for interviewing) or situation (providing the student taking the role of patient with some directions addressing one of her concerns) and directs the groups to communicate for 10–15 minutes. The observer makes note of the effective and ineffective communication techniques, blocks to communication, and nonverbal behaviors. At the conclusion of the exercise, the observer and student–patient share their observations with the student who has taken the role of nurse. Then roles are switched until all three students have had a chance to experience each role (Arnold & Nieswiadomy, 1997).

Games are another alternative activity that can be used in the college laboratory. While many educational games covering nursing content are available commercially, they are expensive and the nursing program may not have elected to purchase these resources. Two types of games are suitable for use in the college laboratory: those that provide opportunities for drill and practice in the recall and application of facts and principles and those that involve role playing to foster affective learning. The resourceful and creative instructor can design her own games along the lines of popular board games or television shows for use in drill and practice exercises. The range of content that can be covered is limited only by the instructor's imagination. For example, one instructor devised a "Jeopardy" game to review clinical pathophysiology, and another adapted this idea to incorporate principles and rationales involved in performing the various technical skills covered in the lab.

Role playing games tend to be more intricate. One game intended to sensitize students to the problems elderly people have in living on a fixed income involves creating a basic budget for an elderly person or couple using information provided by the scenario. The budget (and the elder's ability to continue to pursue activities of special interest) must be adjusted as successive problems are introduced. All scenarios end with the need for the elder to enter an assistive living or long-term care facility, providing students with some insights into what factors may cause an elder to lose his or her independence. Another game designed to sensitize learners to the sensory and motor deficits experienced by the elderly uses a series of props to simulate common problems (magnifying glasses that have been clouded to create "cataracts," cotton plugs for ears, gloves to decrease tactile sensations) and then has learners perform simple tasks, like opening a medication bottle.

Corder (1991) describes the "campus clinical" as a way to enable all students to practice all the skills they have learned in a semester, whether or not the opportunity to perform the skill has occurred in the clinical setting. The group is split in two, with one half taking the role of "patient" one day and "nurse" the other day. (With a small student group, the campus clinical might be completed on a single day.) Clinical situations are created, with separate information provided to each learner. The "nurse" is given biographical information, signs and symptoms, and procedures to be done; the "patient" is given additional information to be elicited by the nurse, such as an ache or itch, difficulty breathing, or a concern about some issue. Name tags, patient wristbands, charts, and order sheets are created for the exercise. At the start of the "clinical" the students in the role of nurse are given the appropriate information on their "patients." The "nurses" then complete the assigned tasks, including necessary communications, observations, and assessments, and record their actions in the patients' charts. Students in the role of "patients" are coached to respond appropriately to their "nurses'" errors, such as lying on the floor if the bed rails have been left down. At the conclusion of the day, a postconference debriefs both "nurses" and "patients." Similarity in their experiences permits students to learn from each other as each shares her perspective on the experience. As skills are added throughout the semester, additional campus clinical sessions can include medication administration, care planning, and patient education to create the desired experiences.

Alternative college laboratory activities, such as gaming and simulations, are time-consuming to create. They do provide a novel approach to learning and to practice that is engaging to learners and opens up new dimensions to their understanding of the skills of nursing practice.

The Process of Learning a Psychomotor Skill

Two schemes for analyzing the process of skill mastery are shown in Tables 5–2 and 5–3. Each describes a roughly similar sequence of progressive learning that starts with beginning awareness of the key elements involved in the skill, moves to a process of acquiring a beginning sense of what it feels like to perform the skill, practice that creates a similar performance with each repetition, and eventual "ownership" of the skill to the point where necessary adaptations and alterations in the skill can be incorporated when necessary.

TABLE 5–2   Gronlund's Hierarchy of the Psychomotor Domain

Perception

    Characteristic behaviors

    Awareness of a stimulus

    Selection of task-relevant cues

    Translation of cue perception to action in a performance

Set

    Characteristic behaviors

    Mental readiness to act

    Physical readiness to act

    Willingness to act

Guided Response

    Characteristic behaviors

    Imitation of instructor's demonstration

    Continuous referral to model performance

    Trial and error

Mechanism

Complex Overt Response

    Characteristic behaviors

    Performance without hesitation

    Movements exhibit ease and good muscle control

    Coordinated, fluid, timely, and automatic performance

Adaptation

Origination

Source: Adapted from Gronlund, N.E. (1991). *How to write and use instructional objectives* (4th ed.), p. 36. New York, NY: Macmillan.

TABLE 5–3	GUINEE'S HIERARCHY OF THE PSYCHOMOTOR DOMAIN

Acquisition

    Reacting

    Modifying

    Coordinating

    Habituating

Application

    Anticipating

    Manipulating

    Adapting

Integration

Source: Adapted from K.K. Guinee. (1978). *Teaching and learning in nursing: A behavioral objectives approach*, p. 36. New York: Macmillan.

Perception—the identification and selection of task-relevant cues—begins with the student's first introduction to the skill, and is facilitated by the instructor's pointing out critical elements to be performed. The student is able to break down the skill into its component units on the basis of these critical elements, especially when the rationale or principle underlying the "criticalness" of the element is explained. Repetition of the sequence of movements comprising the skill through the student's reading and observing the performance on film or video and via the instructor's demonstration, reinforces the elements involved and the order in which they are to be performed.

Set—the readiness to act—involves mental and physical readiness plus a willingness to attempt the skill. Set occurs as the student approaches the materials to be used in performing the skill and positions herself in relationship to these materials and the mannequin or student-model to be used for practice. The observant instructor is likely to recognize the small physical cues that signal the student's preparation to act: a squaring of the shoulders, taking a deep breath, briefly closing of the eyes. (Similar behaviors can be observed in athletes before they undertake a competition involving individual prowess.) This brief moment—most visible with a student's first injection–signals entry into skill performance, and should not be interrupted.

Guided response—action that occurs with reference to written criteria or a model performance—involves the stepwise imitation of the instructional model of the skill. The performance is likely to be rigid and halting, as the student refers to guidelines or attempts to recall the appropriate sequence involved in the skill. The student often stands at a distance from the task—

a signal of her initial discomfort in performing the skill—and uses her fingers and hands awkwardly. Observations of this body language should prompt the instructor to have the student take a deep breath, shake out and relax the hands, and recognize that practice is without consequences. The student may backtrack to undo and redo elements of the task, initially feeling a need to begin at the very beginning of the procedure, and later redoing elements within the procedure. The instructor's coaching to prompt the student to move to the next step is especially valuable in helping the student to begin to put together the elements of the task. Making it through the entire procedure, however clumsily and slowly, gives the student a sense of empowerment, and she is usually eager to try it once more. Subsequent attempts may involve trial and error approaches to organizing or holding materials as the student begins to develop kinesthetic sensitivity to the movements involved in the task. The instructor's positive feedback as the student's performance approximates the model is important for reinforcing this mind-body connection that underlies all skill mastery.

Mechanism—habitual response in performing the skill—occurs when the student can demonstrate some proficiency in movement. It is essential that the instructor verify that the skill is being performed correctly when the student reaches this level of learning, because errors can become a fixed part of the routine if they are not corrected early. It is at this point in skill development that the student is ready to perform the skill in the clinical area. Although she may experience some brief setbacks when confronted with the real-life situation, the student usually is able to make the necessary adjustments in her technique with the instructor's guidance. For example, in her anxiety about performing the skill with a patient the student may forget basic steps in assembling supplies. The instructor's gentle prompting usually is sufficient to get the student back on track again. Review of the procedure prior to entering the patient's room is a good approach to forestalling such blocks.

Complex Overt Response—a quick, smooth, accurate performance of complex movements using a minimum of energy—signals the student's achievement of proficiency in the skill. She is able to perform the skill without instructor supervision, and is comfortable in doing so.

Adaptation—ability to modify the technique as necessary—occurs when the student has sufficient mastery of and comfort with the skill to recognize how the technique can be modified to adapt to presenting circumstances without violating key principles underlying the skill.

Origination—the development of new approaches to a task—occurs when the student's understanding of the rationale underlying the basic skill enables her to not only modify the technique but develop an entirely different approach to achieving the goal of the skill. Nurses' ingenuity in dressing awkward wound sites is a good example of this level of skill development.

INTEGRATING THE COGNITIVE BASIS FOR PSYCHOMOTOR SKILLS

Almost anyone can be taught the "how" involved in the technical skills of nursing practice. It is the "why," the integration of the conceptual pieces, that enables the student to become a flexible, adaptive nurse who is responsive to technological changes and is able to function in a variety of environments. The nurse who is well grounded in the principles underlying her actions in performing a skill is better able to adjust technique when this is necessary. Such knowledge is also critical to successful patient teaching when psychomotor skills are involved.

Smith (1992) contrasts rote learning, which is "a verbatim incorporation of new knowledge into the cognitive structure and is not related to experience with events or objectives" with meaningful learning, defined as "a process of consciously integrating new knowledge with one's previous knowledge in ways that strongly link the two" (p. 17). She advocates using concept mapping and the Vee heuristic as approaches to making explicit the theoretical components underlying basic nursing skills.

Concept maps are schematic depictions of the learner's knowledge related to the identified skill. Concepts are linked logically, with the broadest concepts placed at the top of the map and subconcepts connected to these to demonstrate relationships and interplay. When students complete concept maps for assigned skills, the instructor can readily identify both gaps and misconceptions in their theoretical knowledge base. Smith's example of a concept map for dangling a patient is reproduced in Figure 5–1.

Vee heuristics link theory and practice elements of a skill by asking a focus question that is answered from both theoretical (why) and practice (how) perspectives. Theory elements are listed sequentially on the left side of the diagram; practice elements appear on the right side. They are joined in the activity represented in the skill. The instructor creates these heuristics to guide students' efforts to integrate theory and practice. Smith's example of a Vee heuristic for dangling a patient is reproduced in Figure 5–2.

The instructor can achieve a similar result by consistently asking "why" and "what if" questions as she teaches nursing skills. Questions such as the following stimulate students to reach into their store of cognitive information to problem-solve potential clinical scenarios.

"What would happen if an intramuscular injection entered a vein (or nerve)?"
"How can the nurse prevent this from occurring?"
"What if the patient is immobilized on his back? How would you go about selecting an alternative site for an intramuscular injection?"

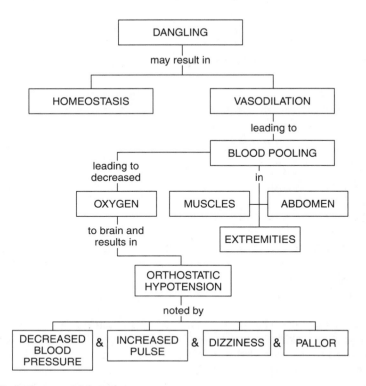

Figure 5–1 Concept Mapping
Source: From Smith, B.E. (1992). Linking theory and practice in teaching basic nursing skills. *Journal of Nursing Education*, 31, p. 18. Used with permission.

At the same time, exploring these issues often stimulates student questions reflecting their unspoken concerns about applying their technical skills in the clinical setting. It is the occurrence of such a dialogue that really represents meaningful learning.

SUMMARY

Just as learning can be rote or meaningful, the college laboratory experience can be a dull series of exercises or a dynamic learning environment. It is the instructor's ingenuity and effort that make the difference in maximizing the use of this potentially powerful resource for clinical nursing education.

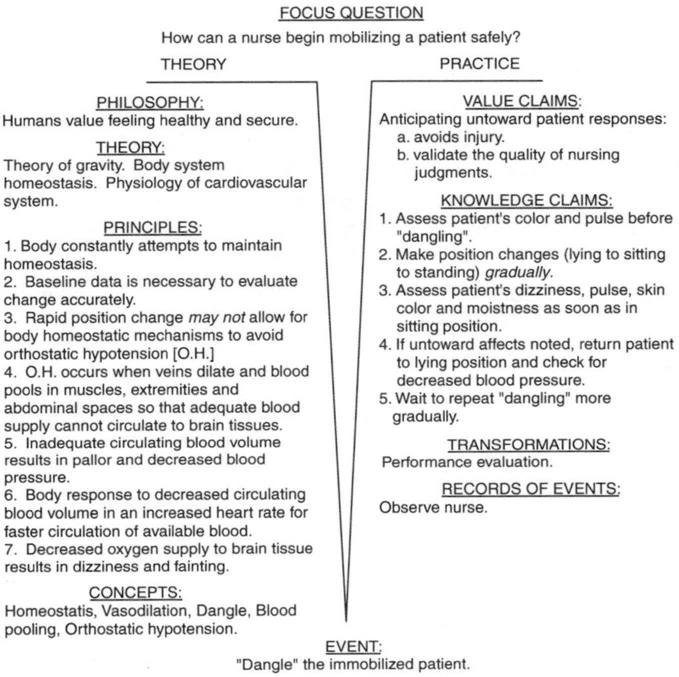

FOCUS QUESTION
How can a nurse begin mobilizing a patient safely?

THEORY	PRACTICE
PHILOSOPHY: Humans value feeling healthy and secure.	**VALUE CLAIMS:** Anticipating untoward patient responses: a. avoids injury. b. validate the quality of nursing judgments.
THEORY: Theory of gravity. Body system homeostasis. Physiology of cardiovascular system.	
	KNOWLEDGE CLAIMS: 1. Assess patient's color and pulse before "dangling".
PRINCIPLES: 1. Body constantly attempts to maintain homeostasis. 2. Baseline data is necessary to evaluate change accurately. 3. Rapid position change *may not* allow for body homeostatic mechanisms to avoid orthostatic hypotension [O.H.] 4. O.H. occurs when veins dilate and blood pools in muscles, extremities and abdominal spaces so that adequate blood supply cannot circulate to brain tissues. 5. Inadequate circulating blood volume results in pallor and decreased blood pressure. 6. Body response to decreased circulating blood volume in an increased heart rate for faster circulation of available blood. 7. Decreased oxygen supply to brain tissue results in dizziness and fainting.	2. Make position changes (lying to sitting to standing) *gradually*. 3. Assess patient's dizziness, pulse, skin color and moisture as soon as in sitting position. 4. If untoward affects noted, return patient to lying position and check for decreased blood pressure. 5. Wait to repeat "dangling" more gradually. **TRANSFORMATIONS:** Performance evaluation. **RECORDS OF EVENTS:** Observe nurse.
CONCEPTS: Homeostatis, Vasodilation, Dangle, Blood pooling, Orthostatic hypotension.	

EVENT:
"Dangle" the immobilized patient.

Figure 5–2 Vee Heuristic
Source: From Smith, B.E. (1992). Linking theory and practice in teaching basic nursing skills. *Journal of Nursing Education*, 31, p. 18. Used with permission.

REFERENCES

Arnold, W.K., & Nieswiadomy, R.M. (1997). A structured communication exercise to reduce nursing students' anxiety prior to entering the psychiatric setting. *Journal of Nursing Education*, 36, 446–447.

Bell, M.L. (1991). Learning a complex nursing skill: Student anxiety and the effect of preclinical skill evaluation. *Journal of Nursing Education*, 30, 222–226.

Corder, J.B. (1991). Campus clinical: An alternative clinical activity. *Journal of Nursing Education*, 30, 420–421.

Doheny, M.O. (1993). Mental practice: An alternative approach to teaching motor skills. *Journal of Nursing Education*, 32, 260–264.

Gronlund, N.E. (1991). *How to write and use instructional objectives* (4th ed.). New York, NY: Macmillan.

K.K. Guinee. (1978). *Teaching and learning in nursing: A behavioral objectives approach*. New York: Macmillan.

Infante, M.S. (1985). *The clinical laboratory in nursing education*. New York: Wiley.

Kolb, D. (1976). *Learning style inventory: Technical manual*. Boston: McBer.

Nabokov, P. (1978). Peer instruction. In Klevins, C. (Ed.). *Materials and methods in continuing education*. (pp. 249–255). Los Angeles: Klevens Publications.

Richardson, V. (1998). The diverse learning needs of students. (pp. 17–33). In Billings, D.M., & Halstead, J.A. *Teaching in nursing; A guide for faculty*. Philadelphia: W.B. Saunders.

Smith, B.E. (1992). Linking theory and practice in teaching basic nursing skills. *Journal of Nursing Education, 31*, 16–23.

CHAPTER 6

ORGANIZING AND MANAGING INSTRUCTION IN THE CLINICAL PRACTICE SETTING

Expectations, Hopes, and Fears   87
    Causing No Harm to the Patient   87
    Helping Patients   88
    Integrating Theory into Clinical Practice   89
    Learning Clinical Practice Skills   89
    Looking Good as a Nurse and as a Student   90
Selecting Clinical Learning Experiences   91
    Curricular Goals   91
    Learning Environment   92
    Instructor Expertise   93
    Learner Characteristics   95
    Other Considerations   96
    Alternative Approaches   97
Techniques to Help Students Prepare for Clinical Learning Experiences   97
    Teacher-Created Data Collection Forms   98
    Daily Nursing Care Plans   99
    The "Verbal Connection"   99
    Clinical Focus Guidelines   100
    Clinical Concept Mapping   100
The Clinical Preconference   103
Guiding Student Learning in the Clinical Setting   104
    Teaching–Learning Principles Underlying Instruction   105
    Modeling the Professional Nursing Role   109
Managing Off-Unit Experiences   112
Taking Advantage of Serendipitous Opportunities   114
The Clinical Postconference   114
Summary   116
References   117

The clinical practice setting provides students with opportunities to develop the knowledge, skills, and attitudes of a professional nurse within the realistic work settings in which they will eventually practice. Although the structure and process of clinical nursing education has changed over time, the critical role of the clinical setting in preparing students for the challenges of practice has remained a central component of nursing curricula. The original apprenticeship model, in which students' work in the hospital was supplemented by occasional classes and the processes involved in delivering nursing care were passed on to students by graduate nurses, was abandoned decades ago for a more structured and organized approach to guiding the transfer of theoretical knowledge to the practice setting.

To succeed in the clinical practice setting, the clinical nursing instructor needs to be well grounded in the clinical specialty in which she is teaching and comfortable in the clinical environment in which she will be providing instruction. A thorough understanding of the systems and procedures adopted by unit personnel for the management of patient care allows the instructional process to proceed with a minimal disruption of the routines that characterize the unit's operations. A rapport with staff members that fosters trust in the instructor and her approaches to teaching students creates a positive learning environment for everyone. The clinical instructor paves the way for students' clinical learning experiences. The relationships she forges with staff—on the basis of her clinical know-how, her willingness to adapt to the culture and flow of the unit, and her enthusiasm for and delight in the work of nursing—result in an atmosphere of collegiality that enhances the students' experience.

Having spent sufficient time on the unit to learn its routines, the clinical instructor is in a good position to orient students to the unit when they arrive for their first clinical day. Sensitivity to fostering collaboration with staff may lead her to ask the nurse manager to perform this task. Such a request consolidates the alliance with staff that the instructor seeks to establish, and makes students feel a part of—rather than apart from—the life of the clinical unit.

For the most part, the initial clinical day is spent in establishing expectations for the clinical experience and for student behaviors in relation to that experience, reviewing routines and procedures used on the unit, and providing students with the opportunity to develop some familiarity with the layout of the unit. This initial day should include a discussion of the types of patient problems that usually are encountered on the unit, the level of acuity involved, and the customary focus of nursing interventions. If appropriate to the setting, nursing rounds may be conducted to enable students to have some initial connection with the patients and the setting in which they are receiving care. Students may be encouraged to review nursing care plans and the Kardex or read patient charts, if this will not be disruptive for staff, to gain a sense of how these documents are organized and where information they will need in preparing for future assignments is located. More advanced students who have some familiarity with the clinical setting may be given a patient assignment in coordination with a staff nurse as a means of introducing students to the clinical environment and its rhythms.

EXPECTATIONS, HOPES, AND FEARS

Students and instructor both approach the clinical learning situation with numerous expectations, hopes, and fears. The ultimate aim of teaching is to skillfully select and apply strategies and techniques that will enable students and instructor to find common ground that will foster learning. Once they have found that common ground, students and instructor are able to develop collaborative approaches to teaching, learning, and providing nursing care that are the essence of a professional nursing education.

One purpose of Wilson's (1994) qualitative study of baccalaureate nursing students in a senior-level clinical course was to identify goals for the clinical practice experience as perceived by the student. Six major goals emerged from the analysis:

- to cause no harm to a patient;
- to help patients;
- to integrate theory-based knowledge from lecture and reading into clinical practice;
- to learn nursing clinical practice skills;
- to look good as a student; and
- to look good as a nurse. (p. 83)

An exploration of the dimensions underlying each of these identified goals is a useful means of uncovering the expectations, hopes, and fears carried to the clinical learning situation by students and instructors.

Causing No Harm to the Patient

Students in Wilson's study identified their responsibility for patient care assignments as quite different from their responsibility for learning. As learners, they expected to make mistakes as part of the process of learning, and to use trial and error approaches in mastering a learning task. This approach was viewed as unacceptable when learning carried with it the responsibility for another person's well-being. Because "doing no harm" was superordinate to other goals for the clinical experience, students were highly motivated to prepare adequately for clinical assignments. They identified any lack of knowledge and/or skills related to patient needs as inherently dangerous to patients in their care, and became anxious when they felt their knowledge and/or skills were insufficiently developed to meet the demands of the assignment.

In reality, however, a student cannot make progress if increasingly difficult assignments, which by their nature contain demands for knowledge and/or skill the student has not yet mastered, do not challenge her. If the learning experience is well designed and the instructor is taking full advantage of the clinical material available in the setting, it is very likely that even the best-prepared students will encounter situations that appear to be beyond their ability. The challenge to the instructor is to make learning safe for the student, while ensuring that no harm comes to the patient because, of course, the instructor shares the students' fear of harming patients. This fear often is the driving force behind the instructor's vigorous quizzing of students prior to their providing care and close supervision as they perform various procedures. Such practices tend to increase students' distrust of the instructor as well as increasing their anxiety. Distrust causes students to avoid interactions with the instructor, particularly those that might reveal any lack of certainty regarding how to proceed with the clinical assignment. This behavior further jeopardizes patient safety.

Practicing nurses are able to tolerate the "messiness" of the clinical area, where it's "okay" not to know immediately what is going on with a patient, as long as the nurse knows enough to know what *might* be going on, what to look for, and what the patient needs from the nurse in the meantime. Is it possible to transfer this tolerance for uncertainty to clinical teaching, to enable students to achieve the goal of doing no harm while also engaging in learning that might result in mistakes? Making mistakes, and overcoming their consequences, has great educational value, and should not be avoided at all costs. Further, in the rapidly changing situations that occur in most clinical settings, things quickly can move beyond the student's ability to manage, and this does not necessarily mean that the student is inadequate or at fault.

The key to accomplishing this involves three steps. First, the instructor must verify with students the level of knowledge and skills they are bringing to each clinical experience, to reinforce the need for adequate preparation for assignments, and to fill in gaps in knowledge when these occur. Second, the instructor must develop a climate of trust with students so that students recognize that perfection is an unrealistic expectation, are able to ask questions freely, and feel that they can acknowledge mistakes when these occur without fear of embarrassment or reprimand. Third, the instructor must be prepared to calmly step in to correct mistakes and address their consequences without distressing the patient or undermining the student's confidence.

Helping Patients

Students in Wilson's study viewed the help they were able to provide for patients as somehow compensating for their "use" of these patients for learning. The instructor can take advantage of this desire to help patients by reinforcing the positive benefits for patients to having students care for them, and encouraging the student to plan care activities so as to maximize the benefits received by the patient. By helping the student to consider what "value added" she might be able to provide for the patient during the clinical experience, the instructor encourages the student to look beyond her own learning needs to consider the larger context of patient care needs. For example, the patient's daily care may be rushed or fragmented when staffing is short; the student is able to provide care calmly and with minimal interruption, *if* she plans and manages her time properly.

The time constraints associated with clinical learning often impede the student's ability to fully help patients. The student's position in the system makes it difficult for her to follow-up on issues that might arise as she cares for a patient, and her sporadic presence on the unit (often only once a week) is disruptive to any continuity of care that might be provided, excepting in long-term care and community health settings. This reality also must be addressed by the instructor, who needs to set boundaries on students' activities with patients once the students have left the clinical learning situation while still providing the mechanisms necessary to ensure that issues identified during the students' work with the patients are addressed by staff after the students depart. The frustration the student feels at not being able to complete the work she has begun in helping the patient can be channeled into equally important lessons concerning the role of teamwork and communication in ensuring continuity of care.

Integrating Theory into Clinical Practice

For some students in Wilson's study, observing or practicing the clinical application of content presented in class provided the means by which they could understand the material. Others found clinical practice experiences to reinforce learning, and so aid their retention of material. For many instructors, such integration is serendipitous, since the clinical situation rarely matches classroom content with a great deal of fidelity. Students are able to identify fragments of the clinical experience that provide the illustration for a theoretical concept (perhaps because they are searching for such connections) and become quite adept at pointing these out to their fellow students and the instructor. It is important for the instructor to validate such integration, and elaborate on the example by distinguishing the theoretical ideal from the observed reality in the clinical setting. It is equally important for the instructor to identify flaws in integration, as when the student misreads the clinical situation as illustrating a theoretical concept or erroneously applies theory in practice. Correcting these errors by explaining the distinctions between the student's application of theory and the correct application in this situation helps the student to fine-tune her understanding of theory through the use of clinical examples.

Learning Clinical Practice Skills

Students in Wilson's study tended to equate learning with the first-time performance or mastery of a growing list of psychomotor skills. Instructors ignore this student goal at their peril, since students seem unable to concentrate on the larger patient care situation until they feel comfortable with the hands-on care they are providing. This focus on skilled clinical performance in accomplishing patient care procedures is likely to be related to the goal of looking good as a nurse. The instructor can accelerate the students' shift in perspective to include larger goals for patient care by identifying those technical skills that are likely to be encountered in providing care in the particular clinical setting, providing opportunities early in the clinical experience for each student to perform these skills, and tracking each student's accomplishments with respect to skill development and mastery. By focusing on a limited list of skills appropriate to the setting, the instructor can satisfy the strong need students have to develop clinical expertise through technical skill performance while limiting the amount of attention and effort expended on technical skill mastery to the detriment of the development of other nursing skills.

Looking Good as a Nurse and as a Student

For the students in Wilson's study, looking good as a nurse involved achieving the goal of helping patients, as affirmed by the patient and his family members as well as by staff members (the instructor's comments on student performance with patients are evaluated differently by students, who judge these in terms of how they affirm or disaffirm looking good as a student); mastering new aspects of nursing care; being organized; and feeling confident and competent in performing nursing care. A different set of behaviors were identified for looking good as a student. Looking good as a student involved answering all questions correctly, performing all skills flawlessly, being involved in clinical learning activities at all times that the instructor is present, and having the right answers in instructor–student interactions. Because such perfection is an impossible feat, students modified their interactions with the instructor based on the confidence they felt in their knowledge and/or skill base. While the instructor struggles to create "teachable moments," in which student learning can be maximized through skilled questioning by the instructor, students view these moments as an examination that will make or break their careers as nursing students. They stop relating to the clinical situation as a learning opportunity, and retreat into their classroom response style. Similarly, students generally avoid asking questions of the instructor (relying instead on fellow students and staff) in order to avoid looking bad as a student.

Despite the instructor's assurance that evaluation is not the central goal of all instructor–student interactions, students remain unconvinced. Consequently, the instructor must structure such interactions to look as little like an examination as possible. In her provocative discussion of thinking in nursing education, Ironside (1999) describes one instructor's approach to stimulating students to think about the process of patient care by sharing her own thinking about the presenting situation and engaging the student in a dialogue about the meanings embedded in the situation as well as the various possibilities for nursing response. Sharing one's own thinking provides the student with insights as to how nurses view and analyze situations; it also reveals the constant interplay of observations, selection of what is relevant in the situation, hypothesis generation, and hypothesis testing—all with the clear potential for "error"—that characterizes nursing in action. Students' usual response in interactions with instructors—to provide the right answers—reinforces a too-rapid closure on a single solution to a problem, forestalling consideration of alternatives or confounding issues. Nursing's particular art is in tolerating a certain lack of closure on problems or answers without losing track of the patient's situational response and corresponding needs for care. Teaching in the clinical setting requires an approach that prevents such premature closure and the resulting simplistic, incomplete responses to the complexities being presented by clinical material.

SELECTING CLINICAL LEARNING EXPERIENCES

The clinical setting is both a stimulus environment for the application of learning and an environment rich in its own opportunities for learning. It is the instructor's job to select the most appropriate "stimuli" for students' application of theoretical knowledge and to capitalize on additional learning opportunities. It is the instructor's use of and response to the complex interplay of educational goals, learner abilities and needs, and the clinical environment that determines the success of the clinical experience.

Fothergill-Bourbonnais and Higuchi (1995) identify four factors that should be considered in selecting clinical learning experiences: curricular goals as determined by the nursing program, the learning environments that have been identified as the places where these goals will be pursued, the clinical expertise of the instructor, and characteristics of the students.

Curricular Goals

Curricular goals are expressed in the objectives that have been developed for each course in the program. These objectives flow from a set of outcomes desired for graduates of the program, and expectations for progressive student growth in knowledge, skill, and attitudes in relation to professional values as they pursue these outcomes throughout their educational experience. Commonly identified curricular goals include the development of

1. clinical judgment through critical thinking in the use of problem-solving and decision-making skills;
2. technical expertise in the delivery of nursing care, based on scientific rationales;
3. communication skills in interactions with patients, their families, and other health care providers;
4. caring behaviors in the provision of nursing care;
5. the full professional nursing role through such activities as advocacy, initiation and response to change, and clinical leadership;
6. operational familiarity with the organizational contexts in which health care is delivered;
7. autonomy in decision making and accountability for actions; and
8. the ability to identify learning needs and plan approaches to meet them.

Course objectives reflect one stage in the sequence that students follow in pursuing program outcomes. Course objectives may apply to both classroom and clinical learning in the course, or a parallel set of objectives may be developed for each area. In some programs, objectives for each clinical experience are created; in others, the approach to be used in addressing the overall objectives for the course is left to each clinical instructor. (Sample course objectives appear in Appendix A.)

From one perspective, any separation of classroom and clinical objectives makes no sense, since all theoretical knowledge should eventually be applicable in the clinical area. From another, the level of learning represented in "knowing that" is different than that involved in "knowing how," justifying the creation of two sets of objectives. The instructor must provide experiences for students that enable them to reach the objectives, and hence move toward achieving the curricular goals; but she has considerable latitude in how to accomplish this. It is entirely appropriate to broadly interpret the objectives provided for the experience so that the richness of the clinical setting can be exploited for student learning. The instructor must, however, be aware of what has been covered in the classroom, so she can provide the relevant theoretical background for the activities in which students are engaged in the clinical setting. Eventually, the two will merge in a synthesized whole, particularly if the instructor is consistent in guiding such integration.

Learning Environment

The clinical environments in which students learn nursing vary enormously in such characteristics as

- acuity versus chronicity;
- pace of unit operations;
- nature of the patient;
- trajectory of a usual episode of illness;
- nature of the patients' needs for nursing;
- level of nursing intervention required (prevention, rehabilitation, etc.);
- length of stay;
- applications of technology;
- intensity of staffing, both nursing and other health care providers;
- relative autonomy and independence afforded the nurse in determining the course of care; and
- impact of financial constraints on the quantity and quality of patient care.

These varied environments expose students to numerous perspectives on the phenomenon of nursing, human responses to illnesses and their treatment, and the processes involved in professional nursing care. As a result of these multiple exposures, students gain much more than a series of snapshots of nursing in action. They begin to recognize the full impact of an episode of illness and the cycle involved in restoring health or promoting optimal functioning or comfort in the face of ongoing chronic illness or death, as well as the nurse's role in assisting the patient through that cycle. In the course of these experiences, students also master an array of technical skills associated with the nursing needs of the patients for whom they care. With time, students' caring for patients involves the selective application of appropriate technical skills, rather than a focus on the skills themselves.

Caring for a variety of patients increases students' sensitivity to the different ways in which people respond to illness and its treatment, enabling them to begin to develop the "skilled clinical knowledge" and "perceptual awareness" that marks the expert nurse (Benner & Wrubel, 1982). Learning about a disease process, treatment, or drug therapy in the classroom becomes enriched by the depth and variety of knowledge that is developed in interaction with patients. In comparing and contrasting the human responses they witness, students begin to integrate the theoretical with the practical. This only can occur if the clinical instructor recognizes these nuances and the subtle distinctions presented in clinical situations chosen for student learning, and deliberately selects assignments to develop this awareness in students. This means that the instructor approaches the clinical setting as a learning environment that presents multiple opportunities for students to observe postoperative healing, with less concern about whether each student has been exposed to a patient who has undergone major abdominal surgery.

As unit staff observe the types of patient situations the instructor selects for student learning, they add to the mix their own perspective on what is significant in the particular clinical setting in which learning is occurring. When the instructor has established positive relationships with staff, they support the instructor's efforts by making suggestions regarding patient situations that would provide good (or negative) learning experiences for students. This collaboration further refines the instructor's ability to capitalize on the richness of the clinical learning environment.

Instructor Expertise

While the instructor must be an excellent role model of professional nursing, the expertise required for clinical teaching, especially with respect to selecting learning experiences, is different and far more complex than that required for bedside nursing. Three areas of knowledge essential for clinical teaching are subject matter content, the teaching-learning process, and the curriculum content (Shulman, 1986, cited by Fothergill-Bourbonnais & Higuchi, 1995).

Expertise in the specialty area represented by the learning environment is essential in order for the instructor to recognize the educational potential that exists within the available patient situations and to guide the student learning that should be taking place. Additionally, the instructor must be able to predict the likely course for each patient being cared for by students, so they are not overwhelmed (or too minimally challenged) by the assignment. While any patient can crash—or be unexpectedly discharged—this will occur infrequently if the instructor has a well developed sense of typical trajectories of response to illness and treatment in her specialty. The instructor must also feel confident in managing multiple patient variables without becoming ruffled or confused. When more advanced students are assigned to care for two or three patients, the instructor's responsibility multiplies to as many as 24 patients whose care must be tracked and safety assured. In acute care areas, even expert instructors will vary assignments by having some students care for the most complex patients on one clinical day, while others have a lighter assignment, and then reversing this on a subsequent clinical day (Fothergill-Bourbonnais & Higuchi, 1995).

Pedagogical expertise is necessary to enable the instructor to help students to make the intellectual connections between classroom theory and the clinical material that comprises their learning experience. The instructor also needs to understand the progressive nature of learning, and be able to track the individual learning needs of students as they develop the necessary knowledge and skills involved in achieving course objectives. The instructor must be as adept at diagnosing and responding to educational needs of students as she is at diagnosing and responding to nursing needs of patients, because each is likely to progress at a different rate.

Curricular knowledge is necessary to understand where in the "vertical curriculum" the course is positioned—what content and experiences have preceded the course and which will follow the course. This way, the instructor won't expect too much or too little from her students. (It is entirely possible that some students in a course will have had a prior course in, for example, maternal-child nursing while others will have this course next. This creates a real challenge for the instructor who would like to draw on this content, for example, in a community nursing experience, but must vary assignments based on individual students' actual experiences in the curriculum.) Placement of content in another course does not mean that the instructor cannot include an experience if it arises, but that she will recognize the student's need for background information to maximize the learning potential of the experience. At the same time, much content in the curriculum—the management of the diabetic patient, acid-base balance, and the like—merits repetition in successive courses. The instructor also must be familiar with the "lateral curriculum," the theoretical content of courses that are being taught simultaneously with the clinical component in which she is teaching. This is necessary so that students can experience the necessary clinical examples of the theoretical as a means of integrating and reinforcing theory and practice (Shulman, 1986, cited by Fothergill-Bourbonnais & Higuchi, 1995).

The instructor also must be skilled in human relations, not only with students and staff, but also with patients and their families. It is the instructor who introduces patient and student and, in the process, helps to build the patient's confidence in being cared for by the student. This introduction assures the patient that there is an expert guiding the student and that the patient has recourse to the instructor.

Learner Characteristics

The clinical instructor must consider the individual abilities of the students in the clinical group, and select learning experiences accordingly. While all students are expected to achieve course objectives by the end of the semester, each will achieve these at different rates and levels of competence. The instructor must tailor assignments to allow each student to progress steadily and comfortably toward the final goal. By sharing with each student her rationale for making specific assignments, the instructor enables the student to focus on the key learning opportunities the assignment presents.

Advanced awareness of each student's academic progress as well as her performance in previous clinical experiences gives the instructor some basic information upon which to base initial assignments while she completes her own initial assessment of each student's strengths and weaknesses (Hill, 1993). In using this information, the instructor must be careful not to allow grades or another instructor's comments on a student's performance to unduly bias her own judgments. Many students whose academic performance has been mediocre excel in the clinical arena, and should be given the opportunity to demonstrate their unique abilities.

"A sequence of experiences that has both continuity and connection is important." (Fothergill-Bourbonnais & Higuchi, 1995, p. 40) The design of successive assignments should build on each student's progress in

- technical skill development;
- ability to manage increasingly complex care demands;
- responsiveness to an increasing number of patient variables;
- ability to recognize typical, then atypical patterns of response;
- ability to organize and manage a complex assignment; and
- achieving independence in making decisions and clinical judgments.

The instructor must tap into the student's knowledge base as it expands, so that the student is continuously challenged to access and utilize prior learning.

The student's level of anxiety or confidence must be considered in selecting learning experiences. The anxious student will need a patient assignment that will enable her to have a positive experience and so reduce some of the anxiety she is experiencing in the clinical area. Often, one or two satisfying experiences are sufficient to enhance the student's level of confidence and lower dysfunctional anxiety. The overconfident student must also be managed carefully, because the student's bravado may mask high anxiety.

The student's ability to function safely in providing care is a major concern in selecting learning experiences. The instructor will not want to "dumb down" an assignment for the student who may pose a safety problem, but she will want to consider her own ability to provide adequate supervision for this student while still attending to the learning needs of others in the group. This is a situation in which the instructor's rapport with staff, who can provide the necessary backup either for the problem student or the remaining student group, is a major contributor to the success of the experience.

The instructor will want to capitalize on a student's unique abilities—for example, language skills in caring for a patient who speaks no English—but not at the expense of the student's exposure to a variety of experiences.

The instructor will need to keep track of various aspects of each student's assignments to ensure that the learning opportunities experienced by each student are relatively equivalent. It's important to track the student's array of psychomotor skills and other, nontechnical skills, such as patient teaching, preparing the patient for a procedure, and conducting an admission interview and assessment. Students also should have equivalent exposure to the typical patient problems encountered in the specialty area, and to managing the care of more than one patient.

Student requests for specific experiences should be honored to the extent that this is possible. Students develop a good sense of their own needs for learning, and this awareness should be reinforced.

Other Considerations

Contingency planning is essential in the rapidly changing environment of health care delivery. A well-conceived assignment can evaporate when a patient is transferred or discharged. A unique experience may be missed because the student who was given the assignment has called in sick, or a magnificent experience may arise just as the students are leaving the unit. A usually busy unit may have a fallow period, with only a few extremely routine patient care situations available for students. Educationally sound backup plans are essential to ensure that each clinical experience offers each student the opportunity to continue her progressive development of knowledge and skills. When the acuity level of patients is unusually high, students can be paired in completing assignments. When acuity is unusually low, students might be given a multiple patient assignment to develop their organizational and time management skills. Case studies can be developed for review to reinforce the application of theory to practice. "Worst case scenarios" can be imagined for stable patients, with students identifying various problems that could develop given the patient's underlying illness, and the appropriate response to each of these. Off-unit experiences, such as observing major diagnostic procedures or becoming involved in outpatient clinic routines, are a good alternative activity if planned in advance.

Needs particular to the clinical setting in which students practice also should be considered in planning learning activities. Assisting with unit routines—such as feeding residents in the long-term care setting—reinforces the concept of teamwork in addition to providing opportunities to witness the problems that may be encountered by the elderly and disabled in managing utensils, or swallowing and chewing food. Any activity can be transformed into a learning opportunity by the clinical instructor who recognizes students' need for socialization into the role of the professional nurse, which involves more than providing patient care. Indeed, Hill (1993) notes, "it is impossible to provide nursing care without processing knowledge in some way" (p. 133).

Alternative Approaches

One scheme for selecting clinical learning experiences is to break the routine practice of assigning each student to care for one or two patients and, instead, have some students engage in a different pattern. Assessment skills can be fine-tuned by having two or three students make "lung" rounds, to listen to the breathing patterns of a variety of patients and develop a sense of the distinctions that are encountered in the clinical setting. It is not necessary for each student to provide all care for a patient for whom a procedure is required in which students need practice; a succession of students can perform the procedure with one patient if the patient is consulted first and agrees to this.

Heims and Boyd (1990) advocate the use of concept-based learning activities as a substitute for traditional clinical assignments that give students responsibility for total patient care. In this approach students receive guidelines developed for each major concept to be addressed in the course. The student's task is to analyze the concept as it plays out in the clinical area. Heims and Boyd assert that this approach enables students to pursue nursing care planning creatively and frees them from repetitive care activities. Missing, however, is the accountability inherent in accepting a total care assignment, as well as the opportunity for the student to develop in the full role of the nurse through clinical activities and to learn through repetition.

The development of integrated health care networks, offering a single system of health services along the continuum of care needs, has been one response to managed care. Within such networks, critical pathways track patient progress in recovery from a health problem and nurse case management is a predominant approach to the delivery of nursing care. Mundt (1997) argues that nursing education programs must keep pace with this development by restructuring students' clinical experiences to enable them to "provide nursing care to and follow patients and families through the continuum of their health-related experience" (p. 312). This approach requires a transformation in the usual configuration of clinical educational experiences, as more responsibility for instruction is given to clinically based preceptors, who are well positioned within the network to guide student learning. Some nursing programs attempt to emulate this model on a small scale, by providing opportunities for students to visit patients in their homes after caring for them in the hospital or subacute setting.

TECHNIQUES TO HELP STUDENTS PREPARE FOR CLINICAL LEARNING EXPERIENCES

Students need some guidance in organizing for the clinical day, although the nature and degree of assistance needed will change as students progress through the nursing program. More advanced students will be able to prepare adequately for an assignment in the period just prior to embarking upon it, much as does a graduate nurse. Beginning students need more time to prepare, and usually are given the clinical assignment the day before the clinical experience to provide the opportunity for adequate preparation.

Structured assignments can be used to guide the student in accessing prior knowledge and identifying gaps that need to be filled before engaging in the clinical experience. Such assignments create an "anticipatory set," or readiness to learn, by helping students to identify important elements of the situation and to do any necessary reading, review, or thinking related to completing the assignment successfully. In making such assignments, however, the instructor must be clear as to how she expects the assignment to contribute to student learning.

Teacher-Created Data Collection Forms

These forms attempt to guide the student's identification and organization of data relevant to patient care. (Sample forms can be found in Appendix F.) The student abstracts data from the patient's chart and inserts the information into the appropriate categories on the form. Then the student consults her class notes and textbooks to review information pertinent to data elements—for example, the normal range of laboratory values given the laboratory test results for this patient; the indications, actions, and side effects of the drugs the patient is receiving; and so forth. As the student proceeds with patient care activities, she may consult the form for information rather than returning to the chart to retrieve it, or she may consult the form to answer the instructor's questions. Rarely is the student asked to verify the data she has collected through her own assessment of the patient, or to add to the patient's database as she works with the patient.

Teacher-created forms have the advantage of providing a format or framework for data collection that ensures that the student's preparation is comprehensive. However, it is difficult for the instructor to thoroughly evaluate each student's preparation in a timely manner in order to guide the student's use of the data or point to areas in which data are missing or incomplete.

A major problem with this approach to preparing for clinical is that the form does not direct the student to what is most relevant in the situation from either a patient care or a learning perspective. Rather, the student is faced with an overwhelming amount of data with no real notion of what matters and what doesn't. The data from the clinical situation initiate the quest for the related theoretical components, but there is no mechanism for reflection of this theory back into practice. The student dutifully records the patient's lab data and notes the normal range for these values, but is not challenged to take the next step to compare the two and identify what might be going on to create abnormal lab findings or, more significantly, the consequences for patient care that might accompany this.

Daily Nursing Care Plans

The student may be required to prepare a plan for the care of the assigned patient based on data drawn from the patient's chart, the existing nursing care plan, and other sources. Such plans are intended to guide the student's intellectual preparation for the clinical experience by encouraging review of relevant theoretical information and procedural guidelines. The student's "planning" takes place apart from the patient, and so does not incorporate much that is relevant to actually implementing the plan.

The format for the care plan usually follows the nursing process, but includes a space in which the student is expected to provide rationales for planned activities. This approach attempts to connect theory to practice in the student's preparation by requiring her to think through the reasons for various actions that she plans to take. As students search for appropriate rationales for planned actions, however, they tend to copy textbook explanations, and rarely consider their applicability to the actual situation or how the theory might guide their interventions with the patient.

As with teacher-created data collection forms, daily nursing care plans are time-consuming to correct, and such correction usually takes place after the day's clinical experience is completed and the plan no longer is a relevant source of learning for the student.

The "Verbal Connection"

Emerson and Groth (1996) describe an alternative to teacher-made forms and daily nursing care plans that is intended to assist the student in analyzing and synthesizing clinical data rather than merely collecting and recording facts and associated theory. The student is encouraged to gather data using a format that works for her. Guidelines that identify what the student needs to know in the specific clinical setting assist the student in her preparation. These guidelines help to direct the student's attention to relevant areas of inquiry (e.g., demographics, diagnostic information, prior history or concomitant health conditions) and a beginning synthesis of information (e.g., by asking questions about the interrelationships among laboratory trends and dietary and fluid status). The student is free to record as much or as little information as she chooses in preparing for the clinical assignment. This is intended to free the student from a focus on paperwork while stimulating a focus on mind work. The approach certainly frees the instructor from the need to review and correct students' written preparation for the clinical.

At the start of the clinical experience, the student and instructor discuss the student's plan of care; this is the "verbal connection." At this time, the instructor is able to verify the adequacy of the student's preparation, the student is able to ask questions, and the instructor is able to guide the integration of complex information gleaned from the student's preparation.

Beginning students may need some guidance in developing a format for seeking and recording data, beyond the structure provided by the familiar nursing process. The concepts identified in the nursing program's conceptual framework are a useful device for ensuring that students consider the full array of nursing issues that are likely to emerge in providing care for the assigned patient.

Clinical Focus Guidelines

Clinical focus guidelines are another approach to both streamlining and focusing students' preparation for clinical assignments (Blainey, 1991). The guidelines are developed for each clinical experience in the semester, and are tied to course objectives. They state expected learning outcomes, the activities in which the student should engage (observations, assessments, interventions, written assignments) in order to achieve outcomes, as well as the criteria that will be used in evaluating learning at the end of the semester. Suggestions for how the student might evaluate her own progress toward learning outcomes also are contained in the guidelines. Students receive all of the guidelines for the semester at one time, so they're able to capitalize on a full array of learning experiences in meeting objectives and completing assignments. The guidelines also assist in communicating with staff nurses who may be called upon to facilitate student learning.

Clinical focus guidelines appear to have the benefit of orienting the student to the content of clinical learning, and providing the means to probe and work with that content on an appropriate level, because the guidelines evolve from course objectives. However, the guidelines may so tightly focus the student's attention that she will seek the "fit" between the guidelines and the clinical material, and miss much that is present in the clinical situation because it has not been explained in the written guidelines or is not a stated focus for learning. If the clinical instructor is aware of this drawback to the use of clinical focus guidelines, and makes continual efforts to encourage students to look—and see—beyond the demands of the guidelines, this approach to preparing for clinical learning experiences can be very fruitful, and certainly promotes a degree of independence and flexibility in learning.

Clinical Concept Mapping

Concept mapping is a "hierarchical graphic organizer" that illustrates students' understanding of the relationships among concepts. In the clinical context, concept mapping demonstrates the linkages that exist between a patient's health conditions, their clinical manifestations, the therapeutic interventions prescribed for each, and any interrelationships that might exist among these (for example, the contraindication of a drug used to treat one of the conditions when another of the conditions is present).

Baugh and Mellott (1998) describe the use of clinical concept mapping with advanced medical-surgical students, who can be presumed to have mastered many of the subconcepts to be dealt with in completing concept maps.

Practice in constructing concept maps is provided in the classroom setting using case studies. Figure 6–1 illustrates the construction of a concept map for a patient with multisystem involvement. First, the student identifies the patient's relevant conditions, with an emphasis on the presenting condition. (Medical terminology is used in this illustration, but nursing diagnoses can easily be substituted.) Then the student clusters the clinical manifestations related to each condition. She adds therapeutic interventions to the map. Finally, the student links the clusters of conditions, manifestations, and interventions as these interact, and explains any relationships among them. Although Figure 6–1 reflects complex interactions, simple maps of single concepts can be developed as a teaching–learning approach to linking theory and practice with beginning students.

Once they have become familiar with the process, students develop one concept map each week for their assigned patients. In order to construct the

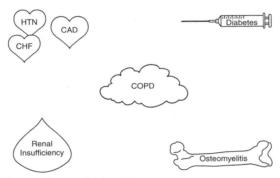

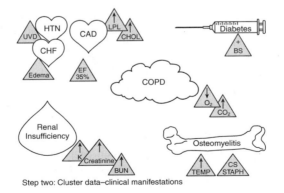

Figure 6–1 Clinical Concept Map Development
Source: From Baugh, N.G., & Mellot, K.G. (1998). Clinical concept mapping as preparation for student nurses' clinical experiences. *Journal of Nursing Education, 37,* 255. Used with permission.

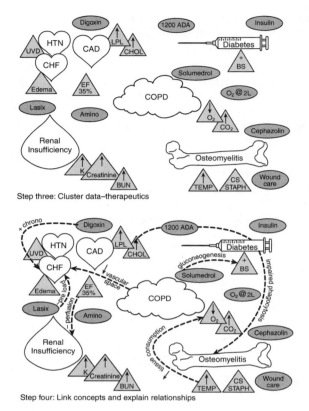

Step three: Cluster data–therapeutics

Step four: Link concepts and explain relationships

Figure 6–1 Continued

map, students must review the pertinent data from the patient's chart as well as the relevant theoretical information to support proposed linkages. As the student interacts with the patient in the clinical area, the map is revised and updated. This process enables the student to reflect theoretical knowledge back into practice, and vice versa, as she deepens her personal understanding of the connections among the clinical elements that are pertinent for the patient for whom she is providing care.

One advantage of clinical concept mapping is that it provides a very accessible means through which the instructor can evaluate student preparation and detect any gaps in her knowledge base or logical flaws in her reasoning concerning clinical connections. Another advantage of clinical concept mapping is that, while focused on a single concept chosen by the student, the map will inevitably encompass more holistic concerns, given the interacting nature of physiological (as well as psychological) processes, their manifestations, and their treatment.

THE CLINICAL PRECONFERENCE

The tradition of preconferences and postconferences as a component of clinical learning experiences persists despite little documentation as to their effectiveness (Packer, 1994). The preconference is intended to prepare both students and instructor for the clinical experience by providing anticipatory guidance for the day. Students are oriented to the objectives or focus for clinical activities, as well as any noteworthy situations or events they should be aware of. The instructor may use the preconference to check on each student's preparation, and to articulate the building nature of successive clinical experiences and the progress that the student group is making.

Each instructor must determine for herself the utility of the preconference in the setting in which she is teaching. Some instructors find that having students attend the change-of-shift report serves as a worthwhile substitute for the preconference. In addition to providing information about the status of the patients for whom students will be providing care, the shift report introduces students to the communications strategies used by nurses to relate complex information clearly and succinctly to one another. Students begin to develop sensitivity to what needs to be communicated to ensure continuity of care (Yurkovich & Smyer, 1998). However, the format and timing of the shift report, or physical limitations of the setting, may make student participation impossible. Many instructors elect to attend report prior to students' arrival on the unit, and then use the preconference time to deliver a modified shift report on students' patients. Others attempt to preserve the positive professional socialization inherent in nurse-to-nurse reporting by having students receive report on their patients from the nurse who will be responsible for the patient that day. Regardless of the approach used, students will need to have the most up-to-date information on their assigned patient(s) prior to beginning care activities, and the instructor must build the means to gain this into her plans.

Many instructors find preconference quizzing of students on their preparation to be tedious and time-consuming, because the group usually "tunes out" while their classmate is on the firing line. The anticipation of being grilled by the instructor (and possibly embarrassed in front of peers) probably magnifies the normal anxiety students bring to the clinical setting. An alternative approach to verifying that each student is adequately prepared for the clinical day is to conduct a form of rounds, visiting each student–patient pair and discussing with the student her plans for the day. Spot checks on essential information ("Are you aware that Mr. D's antibiotic was discontinued? Do you know why?") and the student's familiarity with procedures that must be performed in conjunction with providing care ("When do you plan to check Mrs. P's blood sugar? Do you know where the equipment is?") provide a sense of the student's level of preparation, and also give the student a chance to ask questions about aspects of care to be provided. The instructor also can use this opportunity to remind a student to call for the instructor when she is ready to perform a new skill that the instructor wishes to observe.

The instructor may find preconferences useful at the beginning of a clinical experience and with inexperienced students, and then may discontinue their use as the semester progresses. As long as there is a mechanism for verifying student preparation for the experience and awareness of the goals for learning, it is unimportant what format or approach is used in getting students off to a good start in the clinical setting.

GUIDING STUDENT LEARNING IN THE CLINICAL SETTING

The clinical setting presents students with experiential, practical learning opportunities that involve different processes than the depository–repository approach (so named because the instructor "deposits" knowledge in the students' brains, where it "reposes" until accessed by the student) common to classroom teaching and learning.

First, the clinical setting demands interaction with content. Diekelmann's (1993) study of the lived experiences of baccalaureate nursing students and their teachers uncovered a pattern which she labeled "learning-as-cognitive-gain." This pattern, which emerged in the analysis of stories respondents told about a situation that captured for them what it means to be a student or teacher in nursing, contained two themes: "applying content as thinking" and "content as neutral, unproblematic, and consensual." Diekelmann comments,

> The danger in the view of 'learning-as-cognitive-gain' is that what matters, which is thinking in particular situations, becomes lost as students are schooled to enter practice with a correspondence view of applying content (rules) to practice. (p. 247)

The content of the clinical setting is more subtle, and more embedded within the complexity of the patient's situation, than that presented in the classroom. Unless the student interacts with this content, she will have no means of developing a *working* knowledge of the rules she has learned in the classroom.

Second, the clinical setting is dynamic, with much of the content out of the direct control of the instructor. Clinical content is not organized in sequential packages that match the classroom syllabus, nor can the classroom syllabus be rearranged to adapt to the clinical reality. Like a map, classroom content will have given the student a general sense of the terrain to be traveled in the clinical area, but the student is still apt to get lost in the woods and have to work her way around fallen trees.

Third, the clinical setting invites independence in learning. Because the instructor cannot be everywhere, students are challenged to step into the unknown, assess their need for assistance, and seek assistance when it is needed. To accomplish this, they need broad guidelines for determining when they need help and in identifying whom to turn to if the instructor is unavailable. The instructor also is challenged: to accurately assess each student's readiness to function independently; to accurately forecast her own expectations regarding both student performance and patient responses, so as to anticipate the need for her timely presence or intervention; to adapt to rapidly changing circumstances with respect to student learning needs and patient responses; and to learn to let go.

Finally, while the clinical setting does not preclude reflection on learning, it doesn't invite this without the instructor's assistance. Students who are truly engaged in clinical learning tend to disengage (at least temporarily) from thinking about learning. While the student may mull over a point made during a lecture, or reread a passage in her textbook, similar reflections on the meanings embedded in the practice situation with which she is engaged are not automatic. Rather, the instructor must devise approaches that encourage reflection on practice, both during and after the clinical experience.

Teaching—Learning Principles Underlying Instruction

Several general principles are central to effective instruction in any setting. These concern students' readiness to learn, variety in instructional content and technique, repetition of content and experiences, promotion of transfer of learning to new situations, and making learning meaningful.

Readiness to Learn.   While readiness to learn involves being motivated to learn as well as demonstrating prior mastery of the necessary knowledge and skills upon which clinical objectives are predicated, it also involves being "fully present" in the clinical setting, focused on achieving the goals for learning and for patient care. Ideally, students' attention should not be diverted by concerns about an upcoming examination, family issues, or social affairs while they are in the clinical setting. Yet the reality is that everyone comes to work, educational, and other activities burdened with personal concerns that tend to divert attention from the task at hand. To deal with this reality, the instructor must be prepared to create an "anticipatory set" that invites students to become interested in the content and eager to participate in mastering it (Rowles & Brigham, 1998, p. 253).

Preconferences, preliminary nursing rounds, and listening to reports are commonly used approaches to bringing students' attention into focus as they begin the clinical experience. Regardless of the approach used, the instructor must establish an anticipatory set by clearly identifying the goals and objectives for the day's activities; bringing into the students' awareness the prior knowledge they have that will be needed to achieve the objectives; and identifying the specific content areas that will be the focus of the assignment. In identifying goals and objectives for the clinical day, the instructor should not ignore the students' own goals for the experience. The tendency to focus on the assigned patients' needs, while appropriate, should be balanced with equal attention to what the student hopes to gain from the experience. This helps to further engage the student in the assignment and the possibilities for learning that it presents. Another aspect of identifying goals involves sharing with students the instructor's rationale in making specific assignments. By revealing what she has identified as the "content" inherent in the assignment, and the related learning opportunities to be realized in engaging in the assignment, the instructor makes explicit aspects of the assignment that may have eluded the student.

During the clinical experience, the instructor needs to remain aware of the periodic need to reengage students in learning. Wagner and Ash (1998) describe approaches to create "the teachable moment," when the student will be "receptive to new understandings" (p. 278). As the clinical experience proceeds, the instructor seeks opportunities to interact with the student around the student's immediate concerns or a readily recognizable situation that is clearly important to the student. Student concerns are elicited through open-ended questions ("How is the day going for you?"), sharing of observations ("You seemed to be perplexed when Mr. G. asked about his prognosis"), an invitation to share a professional concern ("Has Mrs. L's early discharge raised any concerns for you?), recognizing a student accomplishment ("Baby G seemed less fussy during his feeding today; how did you manage that?), or when the student discloses a concern. In her dialogue with the student, the instructor structures her teaching to focus first on any expressed student concern. Realizing that her issues have been recognized and validated by the instructor captures the attention of the student and creates the "teachable moment" that signals readiness to learn.

Variety.   Students (and instructors) easily can become bored with learning experiences that become predictable in their pattern. By introducing a change of pace occasionally, the instructor reengages students in the learning. For example, planned rotations off the assigned unit, to participate in alternative experiences (e.g., a rotation through a step-down unit for students in an acute care setting), observational experiences (as of a surgical intervention or invasive diagnostic test or the opportunity to shadow a nurse manager or clinical specialist), and attending a conference, can provide variety that broadens the students' perspective on a clinical specialty. Alternative instructional approaches, such as the use of gaming, case studies, nursing rounds, or other ways of interacting with content, can lend the variety that stimulates learning.

Variety in the ways in which concepts are explained or procedures taught also is necessary to promote learning. A change in the vocabulary of instruction may be the single element that enables a student to grasp a concept. Drawing a picture rather than persisting in a verbal explanation may do the trick. Offering students alternative approaches to performing procedures, while maintaining a focus on the critical elements that remain the same, may enable the seemingly inept student to master a technique. While students become skilled at manipulating content to satisfy their own styles of learning, the ability of the instructor to offer alternative presentations of concepts increases the chances that learning will occur.

For many instructors, variety in clinical teaching means ensuring that students are exposed to patients of different ages, ethnic and social backgrounds, as well as to multiple disease processes. Students should have experiences involving the major health problems encountered in each specialty area, as well as the opportunity to work with diverse patient populations. However, variety involves more than attention to the patient and diagnosis variables. Because skilled nursing knowledge only can be developed through multiple exposures to multiple instances of a concept, students also need to experience variety in clinical assignments that appear to be redundant. While closely related to the principle of repetition, this application of the principle of variety seeks to broaden the student's perspective on a phenomenon through the planning of clinical assignments to include elements that have been encountered by the student before, but in a somewhat different context, so the student can begin to appreciate the differences in patients' responses to similar health conditions and treatments. The instructor may need to point this out to the student. For example, the student's attention might be drawn to the factors that may be contributing to different recuperative trajectories for two patients with similar diagnoses.

Repetition.   Few people are able to master concepts without revisiting them several times and in different contexts. In order for a student to "own" content, she must be able to revisit it frequently, testing out her understanding. While it is easy to interpret a student's repetitious questions as mental laziness, it is unrealistic to expect that each student will retain every scrap of content and word of wisdom the instructor has imparted. Anticipating that students will repeat their questions is less frustrating for the instructor, who might use the occasion to rephrase the answer or provide additional information. Of course, at times a student's repeated queries covering the same issues *does* represent mental laziness, requiring a response that both invites and facilitates the student's recall of the information. Students need encouragement to trust their memories and their brains rather than continually rely on the instructor's input when they are puzzled. Providing prompts, such as, "Do you remember what you did with Mrs. O last week?" helps the student to recognize that she has encountered—and solved—this issue before, and has the requisite knowledge to do so again.

Multiple exposures to situations involving the same concepts are an example of using repetition to both reinforce and enhance learning. Recognition of the commonalties and the differences among patients with the same condition is an essential element of developing clinical judgment and expertise.

Students also need repeated opportunities to perform technical skills. As with the development of proficiency in athletic or artistic endeavors, repetition of skills gives the student the body sense that helps to reinforce performance. With each successive performance, the skill is accomplished with greater fluidity and ease, moving the student to a higher level of psychomotor learning.

Transfer of Learning.   Despite faculty's careful efforts to create a progressive learning experience that builds upon previously acquired knowledge, students tend to approach each new clinical situation as a unique and isolated event. They have difficulty in recognizing the cues that signal the need to apply information or skills mastered in previous courses or during earlier clinical experiences. This may be because they are unable to distinguish those aspects of a presenting situation that are truly novel, and those that resemble or replicate conditions that have been encountered before. Or, the student may be unable to isolate the aspects of the situation that signal the need for specific information from the student's repository of knowledge.

The instructor can facilitate the transfer of learning in the clinical setting by guiding the student to the appropriate area of knowledge that must be accessed in order to understand the situation, and then allowing her to identify and apply the specific information that is needed. For example, many clinical situations require the application of concepts learned in basic anatomy and physiology classes. By asking the student what she knows about the normal function of the system involved in the presenting situation, the instructor stimulates consideration of the applicable anatomy and physiology related to the case, setting the student on the appropriate path to begin to access and use what she knows to understand the situation. Asking a progressive series of questions—while perhaps tedious to the instructor, enables the student to begin building a model for accessing and using her store of knowledge.

"And what happens when function is interrupted?"
"How might function have been interrupted in this case?"
"How will that affect other organs or systems?"
"How might that be manifested in the patient's signs and symptoms?"

This is a process of verbal content mapping, which might be made explicit in written assignments completed by students. Similarly, students may need prompts to recognize commonalties among clinical cases.

It is *least* helpful to students for the instructor to say, "Look it up!" when they have questions while in the midst of a clinical experience. Students who have prepared adequately for clinical already have reviewed those areas of information they believe will be needed to address the clinical problems they have identified in their assignments. If they have failed in this preparation, it is because they were unable to identify what they needed to know. Being told to look it up during the clinical experience does not help them to locate the information they need. If the clinical problem has arisen unexpectedly, the student will need guidance in thinking through the situation rather than running away from the bedside to read the textbook explanation, which she will have difficulty in applying anyway. It is more helpful to assist the student in reasoning through the problem in the present, and then suggesting further review after she leaves the clinical setting so that she can acquire a better understanding of the phenomenon she has observed, as a means to link theory with practice. The student who is truly unprepared for the clinical should be sent to the library to fully prepare for the clinical assignment.

Transfer of knowledge also can be facilitated by assisting students' understanding of a concept as one example of a broader class of concepts to which knowledge can be generalized. Consider, for example, the clinical management of tubes. By their nature, tubes are susceptible to problems with patency, regardless of whether the tube is an intravenous device, a suction catheter, urinary drainage apparatus, a nasogastric tube, or a tracheotomy tube. While the management of a clogged tube will vary with its type and placement, the potential for a patency problem to develop is common to all of them, and this knowledge can be transferred to broaden the student's understanding of management problems concerning a large variety of similar devices.

Making Learning Meaningful. Learning becomes meaningful when students feel they are making progress toward achieving goals. Those goals include the planned outcomes of the learning experience as well as students' personal goals for the clinical experience. Student goals are related to what they hope to accomplish for the patient or patients for whom they are assigned to provide care as well as what they hope to accomplish in terms of their own learning. Both are legitimate. While research findings and the nursing education literature suggest the potential expectations and goals that students have for clinical learning experiences, it is imperative for the instructor to validate those goals with each student. A review of each student's goals enables the instructor to identify the student whose expectations for her own performance are either too high or too low, and then contribute to revising those expectations. Such a review also helps the instructor to shape the learning experience to assist students in meeting their personal goals. The instructor's reference to students' personal goals—and their progress in achieving them—makes meaningful the learning that is occurring in the clinical setting.

Knowledge of the students' goals for the clinical learning experience can inform the instructor's selection of specific assignments, as well as her communications with students concerning the rationale for assignments. For example, the instructor can remind a student that she had expressed an interest in working with a patient with a specific health concern, and that the day's assignment has been made to provide for that opportunity. This validates the legitimacy of the student's goal, the concern the instructor has that the student have the opportunity to achieve that goal, and also directs the student's attention to the primary content of the assignment. Interactions with students during the clinical day also can be structured around goals, by asking whether the student feels she is making progress in achieving a specific goal for the patient or for her own learning. The sense of movement toward goal achievement makes the continued engagement with the content of clinical learning inherently meaningful and exciting for students.

Modeling the Professional Nursing Role

Because clinical learning is experiential in nature, students search for patterns of performance that exemplify the professional nursing role to which they aspire. Once these models are identified, the student attempts to emulate them as she engages in her clinical assignment.

Citing several authors, Wiseman (1994) asserts, "In nursing education, the faculty member serves as the primary role-model initiating the student into the profession" (p. 405). Is this assertion true? If it is, what are the consequences for instructor behavior, in particular, the balancing of the multiple facets of the instructional role? If the instructor must focus on patient care in order to adequately role-model nurse behaviors, does she do this at the expense of the instructional, supervisory, and evaluative components of her role? If it is not the instructor who serves as the primary role model for students, who does? And how can the instructor guide students' selection of role models?

In reality, students draw from a broad variety of persons in their efforts to identify appropriate role models. If the instructor is an active participant in nursing care, working with students (what Kiger [1993] calls "mucking in") rather than standing at the sidelines observing (from the students' perspective, evaluating), she will be among the role models selected by students. Staff who appear to be knowledgeable and effective in providing care, regardless of their professional status, are equally likely to be selected as role models. The instructor can guide the selection of role models by pointing out to students those among the staff who most consistently demonstrate expertise and professionalism, and suggesting that these nurses be observed and emulated.

In her study of role model behaviors, Wiseman found a high degree of agreement among junior and senior baccalaureate nursing students as to the importance of various role model behaviors, but a perceived inconsistency as to the degree to which students were rewarded for emulating these behaviors. This suggests that instructors must carefully consider what professional behaviors are important, how these behaviors can be demonstrated to students, and then consistently provide positive feedback when students in the clinical setting evidence the behaviors. In developing a picture of the "ideal" professional role model, the instructor should consider how such important professional behaviors as caring, advocacy, leadership, and collaboration might be modeled in interactions with students, patients and their families, staff, and physicians. She also should consider how best to articulate the reasoning behind the behaviors that students observe and seek to emulate. For example, students observe the results of the nurse's thought process, but cannot be privy to that intellectual work unless the nurse reveals her process of thinking as well as her conclusions. Similarly, values that are demonstrated in action may need to be made explicit for students in terms of the analytical process of dealing with value conflicts, reaching decisions that result in value choices, and then determining how best to act in accord with those choices.

The role model behaviors identified in Wiseman's study (p. 407) can be organized into four clusters: technical know-how, interpersonal effectiveness, critical thinking, and professional role behaviors (see Table 6–1). Many of these behaviors (those related to interpersonal interactions with students)

TABLE 6–1   ROLE MODEL BEHAVIORS IN THE CLINICAL SETTING

Technical Know-How

- Demonstrates the use of equipment unique to the clinical setting.
- Demonstrates nursing care procedures.
- Demonstrates up-to-date nursing practices.
- Demonstrates ability to care for patients' needs.
- "Pitches in" when needed to assist students.

Interpersonal Effectiveness

- Uses therapeutic communication skills with each patient.
- Interacts with physicians in a confident manner.
- Displays a sense of humor in appropriate context.
- Demonstrates a caring attitude toward patients.
- Demonstrates a caring attitude toward students.
- Appears to have respect of the agency personnel.
- Provides a positive atmosphere for students to learn.
- Listens to students' point of view.
- Gives positive feedback.
- Gives negative feedback in a constructive manner.

Critical Thinking

- Listens to change of shift reports.
- Asks questions regarding patient's condition.
- Demonstrates problem-solving ability in the clinical setting.

Professional Role Behaviors

- Reports clinical data to staff personnel in a timely fashion.
- Identifies self to patients when first meeting them.
- Is neat and clean in personal appearance.
- Keeps confidential information to self.
- Is organized in the clinical setting.
- Is flexible when the situation requires different approach.
- Respects the patients' integrity.
- Encourages discussion of ethical dilemmas.
- Demonstrates accountability for own actions.
- Demonstrates an enthusiastic attitude toward nursing.

Based on Wiseman, R.F. (1994). Role model behaviors in the clinical setting. *Journal of Nursing Education*, 33, 405–410. Used with permission.

can be readily incorporated into the instructional role; others can be demonstrated while assisting students with care activities (demonstrating the ability to care for patients' needs). Other behaviors might be better modeled by staff (those related to demonstrating nursing care procedures and the use of equipment), who are able to communicate "tricks of the trade" developed in their daily practice. Negative role modeling is also an important source of learning for students. The instructor should not hesitate to point out such negative examples and explain why they fail to conform to the expected behaviors of the professional nurse.

MANAGING OFF-UNIT EXPERIENCES

Assignments away from the clinical unit are commonly used to augment the student's perspective on the clinical specialty that is the focus of learning. For example, students whose regular clinical assignment is on a surgical unit may experience rotations through the one-day surgical unit, the operating room, and the recovery room; some may also have an experience in a clinic setting, where preoperative instruction is given and postoperative recovery is assessed. These off-unit experiences help the student to integrate the various components of the surgical cycle (or whatever specialty is being addressed) in a way that makes the direct care she is providing for patients in the immediate postoperative phase more meaningful. Further, her own observations of patients during various phases of that cycle enable her to communicate confidently with hospitalized patients concerning their experiences and anticipated recovery trajectories.

Off-unit experiences may be tightly linked to the primary clinical setting, as with the example of observations of various aspects of the surgical cycle, or they may involve more "offbeat" experiences. Students have few, if any, experiences with "normal" people, other than their peer-partners in a physical examination lab. Consequently, they have not developed skilled observation of normal function in a variety of people. A trip to the mall or other place of activity can help students to tune in to "normal" patterns of gait, respiration, and so forth as a basis for the often difficult to discern subtle signs of decompensation that they eventually will witness in their patients.

By their very nature, off-unit experiences are largely outside the control of the clinical instructor, who must find ways to make these learning experiences meaningful for the students who are involved in them, enabling them to integrate what has been learned with their learning experiences on the unit. Specific objectives that are closely tied to the course or clinical objectives should be developed for all off-unit experiences. Guidelines and assignments should provide a mechanism for students to demonstrate their achievement of these objectives and link the learning that occurs during the off-unit experience with classroom theory and the care being provided in the associated clinical setting. (Sample guidelines for off-unit experiences are shown in Appendix G.)

Guidelines for the off-unit experience should indicate where and when the student should report and who will be her contact and guide. Students should be briefed about what they can expect to observe during the experience, and what their role is likely to be. For example, most nursing programs have students scrub and garb for an observational experience in the operating suite, but do not involve them in direct care activities. In the recovery room, where the focus is on monitoring the patient's emergence from anesthesia, and the potential rapidly changing situation this presents, the student may be recruited to participate in taking vital signs, checking mental status, and monitoring wound drainage. In a clinic setting, the student may be responsible for conducting an intake interview and providing preoperative instruction for a patient who will be undergoing a procedure with which the student is familiar.

When the experience is entirely observational, students will need guidelines that direct them to specific phenomena to be noted during the experience. For example, an experience involving the observation of preschool children should direct the student to identify pertinent aspects of growth and development and evaluate whether the children being observed are within or outside the guidelines for their age group. Asking students to provide examples to support their conclusions helps the instructor to verify whether learning actually has occurred. When the experience involves participant observation, which might also occur if students were sent to a preschool to observe and interact with well-children, similar guidelines would be needed, as well as encouragement to become involved with preschool activities rather than simply stand to the side and observe. This might be encouraged by requiring students to select one of the children for a focused interaction, with a report to include how the interaction proceeded and what conclusions about the socialization skills of the preschooler might be drawn from the experience.

Provision must be made for the student to report on her experiences in off-unit activities. Such a report may be in writing, as in completing an observational guide that asks the student pertinent questions that relate observed activities to events in the primary clinical setting, or it may be an oral presentation made to other members of the clinical group. While either the written or oral report format enables the instructor to verify the student's participation in the planned activity and her achievement of established objectives, oral reports become a common pool of information that can be used by the group as they proceed with patient care activities on the primary clinical unit.

The instructor should make every effort to refer frequently to off-unit experiences when they relate to events in the clinical setting. A discussion of these experiences "fills in the gaps" in the picture presented by patients in the clinical setting, even for those students in the group who have not yet participated in the off-unit activity. The continuous reference to these experiences as sources of information applicable to the immediate clinical situation encourages students to maximize their participation in these experiences and to value the knowledge that can be acquired through simple observations and interactions that do not necessarily involve the delivery of hands-on nursing care.

TAKING ADVANTAGE OF SERENDIPITOUS OPPORTUNITIES

In a now classic article titled, "Serendipity and Objectivity," Styles (1975) bemoans nursing's focus on behavioral objectives as a means of structuring and guiding learning experiences. Styles believes that this focus has limited the use of learning experiences that arise in the clinical setting but cannot be linked to one of the objectives established for the course. As is true of neophyte nurses, it is easy for neophyte instructors to become so focused on ensuring that students are provided with opportunities to achieve course objectives that they miss some of the richest opportunities for teaching and learning that exist in the clinical practice setting. When unusual, one-of-a-kind experiences become available, the instructor should feel free to take advantage of them. By the same token, when a clinical situation occurs that provides an excellent opportunity for teaching some concept, demonstrating some technique, or discussing some ethical issue, this opportunity should be seized without concern about how it "fits" with the day's clinical objectives or even the overall course objectives. The clinical instructor also should remain alert to those events that provide insight into and opportunities to learn more about aspects of the role of the professional nurse within the organizational context of health care, such as interprofessional interactions, resource management, advocacy, and the like. If the situation is pertinent to nursing practice, it will serve the purpose of fostering learning in the clinical setting.

THE CLINICAL POSTCONFERENCE

As is the preconference, the clinical postconference is a traditional approach to the synthesis of clinical learning that has not been subjected to empirical testing of its effectiveness in enhancing student learning. The postconference has become an integral component of the clinical experience that is intended to accomplish numerous worthy outcomes such as

1. providing a time for both students and instructor to pause and reflect on the day's events, their meaning, and the relation between what has been observed and experienced and what was taught in the classroom or discussed in assigned readings;
2. contributing to the achievement of course and clinical objectives by making explicit the connections between clinical activities and the goals for learning;
3. examining commonalties and differences in patient responses to illness and its treatment within the clinical specialty;
4. permitting students to vicariously share in their peers' experiences, broadening their exposure to the clinical situations they might encounter in practice;

5. promoting affective learning through debriefing that allows students to express feelings and attitudes about the experiences they encountered during the day's activities; and
6. providing students with experience in the effective use of the group process.

Several problems typically encountered in conducting postconferences can limit the usefulness of this teaching–learning strategy in enabling students to achieve these goals. Problems arise when the instructor dominates the conference, limiting (or eliminating) student contributions to the discussion. This can occur when the instructor uses the conference as an occasion for the evaluation of student learning rather than an opportunity to promote learning. Alternatively, the instructor may elect to use conference time to teach content that was not covered in the classroom. While such instruction occasionally is necessary, as when the clinical situation has not been dealt with in class but presents an excellent opportunity for connecting theory and practice, presentation of didactic content should be kept to a minimum and tightly connected to clinical events. When the conference involves sequential individual presentations rather than group involvement in a discussion, students often "tune out" until it is their turn to present. This is especially true if students are not encouraged to ask questions of their peers, or to offer suggestions for alternative approaches to the clinical issues being discussed. When the level of content and questions remain at lower cognitive levels, conferences can become trivial or boring. While it takes effort and planning to move questioning to a level that stimulates students' higher cognitive functions, this is essential to an effective postconference session (Wink, 1993). Finally, low energy levels of both students and instructor after a day of nonstop activity are likely to affect student participation in the conference. This challenges the instructor to identify novel and stimulating approaches to introducing conference topics and keep the discussion lively.

Letizia's (1998) descriptive study of the strategies used in clinical postconferences revealed that most such conferences last for 50–60 minutes, and most involve a discussion of clinical experiences or a presentation by students of case studies involving the clinical assignment. Other approaches used included role play, quizzes, tours of other units, nursing rounds, and guest speakers. Ethical issues arising in practice was a frequent source of content for conferences, as was the coverage of theoretical content.

In planning the clinical postconference, the instructor must identify a focus for discussion and an approach to stimulating students' active participation in the discussion. The focus of discussion might be a significant event that occurred during the clinical day, the clinical objective or focus that had been identified for the session, or commonalties encountered by several students during the experience. The selected content must be converted to one or more questions that the instructor can pose to the group or to identified students to get the discussion going. The questions must be open-ended and nonthreatening, requesting the student to share an observation or an experience with the group. The instructor must prepare for the ensuing discussion by knowing where she wants it to go—what she hopes students will learn through the discussion. Usually the goal of the discussion is the synthesis of learning and the evaluation of events and interventions during the clinical experience. Therefore, the instructor must identify just what theory strands are connected to the practice situation that will be the focus of discussion, and how these strands can be interwoven with the practice reality to promote learning.

In addition to planning the discussion, the instructor must create a climate that stimulates both questioning and thinking. Stokes (1998) lists the following actions instructors can take to facilitate conferences:

- support the sharing of information;
- keep the discussion focused and moving in a meaningful way while remaining flexible and open to alternative paths for learning;
- encourage active involvement of each student by raising questions, proposing ideas, providing cues, and offering leading statements;
- provide nonthreatening feedback;
- assist students to identify relationships, patterns, and trends that span their individual experiences; and
- facilitate the group process by encouraging the participation of each member of the group.

Ideally, the clinical postconference can become a means of shifting much of the control of the learning experience to the students. Wagner and Ash (1998) note that when discussions are based in the clinical experiences of the students, as is the usual approach in postconferences, the discussion becomes rich in possibilities. To accomplish this, the conference cannot be allowed to revert to a classroom session. Second, postconference discussions provide opportunities to affirm students' growth as evolving practitioners of nursing. Finally, the postconference engages students with the instructor as partners in learning, as they use their personal knowledge to inform the situation as well as their own learning (p. 280).

SUMMARY

The instructor's organization and management of instruction in the clinical practice setting brings the student into meaningful interaction with the richness of clinical learning opportunities. Through these activities, the instructor orchestrates an experience in which students' activities become the source of their learning and where the goals of both the students and the instructor for the experience can be realized. A well-designed clinical experience frees the instructor to be selective in her work with those students who need individual attention and instruction. It also frees the students to learn.

REFERENCES

Baugh, N.G., & Mellot, K.G. (1998). Clinical Concept Mapping as preparation for student nurses' clinical experiences. *Journal of Nursing Education, 37*, 253–256.

Benner, P., & Wrubel, J. (1982). Skilled clinical knowledge: The value of perceptual awareness. *Journal of Nursing Administration, 12*(1), 11–14.

Blainey, C.A. (1991). Using clinical focus guidelines to emphasize processes of learning. *Journal of Nursing Education, 30*, 141–142.

Diekelmann, N.L. (1993). Behavioral pedagogy: A Heideggerian hermeneutical analysis of the lived experiences of students and teachers in baccalaureate nursing education. *Journal of Nursing Education, 32*, 245–250.

Emerson, R.J., & Groth, K. (1996). The verbal connection: Effective clinical teaching maximizing student communication skills. *Journal of Nursing Education, 35*, 275–277.

Fothergill-Bourbonnais, F., & Higuchi, K.S. (1995). Selecting clinical learning experiences: An analysis of the factors involved. *Journal of Nursing Education, 34*, 37–41.

Heims, M.L., & Boyd, S.T. (1990). Concept-based learning activities in clinical nursing education. *Journal of Nursing Education, 29*, 249–254.

Hill, J.L. (1993). Perceptions of factors affecting student-patient matching in clinical experiences. *Journal of Nursing Education, 32*, 133–134.

Ironside, P.M. (1999). Thinking in nursing education. *Nursing and Health Care Perspectives, 20*, 238–247.

Kiger, A.M. (1993). Accord and discord in students' images of nursing. *Journal of Nursing Education, 32*, 309–317.

Letizia, M. (1998). Stragegies used in clinical postconference. *Journal of Nursing Education, 37*, 315–317.

Mundt, M.H. (1997). A model for clinical learning experiences in integrated health care networks. *Journal of Nursing Education, 36*, 309–316.

Parker, J.L. (1994). Education for clinical practice: An alternative approach. *Journal of Nursing Education, 37*, 401–403.

Rowles, C.J., & Brigham, C. (1998). Strategies to promote critical thinking and active learning. (pp. 247–274). In Billings, D.M., & Halstead, J.A. *Teaching in nursing: A guide for faculty.* Philadelphia: W.B. Saunders.

Stokes, L. (1998). Teaching in the clinical setting. (pp. 289–291). In Billings, D.M., & Halstead, J.A. *Teaching in nursing: A guide for faculty.* Philadelphia: W.B. Saunders.

Styles, M.M. (1975). Serendipity and objectivity. *Nursing Outlook, 23*, 311.

Wagner, P.S., & Ash, K.L. (1998). Creating the teachable moment. *Journal of Nursing Education, 37*, 278–280.

Wilson, M.E. (1994). Nursing student perspective of learning in a clinical setting. *Journal of Nursing Education, 33*, 81–86.

Wink, D.M. (1993). Effect of a program to increase the cognitive level of questions asked in clinical postconferences. *Journal of Nursing Education, 32*, 357–363.

Wiseman, R.F. (1994). Role model behaviors in the clinical setting. *Journal of Nursing Education, 33*, 405–410.

Yurkovich, E., & Smyer, T. (1998). Shift report: A time for learning. *Journal of Nursing Education, 37*, 401–403.

CHAPTER 7

TEACHING AND LEARNING STRATEGIES FOR THE CLINICAL PRACTICE SETTING

Instructional Techniques for the Clinical Setting   121
    Demonstration   121
    War Stories   122
    Questioning   122
    Listening   124
Supervision of Student Performance of Technical Skills   125
    Process of Skill Mastery   125
    How to Let Go   128
    When to Jump In   129
    Ensuring That Patient Needs Are Met   130
Promoting the Integration of Theory and Practice   132
    Case Studies   135
    Seminars   135
    Nursing Rounds   136
    Written Assignments   137
Developing Critical Thinking Skills and Reflective Practice   139
    What Is Critical Thinking?   140
    The Role of Reflective Practice   144
    Strategies for Promoting Critical Thinking and Reflective Practice   142
The Affective Domain: Fostering Caring in Clinical Practice   147
Summary   148
References   149

The clinical instructor's unique focus is on the personal progress of the individual learner within an environment that is structured so that learning can occur, similar to the approach used by coaches in working with athletes (Grealish, 2000). Some instructional strategies will involve the clinical group as a whole, but most clinical instruction occurs within the one-to-one relationship of instructor and student. Grealish identifies two aspects of the coaching provided by clinical instructors: how to develop the student's psychomotor skills in a way that emphasizes technical skill and a caring approach, and how to ensure understanding of the theory implicit in nursing activities. She outlines two sets of coaching strategies addressing these components.

Goal setting is critical to success in developing the student's psychomotor skills. Short-term goals motivate performance, while long-term goals allow the student to engage in self-evaluation of progress toward the ultimate goal of competent nursing practice. In setting goals, a performance-based approach should be used. The goal is not "to pass" the clinical, but to perform specific skills using clearly observable behavioral indicators that identify the characteristics of a successful performance. Goals must be realistic. This is best achieved by tying goals to the student's past performance, and building on those experiences to motivate a higher or more refined level of performance. Goal setting should be negotiated with the student, to ensure that expectations for performance are clear and that the student's perspective has been included in developing those expectations. When students participate in goal setting, the potential for goal achievement is more evident. Including the student in negotiations concerning goals for clinical performance requires the instructor to be flexible, so that she can respond to salient issues raised by the student. Goals must be challenging to remain motivating. When the bar is set high, students generally rise to the occasion; if it is set too low, students will be content to "get by." Mental rehearsal, another coaching strategy, is a technique used by many athletes. This approach is useful in working with students as they perform skills for the first time. The clinical instructor verbally outlines the steps of the procedure, helping the student to imagine that she is performing the steps, and describing possible patient responses. Visualization of success in performing the procedure builds the student's confidence and smoothes initial performance. Finally, quantitative feedback (do less of that, do more of this, do that the same way) shapes the student's behavior as well as motivating her through recognition of progress toward success in skill development.

Grealish describes the second aspect of coaching, cognitive coaching, as "an activity of facilitation" (p. 232) that helps the student transform into professionally valid frameworks for practice those tentative theoretical frameworks she has constructed to make personal meaning out of the situations she experiences. Assessment through observation provides clues to the student's understanding of the theory underlying a nursing activity. Particular emphasis is placed on observations of student behaviors that suggest how the student is organizing or ranking variables in the situation. Describing observations is the second step in cognitive coaching. The instructor describes the student behavior she has observed and then asks open-ended questions that focus the student's attention on the approach to decision making she appears to have used in the situation. By modeling her own thinking processes through the sequence and nature of questions she asks, the instructor helps to shape the student's pattern of thinking to incorporate components of an alternative theoretical framework than the one evidenced by the student's actions. Questioning has the further benefit of fostering the student's recognition of the validity and importance of classroom theory in addressing clinical practice problems. This recognition enables the student to develop insights into the meaning of clinical situations and motivates the search for additional knowledge to better understand these situations.

INSTRUCTIONAL TECHNIQUES FOR THE CLINICAL SETTING

A major goal of clinical nursing education is to enable students to integrate theory and practice in the development of their critical thinking skills, technical skills, and ethical or value-based responsiveness to clinical situations. The ultimate goal of instruction is to promote experiential learning, where the student is able to synthesize theory and practice while demonstrating skilled performance of cognitive, psychomotor, and affective behaviors. Many instructional techniques are applicable to teaching and learning in any of the three behavioral domains; others are more particularly suited to one or another of these domains. This section focuses on the more generalized techniques; subsequent sections focus on techniques most pertinent to helping students develop skilled performance of hands-on nursing care; fostering critical thinking and reflective practice; and developing and acting upon values in clinical practice.

Demonstration

Demonstration can be considered an elaborated form of modeling nursing actions. Demonstration follows a "tell, show, then elicit" pattern, where the instructor explains the concept or procedure, shows the student how to apply the concept or perform the procedure, and then elicits a comparable performance from the student. Usually associated with teaching technical skills, demonstration can be a powerful tool for all types of learning. For example, the instructor might demonstrate her reasoning in reaching a clinical judgment or responding to an ethical dilemma by articulating the focus of her concern, and then, taking the student through her analytic process in addressing the identified problem. This would involve the instructor's discussion of her observations and her rationale in selecting relevant cues; reasoning toward a tentative diagnosis or hypothesis as a potential explanation of the situation; search through her knowledge base and further assessment of the situation for supportive information; selection of a reasonable working diagnosis;

consideration of alternative best approaches to care; and her rationale for the selection of the approach she would use in the situation. By articulating and elaborating on her own analytical process, the instructor encourages the student to be more attentive to her own mental work when confronted with a clinical problem. In future encounters, the student can be encouraged (eliciting) to talk through her own analytical processes.

War Stories

War stories are a powerful means of communicating nursing in action and the learning that can be derived from practice (Heinrich, 1992). War stories describe particularly memorable events in a nurse's past practice that now serve as paradigms for the nurse's present practice. The events described in war stories usually are so exceptional that the nurse has drawn rules of operation from them that guide her actions in similar situations.

War stories are an excellent approach to teaching in the clinical area because they combine reality-based practice with the theoretical learning that can be extracted from them. The learning becomes salient to students because it arises from a situation that each can imagine encountering in future nursing practice. The lesson contained in the war story tends to be retained because it is embedded in a vivid picture of an actual practice encounter. Finally, the notion that learning can occur from one's clinical practice is made evident as a model for students' own further development. War stories have the additional advantage of dramatically depicting highly charged situations with which the student would have difficulty coping. They enable her to be a vicarious observer of the action, and free to draw conclusions from the content without interacting with it directly.

War stories may involve both positive and negative clinical experiences, but most of them describe encounters with highly problematic and potentially dangerous situations. In many of these stories, earlier action by the nurse (based on her intuitive grasp of the situation) might have avoided the incident or lessened its intensity; in others, the situation was entirely unexpected and unpredictable and required the nurse's quick intervention to avert a tragedy. War stories may be told by staff nurses or by the instructor. To ensure their educational value, the instructor should be certain that the lesson that can be derived from the story is clear to students when a staff member has conveyed the story.

Questioning

Questioning is a constant in clinical learning situations. Instructors ask questions of students, and students ask for guidance from their instructors. For the instructor, questioning students provides some insight into the adequacy of their preparation for the clinical assignment, their ability to manage the care demands of the assignment, and their understanding of the dynamics underlying the patient's situation. Students' questions seek information, but also reveal a great deal about their mastery of concepts and the intellectual processes they are using in transferring and applying content in the clinical situation. While questioning is a major means for acquiring information, it can be a powerful approach to teaching and learning.

Skilled questioning that is focused on helping the student to learn rather than on evaluating student learning is a technique that requires much practice. As opposed to evaluative questioning, Socratic questioning invites the student to reflect on an issue raised by either the instructor or the student. Such questioning demands some baseline expression of the student's understanding of a concept, and invites further consideration of how this theoretical knowledge plays out in the presenting clinical situation. Socratic questioning stimulates the student to think aloud in response to questions that have evolved from the instructor's observation of the situation and the student's response to the issue it presents. Evaluative questioning tends to be structured, sequential, preformatted, and closed.

The process of skilled questioning is best illustrated by the following quotation taken from Ironside's (1999) interview with Ivory, a student whose clinical instructor, Vera, uses a style of questioning that stimulates the student's own thinking:

> Vera really gets you thinking. . . . Vera kind of shares *her* thinking with us and, boy, that really turns me on because she always sees something I miss and then that is what we talk about. . . . Like with this dressing change, she says to me . . . "You know what I worry about? . . . his wife is in there with him and she looks like she has been there all night. This wound is pretty ugly and I wonder if she has even had breakfast. What do you think?" [Ivory motions by hitting her forehead] . . . of course, I thought, now why didn't I think of the wife? So [Vera] says, "what should we say to her?" And she makes me think, but we talk, it's not like quizzing because I know Vera doesn't know either, not really. She gets me *really* thinking about how do I offer for this wife to leave in a way that, you know, . . . is like caring but if she needs to stay, that is OK too. Vera asks me, "how will we know if she can tolerate staying or even should stay or if she needs to leave in order not to faint?" Well, Vera was great because we talked together and it made me think about, well, has his wife been here before to see the wound? And then I remembered she was out of town when he had his surgery and so I now kind of have to read the chart. . . . Then as we are going back down Vera says, "let's check to see how he has responded to his wound?" She offers help and really, it's not just question, question, question. . . . Well, it got me thinking a lot about not just doing the dressing change, but more what it is like for the patient and his wife. I am starting to learn to think like a nurse, not just that critical thinking stuff . . . you know, your care plan and your priorities and rationale. Everyone in the school uses critical thinking a lot! It must really be in! [Laughs] (p. 239)

What is particularly significant in this interaction is that critical thinking is *exactly* what Vera's style of questioning has stimulated in Ivory!

In her classic work on teaching in the clinical nursing laboratory, Infante (1985) warns clinical instructors to avoid conceptualizing patients as problems to be solved or even solvable (p. 38). Yet many interpretations of critical thinking equate this intellectual process with problem solving. No wonder questioning strategies follow the rigid format of the problem-solving process, applied in nursing as the nursing process! And no wonder that students are much more compelled by and responsive to a questioning style that stimulates their interaction with clinical content in ways that further develop their sensitivity to and manipulation of the more subtle and complex issues embedded in the clinical situations in which they are learning nursing.

Listening

Careful attention to the content of students' statements is essential to keeping learning on track. Edwards (1991) proposes the use of several communication techniques, commonly applied by nurses in therapeutic interactions, in interactions with students.

Paraphrasing a student's statement provides feedback to the student on the instructor's interpretation of her statement. This enables the student to correct any miscommunication, or to further elaborate on the statement to help the instructor better understand her meaning. Paraphrasing reinforces not only that the instructor is listening to what the student is saying, but that she wants to understand what the student is trying to communicate.

Perception checks involve the instructor's articulation of her own inferences about what might be going on for the student—based both on the student's statements and her associated behavior—followed by a request for feedback from the student as to the accuracy of the instructor's inference. Because the nonverbal behavior that accompanies the student's statement may reveal more about an issue or concern than the student is aware of, perception checks help the student to gain insight into a situation that may be presenting a problem for her as well as providing an opportunity for the instructor to engage in some problem solving with the student.

Summarizing involves the instructor's identification of the themes that appear to be embedded in the student's statements. When students are puzzled by clinical events, they often have difficulty in organizing their thinking for presentation to the instructor. Summarizing is an effective means of helping the student to identify the linkages among her statements. It also provides additional feedback on what the instructor has heard the student say, allowing the student to correct misinterpretations and fill in any gaps in the total picture she is trying to convey.

I-statements describe the instructor's reaction to a student's statement without placing responsibility for this reaction on the student. Edwards provides the following example of the use of an I-statement: "As I listen to your description, I find myself getting very tense and tight. Is that what happened to you?" (p. 329). Rather than place the burden of alleviating the instructor's feelings on the student, through a statement such as, "This conversation is making me uncomfortable," the instructor is instead owning her own response to what the student has said and inviting an exploration of why these feelings might have been aroused by the statement.

SUPERVISION OF STUDENT PERFORMANCE OF TECHNICAL SKILLS

For most students, the hands-on care of patients is synonymous with being a nurse. Consequently, the development of technical competence is the singular focus of students' attention in the clinical learning situation until they have acquired sufficient comfort in performing these skills to direct their attention to mastering other aspects of the clinical situation. Students mark their progress in the clinical setting by the numbers and variety of technical skills they have performed, and the degree of mastery they have gained in performing them.

Providing hands-on care gives the student access to the patient. Such care constitutes a legitimate reason for the student to be there, and satisfies the goal of helping the patient in a concrete, visible way. At the same time, providing hands-on care opens the student to committing an error that may harm the patient in some way, and so technical skill development carries with it a high degree of anxiety that may interfere with learning.

As a nurse matures in her professional practice, she comes to recognize that technical skills are only one component—and not necessarily the most important component—of providing nursing care. As she develops technical expertise in performing complex technical skills, the nurse may begin to disregard the high degree of technical prowess she has developed. Technique becomes important only when there is a specific challenge to be creative in adapting a routine procedure to a complex situation.

Because technical skills have become routine and secondary in importance to other aspects of nursing care, it is easy for the clinically expert nursing instructor to discount the importance skill development has for students. By joining with students in their focus on technical skills at the beginning of the clinical experience, and helping them to broaden their vision of nursing care from technical skill performance to the more salient skills of assessing and responding to a variety of patient needs, the instructor capitalizes on students' readiness to learn and makes clinical learning meaningful.

Process of Skill Mastery

The progressive development of a technical skill begins with the learner's generalized perception of the task and its salient components. The learner then responds to her perceptions by readying herself—mentally, physically, and psychologically—to perform the skill. Initial skill performance is studied, resulting in an often-stilted attempt to model the ideal that has been portrayed in the instructor's demonstration or a graphic depiction of the skill. The student uses trial-and-error approaches as she struggles to link the behavioral components of the skill, to approximate the model, as well as to develop physical comfort in performing the skill. Subsequent attempts to perform the skill are mechanistic, until the student has had sufficient opportunities to repeat the task in a variety of situations so as to develop a smooth, coordinated flow of movements throughout her performance of the skill.

The process of skill mastery epitomizes the difficulties inherent in translating theory into practice. Theoretical instruction concerning technical nursing skills usually consists of providing students with a list of sequential steps to be followed in performing the skill, accompanied by rationales and caveats. Depiction of the skill, whether through schematic drawings, photographs, or video portrayal, presents a deliberately uncluttered, and hence stilted, picture of the situation in which the skill usually is performed. Live demonstrations of the skill usually involve a cooperative mannequin, student, or patient. There is no urgency surrounding completion of the skill, and few, if any, extraneous factors to be dealt with. The student may or may not have the opportunity to practice the skill in the controlled setting of the college laboratory prior to performing it in the clinical setting. Such practice gives the student a beginning sense of the physical movements required to manipulate materials and proceed through the steps involved in completing the skill—an important component of skill mastery—but still occurs in an artificial and contrived setting.

In moving from the theoretical ideal presented in skill checklists, drawings, and the college laboratory into the clinical reality, students attempt to apply the rules (sequential steps, rationales, caveats) to performing the skill with a patient. What tends to be missing is an awareness of and attention to the patient and the environment in which care is being provided, similar to what occurs when the student attempts to directly apply classroom learning to a clinical situation that is less than crystal clear in its presentation of cues. The focus on rules forecloses the student's ability to attend to aspects of the situation that might ease performance of the skill.

Observations of students as they learn technical skills reveal several commonalties that contribute to the awkwardness they feel in the initial stages of skill development. These observations suggest actions that the clinical instructor can take to ease the process of skill mastery.

In the laboratory setting, the checklist of steps to be performed is kept nearby as the student attempts the skill, and she refers to it frequently. If students are partnered with one another, the observing student may be recruited to verify that the performing student is following the correct sequence of steps. Often, the observing student will read the steps for the performing student. Once in the clinical area, however, the student abandons the checklist (except for a hurried review before entering the patient's room), and has no partner to prompt her through the steps of the procedure. Instead, she attempts to commit the steps to memory and may find herself trapped in the intellectual process of information retrieval while attempting to perform the skill. To facilitate independence from the list of rules, the instructor might cluster the steps in the procedure when she reviews it with the student, labeling each cluster so that the related group of steps can be recalled readily. This clustering minimizes the number of steps the student must remember, freeing her from some of her intellectualization of the task. When she first observes the student performing the skill with a patient, the instructor can substitute for the partner student by providing the performing student with verbal cues (the cluster labels) as she moves from one aspect of the skill to another.

Despite the emphasis nursing faculty place on body mechanics, students tend to exhibit awkward postures while providing bedside care. They also appear oblivious to obvious barriers to skill performance, such as the height of the bed, the interference of the side rails, and the position in which they find the patient. There is a seeming reluctance to "set the scene" for skill performance (as if this, in itself, says something negative about the student's ability) rather than create a comfortable working environment for both the patient and the student. The instructor can help the student overcome this tendency by emphasizing that this component of preparing to perform the skill is as important as gathering the necessary materials and explaining the procedure to the patient. Taking the time to arrange the environment also provides some "breathing room" for the student, during which she can defuse her anxiety.

In early stages of skill development, students tend to hold themselves distant from the equipment and supplies to be used in performing the skill, as well as from the patient. This contributes to their awkwardness in doing the procedure, as well as to the tension they feel as they proceed. It is almost as if the student is attempting to gain some space between herself and the object of her anxiety: the skill to be performed. In addition to remaining at a distance from the patient and the task, the student often holds herself stiffly, in an almost defensive posture, as if readying herself to flee the bedside. In addition to interfering with smooth performance of the skill, body tension interferes with the reception of the signals that help to promote body awareness of the movements necessary to perform the skill. Engaging the student in a relaxation exercise—such as contracting and then releasing her neck and shoulder muscles, rolling her head, and shaking out her arms and hands or taking several deep breaths and letting them out—helps to make the student aware of her body tension and to alleviate it to some degree.

Similar to the body tension that students exhibit in early stages of skill acquisition is a tendency to be extremely conservative in body movements. Students will attempt to perform a complex skill using only one hand, or will use the hand only and not flex or move the wrist and arm. A simple reminder to use the nondominant hand to assist in the procedure, or to maintain physical contact with the patient, may be all that is needed to free the student to use her body more effectively in performing various skills.

Students are so focused on the immediate requirements of the skill they are to perform that they lose sight of the reason the procedure is needed and what should be the result at its completion. Visualizing the end product of the procedure, for example, how a dressing will look and what it will feel like for the patient, enables the student to see the skill as a whole rather than as a sequence of steps to be performed. This awareness of the whole task moves the student forward toward the visualized end, and results in a smoother performance.

Students vary greatly in the pace at which they develop competence in performing various skills. Some students are able to verbalize the steps in any procedure, yet remain inept in actually performing it. Others perform ably, but have no sense of the rationale for their actions, and so are unable to adapt to unusual circumstances. The instructor must continuously evaluate each student's progress in developing technical skills, and modify her approach to each based on her observations. Most students are able to master basic skills after a few trials in the clinical area, and need only a spot check on their technique to ensure that critical aspects of the skill are being performed correctly. Smooth performance will evolve over time, as the student becomes more sensitive to the "feel" of the procedure as she performs it. The student who is genuinely inept may require a gentle shaping of her performance through praise for approximations of a competent performance in order for her to develop a degree of confidence in her ability to eventually master the skills necessary for practice. Another may need to be quizzed periodically on her reasons for doing certain procedures, so that she does not develop a habit of automatic action that is oblivious to the needs of the patient.

How to Let Go

The clinical instructor must develop the ability to remain in the situation with the student and patient while the student performs a new skill without taking over for the student. The instructor's need to teach must not be allowed to intrude on the student's need to learn. For the most part, technical skills only can be learned by doing them. Maintaining a watchful presence, and offering occasional words of encouragement or prompts as to next steps, is a different matter. There is no problem with explaining steps in the procedure to the student in front of the patient, as long as the patient is included and the language used can be understood by the patient and his family if they are present. Indeed, talking the patient through the procedure as the student performs it provides a certain degree of camouflage for the assistance the instructor is giving the student. Alternatively, the instructor may take the role of assistant, by helping the student to organize supplies or fetching items that are needed.

It is essential to allow students to work through the performance of technical skills unless there is a clear reason not to. Taking over for the student is a natural inclination for an instructor, who may feel quite uncomfortable while watching the student's inept, often klutzy maneuverings. Taking over interrupts the student's process of learning. It dashes growing self-confidence. It humiliates the student and can disrupt the trust that has developed between the student and the patient.

When the instructor takes over for the student, the student disengages from the learning and begins to focus on herself as a learner, internally seeking some explanation for why she was inadequate to the task or why her approach was the wrong one. In the few instances where the instructor might need to take over an aspect of the task, it is essential to keep the student fully engaged in what is going on to ensure continued involvement in learning. This can be accomplished by encouraging the student's continued participation in completing the procedure. For example, the student might be prompted to shift to the role of assistant, opening sterile dressings, tearing tape, or reassuring the patient. When the instructor has completed the portion of the task that required her intervention, she should return responsibility for completing the procedure back to the student, who then is able to regain some control over the situation. The instructor should remain with the student until the task is completed, so she can "debrief" the student as to what went on once they are outside the patient's room. At this time, the instructor can explain what went wrong and how the student might have prevented this or clarify that the student was not responsible for the problem she has encountered.

Another approach to letting go is to encourage students to consult with patients about the best approach to performing procedures if the patient has had the procedure done several times in the past. The patient then can be engaged in the interaction in a way that is useful to the student (by providing the cues to next steps that the checklist, observing peer, or instructor would provide) and satisfying for the patient (by ensuring a degree of control over and continuity in the approach used to complete the procedure). By placing the student in the patient's hands, so to speak, the instructor has gained an ally in teaching.

When to Jump In

The clinical instructor must be prepared to intervene when the student's actions, inaction, or ineptitude jeopardize patient safety. The danger must be clear and present to warrant this action, which must be taken before harm occurs. When she must take over a patient care situation from a student, the instructor should do so calmly and assertively. For example, the instructor might say, "I'll finish this irrigation, Sue, while you call housekeeping to mop the floor so no one slips." The patient should be spared any alarm that something might have gone wrong, the student should be spared any humiliation at having erred in her performance, but the situation must be addressed directly and promptly. The instructor should return the procedure to the student for completion if it is safe to do so, and must conduct a debriefing with the student after the patient's well-being has been assured and the student and instructor are away from the patient's room.

The instructor also must intervene when the student is unable to continue with the procedure, even after such prompts as "take a deep breath." It is far better to jump in to complete the task than to have the student freeze, faint, or vomit in the patient's presence. After the patient situation is settled, the instructor must follow up with the student to ensure her well being, and to troubleshoot possible causes for her reaction and ways to avert such a response in the future.

Ensuring that Patient Needs are Met

The instructor can help to ensure that patient needs are met by working with students to plan a schedule of care activities that sets priorities within the multiple factors to be considered in providing care. The instructor can guide students to recognize and respond to patients' safety, comfort, and privacy needs while providing care, and encourage students to build flexibility into planned activities to allow for inevitable glitches.

Priority Setting.   Patients' needs are best met if the instructor works with the student to set priorities for the day's activities. A review of the student's plan for the day, and her rationale for ordering activities in a specific way, will help to reveal potential conflicts that would interfere with meeting the patient's needs if the plan is not reordered. This review also can be used to help the student to identify what must be accomplished and at what times, which activities can be completed more flexibly, and which activities can be foregone if there is insufficient time to complete them. This preplanning also establishes expectations for the day that give the student some latitude in making judgments about what is feasible to accomplish. Following are some of the issues to be considered in helping the student to plan her work and set priorities.

Patient Care Demands.   The student must be guided to consider the patient's entire care plan, not just those aspects involving the nursing activities with which she will be involved. Scheduled diagnostic or therapeutic activities must be coordinated with the timing of nursing procedures. For example, the student will need to consider whether to change a dressing before or after the patient leaves the unit for a scheduled physical therapy appointment.

The preestablished schedule for treatments that need to be administered at periodic intervals often perplexes students when this schedule must be adjusted to accommodate other activities. For example, if a wound must be irrigated every four hours, when should the irrigation be done if the patient will be away from the unit for a lengthy period of time?

The timing of physician rounds, particularly where it is likely that the physician will want to examine the patient, must be factored into planned activities. For example, is it best to leave the old dressing on the wound so the physician can observe the exudate, or to change the dressing so that the physician can see the progress in healing? While the student should not feel the need to vacate the room or halt her activities simply because a physician is present, she should be encouraged to adopt a collaborative planning model in her work with physicians. For example, in setting her priorities for the day the student can be guided to consider what information the physician might need to evaluate the plan of care (for example, the nature of the wound exudate, which the student would need to assess prior to the physician's visit) and what issues need to be raised with the physician in relation to the plan of care (for example, the possible need to change from a dry-to-dry dressing to a wet-to-dry dressing to facilitate healing).

Patients' preferences and planned activities must be balanced within the list of activities to be prioritized, and should be accommodated whenever this is possible. For example, if attending religious services comforts the patient, the schedule for this activity should be built into the student's plan. At the same time, the student's desire to please the patient may cause her to defer necessary care, ultimately to the patient's detriment. Students need help in making these judgments. It is helpful if the instructor is able to talk with patients before the clinical day begins concerning their particular needs related to scheduling care activities. For example, if a patient is expecting a special phone call or an out-of-town visitor whose presence might interrupt the plan for the day, this information might be gleaned during a brief visit with the patient to let him know that a student will be involved in his care. Then, the instructor can include this information in her discussion with the student, and help her to plan around the patient's needs. Awareness of and responsiveness to such needs, which are unlikely to be identified by the student, cements the instructor's relationship with the patient and builds the necessary trust that gives the student freer access in working with the patient.

Unit Schedule. The instructor's awareness of the usual flow of unit activities is vital in assisting students to plan their care activities. For example, despite their frequently disparaging comments about institutional food, patients look forward to each meal and resent activities that interfere with the scheduled delivery of meal trays. Knowledge of the expected times for meal delivery enables the student to plan activities around meal times.

The timing of linen delivery and removal of soiled linens also can impact on care activities, as can restocking of supply closets. Awareness of these schedules can help the student to plan ahead in gathering supplies for patient care prior to embarking on the day's activities.

Planned breaks and assigned meal times must be considered in devising a plan for the day, especially when these will impact on staff coverage of the student's assigned patients. The instructor usually will have negotiated meal-time coverage in advance of the clinical day, and staff expect to adhere fairly closely to this schedule. As members of the team, students become an integral component of the unit. Their delay in taking planned breaks or meals will interfere with everyone else's schedule. Students often become so involved in clinical activities that they want to forego breaks and meals. However, they should be encouraged to take breaks and leave the unit for meals as a necessary element in attending to personal needs.

Coordination of Learning Activities. When the student has been assigned responsibility for more than one patient's care, conflicts in the care requirements of each must be considered in planning activities. In setting priorities, the student should be encouraged to consult with the patient whose care will be deferred to address any immediate needs the patient may have and to inform the patient of the anticipated time at which care will be given.

Planning with students also helps the instructor to set priorities and establish a plan for her own activities during the day. For example, the instructor will need to negotiate with students the timing of activities she wishes to observe or supervise.

Priority setting includes establishing a time frame for the completion of activities and the sequence in which they will be performed. Students should be expected to have completed care activities, including documentation and reporting to the primary or charge nurse, in time to attend postconference when this is built into the end of the clinical day. Even when no postconference is planned, students should be ready to leave the unit at the scheduled time, as a component of expected professional behavior.

Safety, Comfort, and Privacy Needs.   The student's focus on skill performance may make her less sensitive to the potential threats to safety and disruptions in comfort, privacy, and psychological well-being that can occur during nursing care procedures. The extended time it takes for a student to perform a procedure may contribute to these issues. For example, the length of time it takes for the student to complete a dressing change may leave the wound exposed for too long a time. Covering the wound with a sterile dressing both protects the wound and shields it from the patient's gaze without disrupting the student's process of skill development. Acting for the student in such situations (for example, using a draw sheet to cover the female patient's exposed meatus while the student sets up the equipment for a catheterization) protects the patient and sensitizes the student to aspects of care she seems unable to discern.

Flexibility.   Students should be encouraged to allow extra time to perform even the most basic skills. They should be warned to expect interruptions and unexpected difficulties in completing tasks.

Students also should be encouraged to develop a backup plan so that they can switch to other planned care activities when the initial plan goes awry. The ability to make adjustments in routines is a necessary component of patient care and is particularly applicable in the area of skill development, where adaptations in technique often are needed.

PROMOTING THE INTEGRATION OF THEORY AND PRACTICE

Students begin to acquire the theoretical knowledge necessary to the skilled practice of nursing in the classroom setting, and then bring this knowledge to the clinical practice setting, where the stimulus situations to which they are exposed enable them to transform theory into practical knowledge that is applicable in a wide variety of clinical situations.

Knowledge is developed hierarchically (see Table 7–1), beginning with acquisition of information relevant to the field of study. At this, the lowest level of the cognitive domain, the demonstration of knowledge occurs when the student is able to recall information that has been presented previously. It does

---

TABLE 7–1 HIERARCHICAL STRUCTURE OF BEHAVIORS IN THE
            COGNITIVE DOMAIN

Knowledge

> Knowledge of specifics
>
> Knowledge of terminology
>
> Knowledge of specific facts
>
> Knowledge of ways and means of dealing with specifics
>
> Knowledge of conventions
>
> Knowledge of trends and sequences
>
> Knowledge of classifications and categories
>
> Knowledge of criteria
>
> Knowledge of methods
>
> Knowledge of universals and abstractions in a field
>
> Knowledge of principles and generalizations
>
> Knowledge of theories and structures

Comprehension

> Translation
>
> Interpretation
>
> Extrapolation

Application

Analysis

> Analysis of elements
>
> Analysis of relationships
>
> Analysis of organizational principles

Synthesis

> Production of a unique communication
>
> Production of a plan, or proposed set of operations
>
> Derivation of a set of abstract relations

Evaluation

> Judgments in terms of internal evidence
>
> Judgments in terms of external criteria

Source: Adapted from Kibler, R.J., Barker, L.L., & Miles, D.T. (1970). *Behavioral objectives and instruction*. (pp. 44–55). Boston: Allyn and Bacon.

not require the intellectual manipulation of that information. At the second level of the cognitive domain, comprehension, the student is able to interpret the information she has learned. A good measure of this level of learning is the ability of the student to repeat information in her own words. Application of knowledge, the next level of cognitive development, is demonstrated by the student's ability to use the information she has acquired in dealing with concrete problems. The fourth level is analysis. At this level, the student is able to break down components of the knowledge she has acquired so that she better understands the relationships that exist among those components. It is at this level of cognitive development that the student demonstrates the ability to use her knowledge to assess a situation, draw relevant cues from that assessment, and organize the cues in a coherent and meaningful fashion that will guide decision making and actions. At the next level, synthesis, the student is able to create a new conceptualization or expression of knowledge that requires the blending of previously discrete blocks of information. For example, at this level the student would be able to transform "rules of thumb" or protocols for the care of a patient with a single health problem to create a plan for the care of a patient with multiple, interacting health problems. Synthesis requires the student not only to identify the relationships among components of information, but also to select certain components for use. This requires the student to develop new intellectual structures or frameworks of knowledge. The final level of cognitive development is evaluation, which requires the student to apply both internal (value-based) and external criteria to information.

In the classroom setting, students' cognitive knowledge tends to remain at the first three levels. Indeed, most testing of students' cognitive achievement involves recall and recognition of material presented in lectures or readings, with few efforts to evaluate comprehension and application, although these clearly are goals of classroom instruction. Multiple-choice examinations remain the predominant approach to the evaluation of students' knowledge, because the development of questions testing levels of the cognitive domain higher than simple application are difficult and time-consuming to create. Consequently, the further development and reorganization of the student's knowledge for use in clinical practice situations falls to the clinical instructor.

Questioning is the usual approach to beginning the process of integration of theory and practice. In order to respond to the instructor's questions, the student must access the appropriate information from her store of knowledge, and then demonstrate her comprehension of this knowledge through her answers to the instructor's questions. To develop higher-order intellectual skills, it is critical that the instructor's questioning continue beyond the levels of recall and comprehension, to draw the student into applying her knowledge to the situation before her, analyzing the situation, synthesizing knowledge from a variety of theories, and evaluating the product of her intellectual work. Questioning that reveals the instructor's thinking processes as a model for the student's own intellectual work is a powerful means of developing students' higher levels of cognitive function.

While much of the integration of theory and practice will occur in one-to-one interactions with students that are centered on the use of knowledge in the context of patient care activities, a number of more structured approaches to promoting this integration are used in the course of clinical instruction.

Case Studies

A case study presents a real-life situation to students for analysis. The case study can be structured as a written assignment or as a focus for group discussion. Usually, students are asked to analyze the problem or problems presented in the case and their cause, identify ways in which the problem might have been prevented, suggest solutions to the problem, and speculate on possible outcomes in response to suggested actions (O'Connor, 1986, p. 164). The approach stimulates analytical skills, insight development, and creativity. It encourages student analysis of clinical problems without the overriding concerns regarding patient safety and comfort that are present in the clinical setting.

The materials presented for study can be as simple or as complex as the instructor desires, and can be drawn from the instructor's own practice, textbook examples, or the imagination. The flexibility that can be achieved in selecting the focus for the study and variables to include provides control over the issues to be considered by students, although Rowles and Brigham (1998, p. 258) suggest that students are likely to raise questions and make comments that have not been considered by the instructor in preparing the case materials. Because this approach depicts an isolated case or incident involving patient care, irrelevant intervening variables that might confuse the situation but contribute nothing to its resolution can be eliminated. (Alternatively, these might be included as "red herrings" for more advanced students.)

A major advantage of this approach is the capacity to expose students to commonly encountered clinical problems, even if actual experiences with these problems in the clinical setting are not available during the times scheduled for the clinical experience. Students' responses to case materials provide the instructor with valuable insights concerning both the students' knowledge base and thinking processes, which can be used in subsequent one-on-one discussions.

The major disadvantage of this approach is the time-consuming process of creating case materials that are related to the theoretical content being studied by students, relevant to the clinical setting in which they are learning, and at an appropriate level for analysis.

Seminars

Seminar presentations that focus on a clinical case encountered by students during the semester are another approach used to integrate theoretical knowledge into practice. The presentation often is a group effort, contributing to the achievement of course objectives related to the development of group process skills. Each clinical group is divided into smaller units comprising three or four students. Presentations are to the class as a whole, permitting sharing of clinical experiences across the various clinical groups.

Ideally, each student in the small group will have had an opportunity to care for the patient under consideration. This enables students to share perspectives on a common experience, and to track the progress the patient has made during the semester. If this is not possible, the small group selects a patient case for presentation and each group member reviews the clinical data to develop a working knowledge of the background of the case. It is wise for the clinical instructor to meet with the small group to review their work as it progresses. This prevents the presentation of erroneous information that would have to be corrected during the seminar, which would be embarrassing to the group members and detrimental to learning by students hearing the presentation.

During the seminar presentation, students present background information on the case as well as the theory that explains the issues and supports the interventions that were used with the patient. Questions from peers are intended to probe for more information so that the entire class is able to relate theory to the clinical case as it unfolded for the students who were actually involved in the patient's care. Encouraging peer participation can be challenging for the instructor. Without meaningful interaction among the presenters and the rest of the group, the presentation can be a boring rehash of lecture content sparked only by the clinical examples identified by the presenters. The use of a format that demands peer participation in problem solving and decision making, such as having presenters provide baseline data with peers requesting additional input rather than the presenters simply detailing the sequence of events, can enliven the seminar format and engage learners' attention.

Nursing Rounds

Nursing rounds are yet another approach to making theory meaningful in the clinical setting. Nursing rounds involve the entire clinical group, which assembles at the bedside of a preselected patient who has agreed to participate and who has been briefed beforehand as to his role in the learning experience. Either the instructor or the student who is caring for the patient may lead the rounds, which are intended to stimulate problem solving or review an approach to patient care that has proven successful. To minimize stress on the patient, background information can be provided away from the bedside. Students and instructor can then gather around the patient for the middle portion of the presentation, with actual discussion of the case taking place away from the bedside. Following the discussion, the patient must be briefed on the conclusions reached in the remainder of the conference.

The benefit of nursing rounds is the presence of the patient as a means to illustrate assessment parameters or intervention techniques. Input and feedback from the patient can be elicited to clarify issues raised by peers that might not have occurred to the primary care provider. Nursing rounds provide a time to step back and reflect on clinical events, deliberately referencing theory and bringing this knowledge into discussions of the clinical case to inform problem solving.

Written Assignments

Most written assignments connected to clinical learning are predetermined (and, often, prehistoric) and are required of all students in the course. The clinical instructor must have sufficient information about the assignment, its pedagogical goals, student objectives, and how much the grade on the assignment will count toward the student's final grade to be able to intelligently answer students' questions, provide necessary guidance for completing the assignment, and fairly evaluate the completed work. Because the mechanics and rules governing the written assignment should be equivalent for all students, the instructor will need to know what elements are to be addressed in the paper, how the work must be presented (hand- or typewritten), approximate length, need for and style to be used in citations, when the paper is due, and whether students will be given the opportunity to rework an assignment that has missed its mark. Examples of previously completed assignments can provide useful information for the instructor, who should ask for these from the lead instructor of the course.

In the absence of clear guidelines for the written assignment, the instructor may decide to flesh out the assignment with her own amplification of directions for completing it. For example, the instructor might suggest the relative length of various sections of the report ("Provide a brief—2–3 paragraph—description of the patient's situation") or provide grading criteria that identify the relative weight to be given to various aspects of the report ("Your analysis of the case will make up 30% of your grade on this assignment"). As the semester proceeds, students may report that the assignment or its parameters have been changed; this needs to be verified with the lead instructor so that everyone is operating from the same information. If the assignment does not bear any relationship to students' clinical experiences, the instructor might wish to offer an alternative approach that achieves the same instructional goals and learning objectives. This should be discussed with the lead instructor before being presented to students as an option, but the instructor should feel free to make such adjustments, as long as the students are required to complete work that is roughly equivalent to that required of their peers.

Because most written assignments designed to help students integrate theory and practice involve a patient care experience the student has had, the instructor must plan assignments that provide a good fit with the written assignment, and to suggest this possibility to the student.

Major Nursing Care Plan.   The nursing process is a commonly used framework for guiding students' integration of theory and practice. While brief nursing care plans are one means by which students prepare for the clinical experience, the major nursing care plan is intended to be more comprehensive in both depth and scope. The phases of the nursing process guide the student's report and analysis of information related to the care of the patient. The student's interaction with the patient may have been brief (one clinical day) or extended over several weeks of clinical experiences. Although it is labeled a nursing care plan, this written assignment generally involves more reflection about and evaluation of the care provided by the student than planning for future care.

Ideally, students should begin to work on this assignment early in the clinical experience, recording baseline data and then updating information as additional data are gathered while working with the patient. In this way, theory can inform each aspect of the nursing process as it is implemented rather than being introduced as a post hoc explanation of events that have transpired. The clinical instructor can encourage this approach to the assignment by requesting periodic drafts of the plan during the semester. Comments on this draft can guide the learning process and sharpen the student's thinking. In reality, however, students are very likely to postpone work on this assignment until the end of the clinical experience, and then spend many hours reviewing the patient's record and attempting to recall aspects of care that was provided weeks before. This reflection back upon the whole record is not without educational value, since the student's "slice-in-time" involvement with the patient can be enhanced by the opportunity to view the entire episode of care and consider the factors contributing to the final outcome.

Although the goal of the major nursing care plan is to promote the integration of theory and practice, completion of this assignment more often involves laying down theory beside the clinical data and drawing connections between the two. Thus, the student will report on an intervention used with the patient, and provide a supporting rationale for the appropriateness of this intervention, without having used theory as the basis for selecting the intervention.

The evaluation component of the nursing care plan—which can provide the opportunity for high-level intellectual work—often confuses both students and instructor. What is to be evaluated? The patient's response to the plan? The suitability of the plan for the patient's problem? The student's selection of and theoretical rationale for interventions? One approach to this dilemma is to structure the assignment to require students to evaluate all three. First, the student can be required to provide data in support of the patient's response to the plan of care, reflecting achievement of the objectives of interventions and evidencing the outcomes of care. This aspect of evaluation focuses the student's attention on outcome-based assessment of patient progress in response to nursing interventions. Next, the student can analyze whether or not the plan resolved the identified problems and what other approaches to care might have been considered or implemented instead of or in addition to those that were used. This aspect of evaluation involves the student in selecting among alternative approaches to patient care, and considering how each of these might have worked in resolving the patient's problems. Consideration of alternatives—even after the fact—helps the student to recognize that there is more than one "right" approach to patient care problems, although there may be one "best" approach. Finally, in the third aspect of evaluation the student is called upon to make explicit her decision-making processes in formulating nursing diagnoses and selecting and implementing interventions.

Synthesis Paper. This type of assignment takes a broad clinical problem (e.g., medical condition, nursing diagnosis, or other issue common to the clinical specialty in which the student is learning) and requires the student to demonstrate her understanding and analysis of the problem through a thorough review and synthesis of the literature. The assignment often requires the student to integrate current research findings into the analysis and to draw examples from the clinical setting to illustrate specific points. The identification of implications for patient care often is the final step in this type of assignment. This requires the student to reach conclusions as to appropriate nursing actions based on the information gleaned from the literature, involving the synthesis of theoretical knowledge as well as the evaluation of its suitability for application to clinical problems.

Other Written Assignments. Modifications of the nursing care plan and synthesis paper have been proposed as alternatives to these traditional assignments. Delehanty (1996) describes an assignment that is focused on nursing interventions. Students provide background information on a patient, and identify a nursing problem that should be addressed. Data supporting problem identification must be detailed, along with indicators that can be used to monitor the problem and document any improvement or resolution as a result of planned interventions. The major focus of the paper is on the intervention. Literature sources are used to describe the intervention and support its selection as an appropriate approach to the identified problem. Details concerning implementation of the intervention (e.g., safety issues, special precautions) are identified, and steps to be taken are outlined. Finally, approaches to evaluation are described. The focus on interventions, which are selected on the basis of probability of success in achieving desired outcomes, helps students to move from assessment and diagnosis to a consideration of alternative approaches to care and the nurse's role in monitoring progress and outcomes in response to interventions. Delehanty indicates that students are not required to implement the selected intervention, although this is a desirable component of the assignment. A similar approach can be used to integrate the theoretical aspects of pharmacological therapy with the nurse's assessment and monitoring functions in the clinical setting.

DEVELOPING CRITICAL THINKING SKILLS AND REFLECTIVE PRACTICE

Educators have identified the development of critical thinking ability as a primary goal of the educational process. Indeed, critical thinking—along with communication and technical skills, in the delivery of therapeutic nursing interventions—is one of the major educational program outcomes identified in criteria issued by nursing education accreditation bodies associated with the National League for Nursing (NLN) and the American Association of Colleges of Nursing (AACN). Despite this emphasis on critical thinking, the concept remains ill defined and difficult to measure. Still, a major expectation of clinical instruction is that it will contribute to students' critical thinking abilities.

Reflective practice—the process of thinking back on clinical experiences as a means to derive new meanings from the events that transpired—has been identified as a key element in the process of critical thinking. When reflective practice occurs, context enriches and transforms knowledge in ways that instill in theoretical knowing the practical knowledge (know-how) that makes clinical nursing practice so challenging and exciting.

What Is Critical Thinking?

Critical thinking is the transfer and application of knowledge and skills to a new situation. The critical thinking process begins with an open-minded assessment of the presenting situation in order to identify pertinent data and relevant patterns that suggest the nature of the problem to be solved. During this assessment, the critical thinker tolerates ambiguity and questions assumptions in order to avoid premature closure of the assessment phase. Following assessment, the critical thinker formulates a working hypothesis as to the problem(s) suggested by the data. For many critical thinkers, hypothesis generation occurs concurrently with data collection, and guides the assessment process.

Once one or more problems have been identified, the critical thinker then selects from her store of previously acquired knowledge and skills those that are pertinent to the unique elements of the presenting situation. She then decides how knowledge and skills will be applied in resolving the identified problem(s). Where gaps in existing knowledge and skill occur, the critical thinker seeks out the required information.

Following the application of knowledge to the identified problem, the critical thinker evaluates the outcomes of the intervention, the appropriateness of knowledge and skill application, the accuracy of problem identification, and the completeness of the assessment process based both on data derived from the situation and a reflective consideration of the problem-solving process. Table 7–2 lists indicators of critical thinking in nursing practice contexts.

Although critical thinking has been likened to the problem-solving process (scientific method), the nursing process, diagnostic reasoning, clinical judgment, and clinical decision making, it is more a necessary element in these than synonymous with them. Cox (1998) identifies the following elements of the critical thinking process in which students need practice:

- defining a problem contextually;
- maintaining an open attitude of inquiry;

TABLE 7–2 INDICATORS OF CRITICAL THINKING APPLIED TO NURSING CONTEXTS

Breadth of assessment: A broad range of cues is considered in conducting the assessment.

Questioning of assumptions: Assumptions inherent in the situation being considered are challenged.

Cue recognition: Pertinent data and relevant patterns are abstracted from the situation being considered.

Problem framing: One or more potential problems suggested by identified data and patterns are selected for resolution.

Aggregation of relevant knowledge and skills: Knowledge and skills pertinent to problem resolution are identified from the previously acquired store of information; where knowledge or skills required for problem resolution are absent, a search for the necessary information is conducted.

Application: Knowledge and skills are applied appropriately to resolve the problem(s) identified in the situation.

Evaluation: The success and suitability of problem resolution are assessed.

Reflective thinking: The problem-solving process is analytically reviewed and critiqued.

- learning to ask circular rather than linear questions;
- examining underlying assumptions and making theoretically based hypotheses;
- reflexively examining the situation prior to drawing conclusions;
- deciding what to believe and do; and
- evaluating hypotheses, assumptions, and interventions. (p. 40)

The Role of Reflective Practice

Reflection "seeks to make sense or meaning out of [an] experience and to incorporate this experience into one's view of the self and the world" (Baker, 1996, p. 19). Reflective practice requires students to "actively draw on their past experience, describe the experience, work through their attitudes and emotions relative to the experience, and then order and make sense of new ideas and information" (Davies, 1995, p. 167). Emotional distance and "objectivity" have no place in reflective practice. Rather, the feelings and attitudes that are a natural component of new experiences are "allowed in" as a vital component of the intellectual work involved in making meaning from clinical experiences. At the same time, the contextual elements inherent in the experience—those elements that will eventually alter the ways in which the student selects and applies theory-based rules of operation—come into the foreground, and their significance in the situation becomes more evident as their role in defining the problem is clarified.

Baker (1996) identifies the following as aspects of the reflective learning process:

1. A sense of inner discomfort is triggered by a life experience.
2. Identification or clarification of the concern makes the nature of the problem or issue more evident.
3. Openness to new information from internal and external sources exists, along with the ability to observe and take in from a variety of perspectives; there is a willingness to forego a quick resolution or closure concerning the problem.
4. Resolution occurs through insight, where the learner feels she has changed or learned something that is personally significant.
5. A change is experienced in self, as a result of internalization of a new perspective.
6. A decision is made whether to act on the outcome of the reflective process by determining whether the insight can be operationalized. (p. 20)

Whether or not they are invited to engage in reflective practice, students will inevitably do so. The process can become more meaningful, and "feelings of fear, doubt, and inadequacy" (Davies, 1995, p. 172) relieved, if the instructor incorporates reflective practice strategies into the clinical setting.

Strategies for Promoting Critical Thinking and Reflective Practice

Critical thinking is "critical" because it involves continuous engagement in a process of critique or evaluation of both the thinking process and its products while the thinking is going on, regardless of the subject matter or the goal of the thinking. The openness to alternative meanings and the tolerance of ambiguity that are characteristic of critical thinking set the stage for meaningful reflection on practice. Critical thinking and reflective practice are interactive, intertwined processes that enable the student to build upon knowledge acquired in the classroom through thoughtful consideration of and active involvement in the contextual complexity that is present in the clinical setting.

The primary teaching–learning strategy supporting both critical thinking and reflective practice involves making explicit and verbal that which is tacit and unspoken. Writing about and talking through her thought processes enable the student to recognize the connections she is making in processing information (Cox, 1998). When students are encouraged to verbalize their thought processes while engaged in thinking, they reveal their patterns of information selection and decision making. When they record in writing their feelings and attitudinal responses to the clinical situations they encounter, the salience of these feelings for understanding the situation becomes evident. Either approach gives the instructor a base of information that can be used to assist students in making meaning from their clinical experiences.

Higher-Order Cognitive Questioning.   One characteristic of nursing students, who are at the novice stage of developing competence, is the equal weight they assign to all data elements in a situation when making a decision. Selective attention to cues only can occur when context informs the nurse as to what is important in the given situation, and students have yet to learn the vital role that context plays in prioritization of cues. It is this dependence on context that leads the expert nurse to respond, "it depends," when presented with a hypothetical case scenario. Tschikota (1993) argues that the usual method of teaching clinical decision making, which involves "the collection of a comprehensive database followed by summative decision making" (p. 396), should be replaced with techniques that encourage progressive hypothesis generation and testing. This pattern of information processing, in which hypotheses are activated early in the reasoning process, more closely follows that employed by expert nurses. Tschikota suggests the use of case studies of varying complexity and ambiguity as one way to stimulate and develop critical thinking in clinical decision making. However, progressive hypothesis generation and testing also can be stimulated through the instructor's approach to questioning and her sharing of her own thought processes by thinking aloud with the student.

Critical thinking can be developed through questioning that moves beyond "what," which stimulates recall of factual information, to ask students "why" they have reached the conclusions they report or made the decisions upon which they are acting. "Why" questions require the student to analyze both the presenting situation and the relevance of theoretical knowledge in relation to it, as well as to synthesize aspects of theory with the presenting features of the clinical reality. Even if the student's reasoning was accurate and resulted in an appropriate decision, "why" questions stimulate a conscious review of the thought process, which is essential to critical thinking.

In a study of a program designed to increase the percentage of cognitively high-level questions asked by instructors in the clinical setting, Wink (1993) found a dearth of questions reflecting the highest levels of the cognitive domain, synthesis and evaluation, even after the intervention. These levels of intellectual work, involving the construction of new knowledge that incorporates the contextual elements of the clinical experience as well as the evaluation of the accuracy of assessments and the effectiveness of interventions, represent the essence of critical thinking. Unless students are questioned in ways that stimulate this level of thinking, and encouraged to ask questions of the clinical instructor that reflect synthesis and evaluation, their development of the critical thought processes that will enable them to make meaning from clinical situations will be thwarted. Table 7–3 classifies questions according to the cognitive domain, and suggests words reflecting each level of this domain that might be incorporated into questioning.

TABLE 7–3   QUESTIONS REFLECTING THE HIERARCHICAL STRUCTURE OF COGNITIVE KNOWLEDGE

CATEGORY	REQUIRED COGNITIVE ACTIVITY	SAMPLE QUESTION WORDS
Knowledge	*Recall*: Questions, regardless of complexity, can be answered by simple recall of previously learned material.	What; When; Who; Which; Define; Describe; Identify; List; Name; Recall; Show; State; How; Indicate; Tell; Yes or no questions, e.g., Did? Was? Is?
Comprehension	*Understanding*: Questions can be answered by merely restating and reorganizing material in a rather literal manner to show that the student understands the essential meaning.	Compare; Constrast; Conclude; Demonstrate; Differentiate; Predict; Reorder; Which; Why; Distinguish; Estimate; Explain; Extend; Extrapolate; Rearrange; Rephase; Inform; What; Fill in; Give an example of; Illustrate; Relate; Tell in your own words.
Application	*Solving*: Questions involve problem solving in new situations with minimal identification or prompting of the appropriate rules, principles, or concepts.	Apply; Build; Construct; Solve; Test; Consider; Demonstrate (in a new situation); How would; Check out.
Analysis	*Exploration of reasoning*: Questions require the student to break an idea into its component parts for logical analysis, facts, opinions, logical conclusions, etc.	Support your; What assumptions; What reasons; Does the evidence support the conclusion; What does patient seem to believe about; What words indicate bias or emotion; What behaviors.
Synthesis	*Creating*: Questions require the student to combine ideas into a statement, plan, product, etc., that is new for the student.	Write; Think of a way; Create; Propose a plan; Put together; Suggest; Develop; Make up; Formulate a solution; Synthesize; Derive

TABLE 7–3	QUESTIONS REFLECTING THE HIERARCHICAL STRUCTURE OF COGNITIVE KNOWLEDGE (CONTINUED)	
CATEGORY	REQUIRED COGNITIVE ACTIVITY	SAMPLE QUESTION WORDS
Evaluation	*Judging*: Questions require the student to make a judgment about something using some criteria or standard for making the judgment.	Choose; Evaluate in terms of; Decide; Judge; Select on the the basis of; Which would you consider; Defend; What is the most appropriate; For what reasons do you favor.

Source: Adapted from Craig, J.L., & Page, G. (1981). The questioning skills of nursing instructors. *Journal of Nursing Education*, 20 (5), 20. Used with permission.

Debriefing. Debriefing is a group process in which students are invited to share their personal responses to their experiences in the clinical setting. By expressing their doubts and fears with peers, students begin to recognize that their feelings are not unique. From this perspective, the problem that has generated the feeling of unease becomes solvable.

Debriefing sessions usually occur at the end of the clinical day as a component of the postconference. The topic for discussion is patient-centered, and usually is initiated by the students. Initially, the debriefing session is centered on personal responses to the situation and making sense of what has happened as the experience relates to the student as a person, the health care system, and others involved in the situation. Soon, the sessions shift in emphasis to identifying students' individual learning needs, as they encounter and explore problems that they are unable to solve themselves. As these issues are brought to the debriefing session, clinical problems stimulate peer sharing in generating potential problem solutions. The identification of individual learning needs also challenges peers to broaden the scope of their own learning, as the possibilities inherent in the clinical learning experience become more evident. As students mature in their clinical development, debriefing sessions take on the characteristics of collaborative problem solving, as students bring partially resolved issues to the group for input. The collaborative process engages students in the critical appraisal of their own practices as well as those of their peers. As they reflect on a specific clinical problem, students construct new understandings based on their collective knowledge and experiences (Davies, 1995, pp. 169–171).

Debriefing sessions encourage an atmosphere of inquiry rather than inquisition. The role of the instructor is as facilitator rather than as evaluator of the students' clinical performance. Acknowledgment that no one has all the answers and that each clinical situation presents unique problems for solution motivates students to search out possible answers and engage in creative problem solving based on reflection on and analysis of what has been experienced rather than mere reliance on theoretical knowledge. The novice clinical instructor may be both puzzled and dismayed by the apparent ego-centrism of students' initial emotional responses to the clinical situations they encounter. Davies (1995) explains that students gradually shift from a focus on themselves in clinical situations (How am I doing? Why do I feel this way?) to a focus on the patient (How is this working for this patient? Why is the patient responding in this way?) as clinical experiences continue. The sharing that occurs with peers during debriefing sessions facilitates this transition.

Journaling.   The process of writing about clinical experiences structures students' reflections on practice. Journals and critical thinking logs deliberately focus on the student's exploration of the meaning of clinical experiences rather than recording a diary of events that transpired in the clinical setting. Journals can be written as a dialogue with the instructor, or they can remain private. When structured as a dialogue between student and instructor, there is an opportunity for the instructor to better understand the clinical experience from the student's perspective, share perceptions, correct misconceptions, and offer insights into situations that are puzzling to the student. This requires the instructor to thoughtfully respond to each student's entries, and to respect the sensitive nature of the writing as an expression of the student's innermost feelings.

Regardless of the approach used for journaling, the purposes, goals, and format of this assignment must be clearly identified for students, along with an explanation of how the journal will be used as a component of the clinical experience, in particular its contribution to grading, which is a major concern of students (Kobert, 1995). Holmes (1997) cautions that grading clinical journals has the potential to direct students' attention to what the instructor expects from the student rather than provide the freedom to explore the more pertinent question of what is going on for the student. When grading is a required component of journaling for a clinical course, the instructor should focus on the processes the student reveals in her writings, rather than the content. Otherwise, journal entries will simply regurgitate what she thinks the instructor wants rather than what she really thinks and feels.

The stimulus questions for journal entries can be very simple or highly detailed, and can emphasize critical thinking processes or stimulate reflective practice. Because the instructor has been present with the student during the clinical experience, it is not necessary for the entry to provide details concerning the clinical assignment. However, students should be encouraged to provide sufficient information so that they can readily recall the experience when they review journal entries. This process of review is a useful device for demonstrating to students the progress they have made during a clinical experience and helping them to identify the commonalties and links that exist in the student's evolving approach to the nursing care she has provided to a variety of patients.

Andrews (1998) advocates the use of open-ended questions, such as, "One new thing I learned today was . . ."; "I was surprised when . . ."; "I was disappointed when. . . ." Patton et al. (1997) provide discussion points for students, five of which must be addressed in each entry:

1. Describe what nursing interventions you or others did.
2. Describe your decision-making process.
3. Describe what you would do differently when a similar incident occurs.
4. Describe the clinical incident in relationship to the parts and the whole.
5. Identify previously learned knowledge/clinical experience(s) that helped you in this situation.
6. Use Benner's competency statements and describe where you view yourself.
7. Describe your areas of strengths and weaknesses. Include your thoughts, perceptions, and feelings.
8. Describe resources you identified and/or utilized and your rationale. (p. 238)

Baker (1996) encourages students to select an event or experience that will be the focus of the entry. A description of the experience containing both objective and subjective data is included, using poetry, drawings, or other creative expressions. The student then explores the significance of the experience in terms of its inherent meaning, and discusses the implications of the experience for her own clinical practice, her perceptions of herself as a nurse and/or a learner, and her own learning as a human being.

Journaling can be a means to develop holistic practice. It is impossible not to involve the affective domain when called upon to record feelings and responses to situations. Students' tendency to remain focused on the development of technical skills and stuck in the textbook explanations of clinical phenomena can be released by providing a mechanism for exploring their clinical experiences as they are lived.

Process Recordings.   Process recordings are a time-honored approach to teaching therapeutic communication skills, particularly in mental health settings. The student attempts to capture a "snapshot" of the patient with whom she has interacted, and her goals for the interaction. A significant portion of the interaction (beyond the introductory conversation) records both the patient's and student's verbal exchange and makes note of nonverbal behaviors. Following the recording of this information, which tends to paraphrase the interaction rather than be a verbatim record of it, the student analyzes the interaction to reveal her thought processes as the interaction proceeded and to evaluate the appropriateness of various communication strategies. After recording the interaction and her analysis of it, the student briefly summarizes what she has learned from the analysis and how she would alter her approach in future interactions with the same or other patients.

Process recordings are, by their nature, reflective. They provide a structure for the student's review of a situation and her own actions within it, as well as a basis for reflective critique of what was going on in that situation. The insights developed by completing a process recording enable the student to become more aware of their patterns of communicating with patients, so that reflection becomes incorporated into communication techniques as a means to improve its quality.

In reviewing students' process recordings, the instructor often will become aware of nuances expressed in the recording but not recognized by the student. By pointing out these alternative interpretations of the data the student has recorded, the instructor can broaden the student's awareness of the complexity of therapeutic communications.

Self-Evaluation.   Another approach to the development of critical thinking and reflective practice is to invite students to engage in a process of self-evaluation that encourages the examination of their decision-making processes and resulting actions on a regular basis. Instead of the usual checklist self-evaluation in relation to clinical learning objectives, the instructor might require students to provide specific examples of how they have demonstrated achievement of each of these objectives, and what might be improved in their practice in relation to each objective. Having students write anecdotal notes on their own clinical performance is another means of encouraging reflection on practice. As with journaling, the emphasis of any instructor evaluation of this work must focus on process rather than content if students are to be honest and forthcoming in their self-evaluations.

THE AFFECTIVE DOMAIN: FOSTERING CARING IN CLINICAL PRACTICE

Techniques that encourage students to engage in reflective practice access behaviors related to the affective domain, comprising feelings, attitudes, and values. Indeed, it is the student's strong emotional response to the clinical work she is doing that stimulates questions concerning how one *should* respond as a nurse in the situation. These questions lead the student to examine her own system of values and approach to ethical decision making in comparison with the professional ideal. It is the clinical situations with which students are involved that stimulate the issues that make possible a meaningful discussion of ethical dilemmas in professional nursing.

Initially, the student is likely to have difficulty in articulating the ethical issues embedded in the clinical situation, and will focus her questions on an examination of the appropriateness of her emotional response to the situation (Why does this bother me?). By inviting the student to explore her feelings (Can you describe what you are feeling? Anger? Sadness? Despair? What was going on when you first noticed these feelings? What do you think is prompting these feelings?) enables the student to better articulate the dilemma.

Then, techniques for values clarification and ethical problem solving can be introduced as approaches to further exploring and resolving these issues, both now and in the future.

Many of the same concerns that generate students' exploration of ethical dilemmas in practice also provide the stimulus for learning caring behaviors. "Students have the capacity to care and know what it means to care for another human being" (Canales, 1994, p. 416); they need to learn how to act upon the caring impulses they feel in response to patient's needs.

Kosowski (1995) describes five modes of learning caring reported by baccalaureate nursing students. Students most frequently reported *role modeling* by staff nurses and the clinical instructor as the means by which they learned caring as a "way of being" (p. 236) in the clinical setting. They were particularly influenced by caring behaviors of the instructor toward learners in the clinical group. Students also learned caring through negative role modeling, labeled by Kosowski as *"reversing."* Noncaring behaviors stimulated in students a commitment never to behave in uncaring ways. *Imagining* was a third way of learning caring. This learning mode involved picturing oneself or a family member (often a parent or grandparent) in the situation as a means to better understand patient needs and what would constitute a caring response. *Sensing* was the fourth mode of learning caring. This involved attention to the perceptible changes in one's own body in response to the patient's verbal and nonverbal expressions of discomfort or distress. Attention to these "gut feelings," prompted a caring response. The fifth learning mode was labeled *constructing*, and involved building on previous experiential as well as theoretical knowledge to make sense of observations of patient behaviors. Often the previous experience involved events in the personal lives of the student. This framework for learning caring can guide the clinical instructor in developing trigger questions for discussions that focus on caring behaviors of the nurse.

SUMMARY

Much of the teaching and learning that occurs in the clinical setting takes place in one-to-one interactions with individual students. The instructor's ability to stimulate students to share those experiences that contributed to learning with the entire clinical group expands the power of the clinical setting to promote the growth and development of nursing students. Learning in the clinical practice setting is complex and multidimensional, involving each of the behavioral domains—cognitive, psychomotor, and affective—in interaction with the others. As students' knowledge in each of the behavioral domains develops, there is a gradual integration of the component behaviors into an experiential whole that results in the skilled practice of nursing.

REFERENCES

Andrews, C.A. (1998). Engendering community: Writing a journal to clinical students. *Journal of Nursing Education*, 37, 358–360.

Baker, C.R. (1996). Reflective learning: A teaching strategy for critical thinking. *Journal of Nursing Education*, 35, 19–22.

Canales, M. (1994). Clinical education: A caring approach. *Journal of Nursing Education*, 33, 417–419.

Cox, R.P. (1998). IPRs revisited: Using process recordings to develop nursing students' critical thinking skills. *Journal of Nursing Education*, 37, 37–41.

Craig, J.L., & Page, G. (1981). The questioning skills of nursing instructors. *Journal of Nursing Education*, 20 (5), 20.

Davies, E. (1995). Reflective practice: A focus for caring. *Journal of Nursing Education*, 34, 4, 167–174.

Delehanty, L. (1996). Nursing intervention: A student assignment. *Journal of Nursing Education*, 35, 93–95.

Edwards, E.J. (1991). Use of listening skills when advising nursing students in clinical experiences. *Journal of Nursing Education*, 30, 328–329.

Grealish, L. (2000). The skills of coach are an essential element in clinical learning. *Journal of Nursing Education*, 39, 231–233.

Heinrich, K.T. (1992). Create a tradition: Teach nurses to share stories. *Journal of Nursing Education*, 31, 141–143.

Holmes, V. (1997). Grading journals in clinical practice: A delicate issue. *Journal of Nursing Education*, 36, 489–492.

Infante, M.S. (1985). *The clinical laboratory in nursing education*. New York: Wiley.

Ironside, P.M. (1999). Thinking in nursing education. *Nursing and Health Care* Perspectives, 20, 238–247.

Kibler, R.J., Barker, L.L., & Miles, D.T. (1970). *Behavioral objectives and instruction.* Boston: Allyn and Bacon.

Kobert, L.J. (1995). In our own voices: Journaling as a teaching/learning technique for nurses. *Journal of Nursing Education*, 34, 140–142.

Kosowski, M.M.R. (1995). Clinical learning experiences and professional nurse caring: A critical phenomenological study of female baccalaureate nursing students. *Journal of Nursing Education*, 34, 235–242.

O'Connor, A.B. (1986). *Nursing staff development and continuing education.* (pp. 163–165). Boston: Little, Brown.

Patton, J.G.; Woods, S.J.; Agarenzo, T.; Brubaker, C.; Metcalf, T.; & Sherrer, L. (1997). Enhancing the clinical practicum experience through journal writing. *Journal of Nursing Education*, 36, 238–240.

Rowles, C.J., & Brigham, C. (1998). Strategies to promote critical thinking and active learning. (pp. 258–259). In Billings, D.M., & Halstead, J.A. *Teaching in nursing; A guide for faculty.* Philadelphia: W.B. Saunders.

Tschikata, S. (1993). The clinical decision-making processes of student nurses. *Journal of Nursing Education*, 32, 389–396.

Wink, D.M. (1993). Effect of a program to increase the cognitive level of questions asked in clinical postconferences. *Journal of Nursing Education*, 32, 357–363.

CHAPTER 8

SPECIAL TECHNIQUES FOR SPECIAL SETTINGS

The Maternity Setting: Managing Instruction to Capture the Cyclical Nature
of the Maternity Experience   151
The Pediatric Setting: The Problem of a Disappearing Clientele   153
The Mental Health Setting: It's Communication, But Is It Therapeutic?   155
Community Health Settings: Independent Practice in Unstructured
Settings   157

The teaching–learning principles and strategies that are discussed throughout this book are applicable to any clinical setting in which nursing educational experiences occur. However, certain settings require special techniques to address the unique elements within them that have the potential to impact the educational process. These elements include the nature of the health problems of concern in the specialty area, the nature of the patients, and the nature of the setting. This chapter discusses special techniques pertinent to maternity, pediatrics, mental health, and community health settings.[1]

THE MATERNITY SETTING: MANAGING INSTRUCTION TO CAPTURE THE CYCLICAL NATURE OF THE MATERNITY EXPERIENCE

The cyclical nature of the maternity experience, encompassing the antepartum period, labor and delivery, care of the newborn, and postpartum care of the mother and child, is unique to the maternity setting. Students should have

---

[1] I am indebted to my colleagues, Dr. Carol Avery, Dr. Patricia Lund, Professor Sheila Molony, and Dr. Barbara Piscopo at Western Connecticut State University for providing me with insights into the particular issues they have encountered teaching in these clinical areas.

experiences in all phases of the cycle, and need to be actively engaged in the clinical area early in the experience regardless of the sequence of theoretical instruction in the classroom. Ideally, each student should be able to observe a normal vaginal delivery as well as a birth by Cesarean section, and be involved in the care of a mother in active labor. In the postpartum area, students should have experiences with the mother who has had a normal vaginal delivery (ideally, a primipara who is attempting breastfeeding), a mother who has had a Cesarean section, and a mother who is experiencing problems during the postpartum period. Most instructors have students observe events in the antepartum clinic rather than assign students to care for pregnant mothers who are hospitalized, who may decompensate quickly but are otherwise well and require little nursing care.

In order to manage instruction that spans these aspects of the maternity cycle, the instructor must be highly organized. Students will need preparation for each phase of the cycle, so that they understand the processes they are observing. It is particularly important to provide students with guidelines or protocols for learning activities in each area, so that they know what they should be doing—and what should be left to the primary nurse. Because classroom instruction often is "out-of-sync" with the learning opportunities present in the clinical experience, the instructor must be prepared to fill in the blanks for students who are working with a situation that has not yet been covered in the classroom. As the semester proceeds, the instructor should attempt to integrate the content being presented in the classroom with both past and present clinical learning experiences.

Because of the rapid changes in this patient population, particularly with shorter hospital stays postpartum, it is unrealistic to plan specific patient assignments in advance. This means that the instructor must arrive in the clinical area well in advance of the students, get report on each of the patients, and then plan the deployment of the student group. Coordination and cooperation with staff is essential in planning for the clinical day and in obtaining the information relevant to making sound clinical assignments. Report conveyed to students should include details of the patients' histories, so that the students have a sense of continuity in the maternity process even though they will be involved with only one aspect of the cycle with a specific patient. Throughout the clinical day, the instructor must manage her own time effectively, so that she is aware of what is happening in each of the areas of the maternity unit and is able to move quickly between these. It is especially important to keep track of the progress of the laboring mothers with whom students are working, in order to be prepared for the move into the delivery suite to guide students there. Teaching in the maternity setting requires the instructor to do a lot of juggling. She must remain flexible and open to the possibilities that arise during the clinical experience.

In addition to the uniqueness presented by the maternity cycle, this setting involves patients who are essentially well. Students may not know what to do. They need help in prioritizing the issues to be dealt with and in attending to the patient's own priorities for care. In the postpartum area, students can be guided to attend to the following issues:

- the mother's well-being, in particular, her level of pain;
- the infant's well-being;
- the mother's perception of the infant's well-being;
- coordination of care activities;
- preparation for early discharge;
- helping first-time parents with a new role; and
- encouraging parents to try out alternative techniques to see what works rather than worry about how to deal with conflicting information from various sources.

In the labor and delivery suite, students can be guided to

- observe nurse–patient interactions and the different styles of practice these represent;
- observe the interplay with the patient if the father, a significant other, or a duella is involved;
- note differences in patient responses to the labor process;
- note differences in the contextual situation surrounding care;
- note the team approach as transition occurs;
- focus on providing a "good" experience for the mother, with a good outcome; and
- keep active, and then reflect on what was going on.

Because the patients for whom students are providing care are walking, talking, and alert, the instructor must be careful in guiding student learning so as not to alarm the mother. She also must remain sensitive to the level of tension in the environment, where the usual normality/wellness focus can quickly disintegrate, with tragic results.

Another unique characteristic of the maternity setting is that nursing activities involve a mother and child, where two people are the focus of care. (Depending on unit policies, more than mother and child may be involved, if the father or significant other is able to participate actively in care of the newborn.) This requires the student to expand her awareness of issues to include each member of the family, rather than remain focused on the mother or child.

THE PEDIATRIC SETTING: THE PROBLEM OF A DISAPPEARING CLIENTELE

Only a small percentage of children are ever hospitalized. Coupled with a shortened length of stay for those children who do require hospital care, the disappearance of inpatient subjects for pediatric nursing experiences makes the design of meaningful clinical learning involving the care of children difficult.

Alternative placements for student experiences are a necessary aspect of planning for the pediatric clinical experience, and usually involve ambulatory care settings and settings that provide care for the developmentally disabled child or the child with behavioral problems who is in a residential facility. The use of nonhospital-based settings raises issues related to faculty supervision of student experiences if students are in a number of different facilities at the same time. Additional issues arise when schools and well-child clinics are accessed for alternate experiences. These settings have a predominantly public health orientation, to which students may not yet have been exposed.

The clinical instructor must arrange alternative experiences well in advance, and provide ample information to staff regarding the goals for these learning experiences and the activities in which students can and cannot participate. Mechanisms for contacting the clinical instructor in the event problems or questions arise must be in place, and the instructor must be prepared to engage in prompt trouble-shooting to alleviate staff concerns about specific student behaviors. Students will need thorough instructions that describe how to get to the alternate site and what their role will be there. Observational guidelines that require meaningful involvement with the activities that are available at the site can help to structure learning. Students should be expected to report back to the clinical group on what they learned. This requirement reinforces the learning that has occurred and broadens the conceptions of pediatric nursing held by those students who will not be participating in this activity. Feedback on the experience also alerts those students who will follow their peers into the alternate site to the potential learning that can occur there.

In the hospital setting, each student's technical skill proficiency must be checked out by the instructor before the student is allowed to perform the skill with a child. Children will not wait patiently while the student figures out the next step in a procedure. More time must be spent on performing nursing procedures with children than with adults. Even the simplest task will require additional time and planning. The instructor must be prepared to spend time with the student when she first performs a skill with a child. This means that staff members must be relied upon to provide the necessary supervision of other students. Strong relationships with staff are essential if the instructor is to provide the supervision needed by one student without sacrificing the learning needs of the remaining students in the group. Consequently, it is vital that the instructor invest time in learning how the unit operates, and in providing staff with opportunities to witness her expertise in providing care to pediatric patients and her willingness to expend the effort necessary to keep the unit functioning.

Parental involvement is another factor to be considered in planning clinical learning experiences in the pediatric setting. Parents are naturally anxious about the care provided to their children, and this can be intimidating for students. Parental anxiety can escalate rapidly—and infect the student—if the student hesitates in performing a task or seems uncertain about what to do for the child. Suggesting that the student involve the parent in the care of the child is an excellent strategy for allaying both the student's and the parent's anxiety. Another factor concerning parents who are present in the clinical area is the need for caution in discussing the child's condition and nursing needs, so as not to unnecessarily alarm the parent concerning the child's status.

Finally, ethical issues surrounding the care of children may create great emotional upheaval for students. The instructor must remain sensitive to students' reactions to such issues as the dying child, child abuse, and child rape, and provide opportunities for a full discussion of their feelings and concerns. Of particular importance is the exploration of the effect students' emotional responses have on the nursing care they are providing, and how disabling responses can be managed to permit effective care to proceed.

THE MENTAL HEALTH SETTING: IT'S COMMUNICATION, BUT IS IT THERAPEUTIC?

The goals of nursing education in mental health are as varied as the types of health problems encountered in these settings, which may include a mix of medical and psychiatric concerns; clients of all ages; and the nature of the settings in which care is provided. The focus of the educational experience generally includes the development of therapeutic communication skills within the context of a one-to-one therapeutic relationship with a patient who is either recovering from the acute phase of mental illness or is chronically ill but sufficiently stable to participate meaningfully in therapeutic interactions. Application of the nursing process in conducting a mental health assessment, planning both short- and long-term goals, and implementing therapeutic interventions is a second goal of these experiences. Assessment often includes the analysis of family dynamics in the context of mental illness, as well as the identification and description of the patient's use of defense mechanisms, evidence of delusional states, and behavioral manifestations of neuroses or psychoses, applying one or more theoretical frameworks for mental illness presented in the classroom. A third goal of the mental health clinical experience is to develop the student's appreciation of the therapeutic milieu and the varied modalities employed in addressing mental health problems, including neurobiological, psychological, social, occupational, and recreational approaches. The importance of teamwork and collaborative sharing of information concerning patient progress in designing the plan of care is identified as a significant aspect of this goal, and participation in team planning conferences is often a component of the planned clinical experience. A fourth goal of this experience is the student's development of personal insights as a result of her interactions with mentally ill patients.

The clinical experience may involve the care of acutely or chronically ill patients, or both. Patients may present with neuroses or psychoses. Substance abuse, whether involving drugs or alcohol or both, may be a predominant diagnosis for some experiences. Patients may include children, adolescents, adults, and the elderly. Experiences may take place at inpatient facilities or at outpatient rehabilitation or social and recreational programs and residential facilities. This great diversity in problems, patients, and settings requires careful management of clinical assignments by the instructor if students are to develop a working appreciation for the richness of this specialty area and the opportunities for therapeutic nursing interventions that are available in the mental health field.

Students often are fearful when they begin the mental health clinical experience. Their apprehension, often stimulated by portrayals of mental illness in the entertainment media, centers on the anticipation that patients' behavior will be unpredictable and possibly violent. They also question their ability to communicate effectively and therapeutically with patients, and that they will say something "wrong" that will trigger a psychotic response that will be uncontrollable as well as detrimental to the patient. It is important for the clinical instructor to recognize these common responses, and to provide ample time during early conferences to allow students to share their concerns and deal with their fears. As their comfort in communicating with patients increases, the ability to develop a one-to-one therapeutic relationship with a mentally ill patient becomes a satisfying and fulfilling component of the mental health clinical experience.

In most mental health settings, students do not administer medications. The failure of the experience to provide opportunities to practice technical skills often causes students to question the legitimacy of a professional nursing role in mental health settings. This issue may be magnified by competition with students from other disciplines for access to the pool of patients, and by observations of nurses in the setting if they are not actively involved in patient care. It is vital, therefore, for the clinical instructor to clarify the nurse's role in assessment, planning, and intervention with mentally ill patients, and the special skills that are necessary to perform successfully in this setting. This positive role modeling and role shaping encourages students to move beyond social chitchat with patients, and into a therapeutic relationship with them.

In some nursing education programs, the clinical experience may be divided between several locations so students are exposed to a variety of mental health problems at various stages of acuity and chronicity. This arrangement poses problems related to time spent in orientation to several facilities, which detracts from the time in which students can develop relationships with patients. The instructor will need to devise means to streamline the orientation process so that students can become engaged in the clinical setting as quickly as possible. On the other hand, if the clinical experience is confined to a single facility, with a focus on only acutely ill or on chronically ill patients with little potential for rehabilitation, then the students' perceptions of the scope of mental health nursing practice will be limited. In this case, the instructor will need to build into the clinical experience several observational experiences in other settings or discussions of other approaches to the treatment of mental health problems in patients who are at different stages of illness and its treatment.

COMMUNITY HEALTH SETTINGS: INDEPENDENT PRACTICE IN UNSTRUCTURED SETTINGS

The community health settings used for nursing education clinical experiences vary greatly. Some focus almost entirely on public health problems; others focus almost entirely on home nursing. Ideally, students should be exposed to both types of experiences, so that the community health experience includes both the unique experience of practicing direct nursing care in the unstructured home environment as well as the unique perspective on health issues offered by a public health orientation. Many educational programs achieve this blend by placing students in home health agencies for a home nursing experience, and then requiring them to complete a community assessment as an ongoing assignment during the agency placement. The community assessment explores the health of the surrounding community, particularly as it impacts on assigned patients, as well as community resources available to provide services for patients. The assessment might be a group effort, in which different students in the clinical group explore facets of the community and then combine their findings in a final assessment and plan of care for the community. Home nursing visits also may be supplemented by assignments in clinics run by the agency (for example, well-child clinics, flu immunization clinics, and the like) or rotations into special services provided by the agency, such as hospice home care services. Such alternative assignments expand students' perspective on the scope of community health nursing.

Anticipatory guidance that addresses the particular issues encountered in the community health setting is especially important for students, who often enter this experience with a high degree of anxiety. Students recognize that they will be "on their own" during most of the clinical experience. The lack of readily available support systems in the form of the instructor, peers, and staff members, coupled with the lack of institutional structures that provide a "safe haven" for students, is the source of most of this anxiety. Registered nurse students who are returning to school for the baccalaureate degree are particularly susceptible to anxiety prior to the community health experience, because most of them have practiced entirely within a structured institutional setting. Anxiety will diminish as students become actively involved in patient care, but it is important to acknowledge its presence and help students to work through their concerns prior to moving into the community on their own.

Guidance also is needed to deal with the inevitable culture shock that occurs as students encounter lifestyles and living conditions that are very different from their own. They often need emotional support as they work through their feelings and begin to recognize the necessity of setting boundaries concerning what can and cannot be accomplished within a given setting. The need to abide by the patients' decisions as to what care they will accept and what advice they will follow is a particularly important concept for students to learn, as is the notion that students are guests within the patients' homes and must act accordingly. Encouraging students to conduct an environmental assessment that scans the immediate home environment from a safety and sufficiency perspective helps them to come to terms with the differences they observe, and begins to challenge their assumptions concerning the availability of basic services, such as refrigeration and cooking facilities. When considered in conjunction with the community assessment, the home environment assessment can provide a comprehensive, if unsettling picture of the context of health care problems encountered by community health nurses.

Personal safety is yet another issue about which students will need guidance. The instructor will need to be familiar with the community in which students will be functioning, including any dangers that are present in this environment. Students will need to be counseled as to how to dress and behave so as not to invite problems. Students should know when to avoid entering a building and when to call for an escort service or partner if this option is available. Students will need maps and clear directions about how to get to assigned patients and then back to the agency. They should expect to get lost initially, and should know how to manage this. Many students are afraid of dogs, and the instructor should elicit this information before assigning a student to a home visit that will involve an encounter with a dog.

Certain practice issues are unique to home care practice and must be discussed with students prior to the first home visit. Infection control measures and how to manage the nursing bag to avoid contamination of its contents— or the next patient's home—are novel concepts for students. Maintaining a clean or sterile environment while performing such care activities as dressing changes and urinary catheterizations can be a challenge, and students will need pointers on how to proceed. Students will need to know what supplies and equipment can be expected to be available in the home, since few supplies are provided by the agency. They will need guidance in improvising when necessary, so that needed care can be provided even when the expected supplies and/or equipment are lacking.

Students will need to be oriented to the structure of each home visit, including detailed planning of activities. The need for social conversation as a means of gaining the patient's confidence in the student as a care provider must be introduced, as students have been taught repeatedly that such conversation is inappropriate in clinical settings. Here, the rules are somewhat different, and students need to become aware of the nuances of being a guest in the patient's home while still providing therapeutic services. Within the hospital and many other health care settings, the focus of the student's attention is on the assigned patient. In the home health setting, the student must include other family members and care providers in the scope of her assessment and teaching activities. It may be a family member who is best able to provide accurate information about the patient's progress. This same family member may be the person who will translate, interpret, and follow instructions for care. At the same time, the nurse cannot ignore the patient and his response to the nurse's interaction with the family member, for these responses are likely to yield clues about the adequacy of care being provided in the home. The concept of case finding also must be introduced as part of the planning for a visit, because the assigned patient may not necessarily be the person most in need of nursing interventions within the home care setting.

Much of the work in home care nursing involves accessing and connecting patients with community-based resources for health care services. The student will make many follow-up calls to pharmacies, physicians, and the like in the course of the day's activities, and should be briefed on how to conduct and record these calls. Similarly, the student will need ample orientation to documentation procedures in place at the agency, in particular, the necessity for care in documentation to avoid inadvertently disqualifying a patient from receiving Medicare or Medicaid benefits covering home care visits.

Students differ in their responses to the community health clinical experience. Registered nurse students often are delighted to have opportunities to teach patients in the home care setting, since this nursing function is afforded limited time in institutional settings. The opportunity to work with a patient on his "own turf," and to recognize the interaction of environmental factors with health care issues is both challenging and exciting for the RN student once she has defused the anxiety that accompanies her practice experiences in this unstructured setting. Students in the basic nursing program tend to be dismayed by the lack of technical work during home care visits. Because they are task-oriented, they often fail to see the broader health care issues and potentials for nursing intervention that exist in this environment unless these are pointed out by the preceptor or instructor. Many of these issues will emerge in postconference sessions, particularly if RN and basic students are mixed in the same clinical group. RN students tend to focus on compliance issues in the community setting, and use theoretical frameworks to search for reasons why people behave as they do. RN students also focus on teaching as a primary intervention in this setting, and explore different approaches to the challenge of teaching people to care for themselves and family members. They are eager to identify and use community resources, and engage other disciplines in the care of patients. Basic students tend to be more patient-centered in their focus in addition to their concentration on technical skill performance. These students are very aware of family members and other support persons in the home environment, and seek ways to help these helpers. In this regard, they need to be oriented to the distinctions in the roles of the professional nurse, the home health aide, and the homemaker in the scope of services each provides.

Because the setting is unstructured, the clinical instructor's activities are very different than those of clinical instructors in institutional settings. Despite the availability of staff members to serve as preceptors for these initial visits, the instructor must plan each clinical day carefully in order to provide necessary supervision for students who have problems, remain available for emergency consultations by students, make home visits with students on a regular basis, and return to the agency in time to debrief students, review their documentation, and conduct the postconference. The instructor should carry a beeper or cell phone that enables students to contact her at any time during the clinical day. She should also provide students with a list of her anticipated activities for the day, and the phone numbers of homes where she will be at given hours of the day. Providing this access and information lessens both staff and student anxiety concerning the adequacy of faculty supervision during field experiences, and also makes the instructor more comfortable in focusing her efforts on a few students at a time.

Most students will work with a preceptor (usually the primary nurse for the assigned patient) for the first one or two home visits. The preceptor provides an introduction into the home and its residents for the student, as well as guidance in the conduct of the visit. After the student is adequately oriented to the patients she will be seeing, the instructor should review each day's plans with the student, to ensure that the student has a good understanding of the ongoing needs of the patients to whom she is assigned. The community health clinical experience provides an excellent opportunity for students to witness continuity in the provision of nursing care. This is best achieved by selecting patient assignments that involve patients with chronic conditions who are expected to receive nursing services over a long period of time. However, it is always possible that the patient will be rehospitalized or will have a physician's appointment scheduled for the time of day at which the student usually visits. Consequently, it is essential for the instructor to have backup plans for each student's experience. Many instructors achieve this by assigning two patients to each student, so that there will be at least one patient care contact on a given clinical day.

The instructor should take the time to review the academic records of students in her clinical group, to identify those students who may have problems with performing technical skills or in applying theory to practice issues. These are students she will want to work with more closely, or assign to an attentive preceptor for a longer-than-usual period of time.

Evaluation of student learning during the community health experience will be based on a combination of home visits made with students during the semester, review of the students' documentation, and their contributions to postconference discussions. The instructor will want to assess each student's ability to apply the nursing process in interactions with patients as well as her ability to appropriately apply theoretical concepts to decision making regarding patient care, and to assess the relationship each student is able to develop with assigned patients and the relative ease with which each party to the relationship (student, patient, and significant family members) communicates during an observational visit. Awareness of environmental factors that may impact on the patient's health problems is a second area for evaluation. Students should be able to evidence an appreciation for the multiple contextual factors that are present in the home care environment that have the capacity to either promote or impede recovery. Finally, the instructor should assess the student's ability to truly listen to her patient and to hear and appropriately respond to the concerns that the patient expresses. Nursing care in the community health setting is never confined to the presenting issues. It always involves ongoing monitoring for additional issues that may arise during the nurse's visits.

CHAPTER 9

THEORETICAL APPROACHES TO THE EVALUATION OF LEARNING IN THE LABORATORY AND CLINICAL PRACTICE SETTINGS

Philosophies of Evaluation   164
Purposes of Evaluation   166
The Evaluation Process   167
    Goals of Evaluation   168
    Standards for Evaluation   169
    Evaluation Methods   170
    Analyzing Results   172
    Reporting Results and Making Decisions   172
    Using Results   173
    Evaluating the Evaluation Process   173
Summary   175
References   175

Evaluation is the process of collecting and analyzing data gathered through one or more measurements in order to render a judgment about the subject of the evaluation (Bourke & Ihrke, 1998). In the educational setting, evaluation is conducted to determine students' progress toward and achievement of program outcomes; the effectiveness of the educational process in fostering student learning; and the success of the program in accomplishing its mission of preparing professional nurses for entry into practice. Although the clinical instructor has a role in each of these aspects of evaluation, the emphasis in this chapter is on concepts and theories relevant to the evaluation of students' performance in the college laboratory and clinical practice settings. It is assumed that the instructor will engage in an ongoing process of self-evaluation concerning the effectiveness of educational strategies to enable students to achieve the goals and objectives of the learning experience.

PHILOSOPHIES OF EVALUATION

Bourke and Ihrke (1998) identify several philosophical perspectives that influence the evaluation process. Of these, the *objectives* approach, *service* orientation, *judgment* perspective, and *constructivist* view (p. 351) are most salient to the evaluation of students' clinical performance. While one or another of these perspectives is likely to dominate the instructor's approach to evaluation, each will be represented to some degree. Most important is that the instructor become aware of her perspective on evaluation, the issues inherent in that perspective, and the impact of philosophical perspective on the task of evaluating students' clinical performance.

The *objectives* approach is characterized by an emphasis on the achievement of course objectives and program goals as the primary focus of evaluation. In this approach, the learner is assumed to have a deficit in knowledge, skill, and/or attitude that is amenable to education. Learning is represented in movement from the existing level of performance to the ideal level of performance as described in course objectives and program goals. The objectives approach assumes that all behaviors relevant to clinical practice are reflected in course objectives, and that the clinical experience will provide opportunities for all students to demonstrate these behaviors. Whether each objective or outcome is to be considered equal in value to all others is a question each instructor must reflect upon. Most instructors would agree that demonstrating professional accountability is an overarching objective; others would add objectives related to safety or caring as carrying more weight. The objectives approach also suggests that it is the performance achieved at the end of the clinical experience that matters most (i.e., whether the student has, ultimately, achieved the objectives) rather than the student's pattern of behavior over the course of the experience. If this is the case, the instructor will need to determine what behaviors (if any) would warrant removing a student from the clinical area or failing the student clinically before the experience is ended.

The *service* orientation considers evaluation as one means of making decisions about learners and the educational process. In this orientation, the instructor holds a more global or holistic view of the goals of the educational process than is reflected in course objectives. These goals are integrated in a model of performance representing the typical or ideal student at this level of development. The model becomes the standard against which each student is evaluated. It is important for the instructor with a service orientation toward evaluation to reflect on the source of the performance model selected for evaluation purposes to ensure that it represents a realistic portrayal of desired behaviors in the clinical setting in which learning experiences occur. If the model of performance selected by the instructor represents the typical student, then it can be assumed that actual student performance may fall above or below the envisioned level. If the model of performance represents the ideal student, then it is likely that few, if any, students will achieve this level of performance. Consequently, the instructor must consider how short of the mark student performance can fall and still be considered adequate, resulting in a vision of the marginal or borderline student. The two poles—typical or ideal performance and marginal or borderline performance—then serve as markers for determining the acceptable range of student performance. Instructors with a service orientation also view the evaluation process as a means to identify student strengths and weaknesses in the multiple components of the overall clinical experience, and a guide to facilitating student progress toward model performance. Thus, evaluation informs the educational process as well as the assessment of student achievement.

The *judgment* perspective focuses on the end point of the evaluation process: the determination of the acceptability of student performance and the value (grade) that should be assigned to that performance. Two systems of grading students in clinical experiences are used in nursing programs—pass/fail grading and letter or numerical grading—with one or the other approach selected for use in all clinical experiences throughout the program. Of the two systems, pass/fail grading seems to be preferred among nursing educators. The pull toward the discrimination among levels of performance that is possible in the letter or numerical grading system is evident when faculty use such terms as "high pass" and "low pass," creating four levels roughly comparable to letter grading. Use of these terms, even if they are not translated into actual grades assigned to students in the clinical experience, suggests that instructors engage in comparisons among students as well as in relation to course objectives or a model of performance. The pass/fail system allows for the inevitable subjectivity that enters the evaluation process and compensates for differences in students' exposure to various clinical experiences and opportunities to demonstrate competent performance. The judgment perspective enables the instructor to identify and label as unacceptable certain behaviors that warrant removal of the student from the clinical area or the course. The issue that arises is whether the mere absence of negative indicators is sufficient to award a passing grade in the clinical component of the course.

The *constructivist* view gives greatest consideration to those stakeholders who will be affected by the success or failure of the program in achieving its mission of preparing entry-level nurses. These stakeholders usually are considered to be the employers of program graduates and the recipients of their care. (Obviously, others hold a stake in the success of the educational enterprise: the students themselves, those who pay the expenses of education, program faculty, and the college as a whole.) Instructors with a constructivist view ask what is most important to identified stakeholders, and evaluate students in relation to those standards. One colleague states, "My bottom line is, would I want this student to take care of me or a member of my family"; another says, "Mine is safety. I don't want to be responsible for allowing a fundamentally unsafe student to continue in the program." Greater emphasis may be placed by the instructor on those characteristics and abilities perceived to be valued by employers: skilled technical performance or reliability as evidenced by the attendance record and timely performance of tasks.

The instructor with a constructivist perspective often will seek the input of patients and staff in evaluating student performance, and consider this information in making a final determination as to a student's clinical grade. One problem with the constructivist perspective is the limited ability of stakeholders to recognize or articulate the intellectual components of nursing practice, which may lead the instructor to be less attentive to these aspects of the student's clinical performance. Does a student merit a passing clinical grade if she performs tasks correctly, with evidence of caring, and in a timely fashion, but cannot explain the rationale for actions or the reason the patient requires the treatment?

PURPOSES OF EVALUATION

Evaluation serves many purposes. The instructor needs to remain attuned to the purposes for which evaluation data are being collected so that the data are used appropriately. Assessment of the individual learner is likely to involve

- identification of existing ability and aptitude, which provides a base upon which further learning can be built;
- identification of learning needs, or observed deficits or missed opportunities that should be addressed during the clinical experience;
- assessment of progress toward achievement of course objectives; and
- judgment concerning students' achievement of a satisfactory level of performance at the conclusion of the clinical experience.

Assessment of the clinical group as a whole will involve the same areas of concern. While one anticipates that the students will be relatively homogeneous in terms of existing ability and aptitude, for example, this may not be the case. Gearing instruction to a level of ability identified in one or two students but not verified for the entire group may result in overwhelming (or boring) the majority of group members. Assessment of the teaching-learning process should consider both its effectiveness and efficiency. One can be highly effective in coaching the less able student, at the expense of remaining clinical group members. Teaching a skill to each student individually is less efficient than teaching the group as a whole, and then providing support as students practice the skill, addressing individual problems as needed. Efficiencies of this sort are best accomplished in the college laboratory setting. Of concern to program faculty and administrators is the degree to which evaluation outcomes indicate students' progress toward the achievement of course, level, and program objectives. This may require some standardization in the format and timing of evaluation, to permit cross-program comparisons as well as generating longitudinal data concerning program effectiveness. Such assessments rarely, if ever, contribute to individual student grades.

Another way to consider the many purposes of evaluation differentiates among *process, product, outcome, impact,* and *program* evaluation. *Process* evaluation assesses the degree to which students and instructor were satisfied with the experience. This type of evaluation has been labeled a "happiness rating," but serves an important purpose in alerting the instructor and others to flaws in the experience that might be remedied. When students report that an observational experience could be shortened (or eliminated), the instructor should review the objectives for the experience, the degree to which student reports of the experience reflect learning, and whether the same objectives could be met in other ways. When students complain that staff were hostile and unsupportive, steps should be taken to determine what is wrong and how the clinical environment might be improved for both staff and students. Process evaluation also provides feedback to the instructor about her management of the clinical experience and instructional strategies.

Product evaluation is concerned with the immediate results of the educational experience, that is, whether students learned. This type of evaluation is reflected in the clinical evaluation form used to rate students' overall clinical performance, as well as in students' self-evaluation. Product evaluation also may involve some synthesizing written project or oral presentation, such as a major nursing care plan in which the student demonstrates the ability to pull together, analyze, and communicate a wide range of information related to the care of a patient.

Outcome evaluation focuses on changes in behavior that persist after the educational experience has ended, or the retention of learning. This is reflected in the student's success in transferring learning to other clinical settings, and ability to build on knowledge and skills acquired at one level of the program in successive courses.

Impact evaluation attempts to identify changes in health care delivery and outcomes of care that can be attributed to program graduates. This long-term evaluation is difficult to conduct, given the many factors contributing to changes in health care.

Program evaluation assesses the degree to which program goals and outcomes are being achieved. With respect to student outcomes, licensing examination results and employer responses to surveys concerning satisfaction with graduates' clinical performance contribute to the evaluation of program effectiveness.

THE EVALUATION PROCESS

A stepwise approach to evaluation ensures that the process is deliberative rather than haphazard. The use of such an approach enables the instructor to feel confident in evaluating students' clinical performance. The evaluation process involves

- identifying the specific purposes or goals of the evaluation;
- establishing standards against which results of the evaluation will be weighed;

- selecting the methods to be used in conducting the evaluation, including sampling, scheduling, and instrumentation;
- conducting the evaluation;
- analyzing results in relation to established standards;
- reporting results to concerned participants;
- using results to make decisions about student performance; and
- evaluating the evaluation process.

Goals of Evaluation

Students assume that evaluation occurs whenever the instructor interacts with the student or is present during a caregiving event. To some extent, this is true. The instructor continuously gathers data on student performance, building a picture of strengths, weaknesses, abilities, and deficits as a basis upon which to design learning experiences that will enable the student to develop beginning clinical competence. The evolving assessment of each student also alerts the instructor to potential performance problems that should be monitored carefully to ensure patient safety.

Formative evaluation, which seeks information concerning the student's readiness to learn and learning needs, does not contribute to final grading. The assessment of student performance serves as a guide to further shaping the learning experience. Formative evaluation occurs throughout the clinical learning experience and is distinct from *summative* evaluation, which occurs at the end of the experience and indicates the level of performance achieved by the student. Students need to be aware of this difference so that their ongoing interactions with the instructor facilitate the process of learning. A good example of the difference in these two goals of evaluation is shown in the college laboratory setting. As students are introduced to and practice skills in the laboratory setting, the instructor observes and corrects the student as she proceeds with the skill. The laboratory setting allows time for both student and instructor to pause to discuss a fine-point of technique or to backup and begin again. This formative evaluation, which seeks to identify flaws in technique in order to shape and refine the student's skills, has its focus on the educational process. The final lab practicum, where students demonstrate achievement of competence in performing selected skills, exemplifies summative evaluation.

The use of formative evaluation is formalized in a midsemester evaluation, which rates each student's achievement of clinical objectives. The use of the final clinical evaluation instrument for this evaluation alerts students to their progress toward the goals of the experience. During the conference with each student that should accompany the midsemester evaluation, the instructor and student can discuss how the student's performance might be enhanced during the remainder of the experience. If all is going well, the instructor should provide feedback to the student on examples of those specific behaviors in the clinical setting upon which the evaluation has been based, in order to reinforce these and encourage their future development.

Students should be told when the instructor is shifting from formative to summative evaluation. One hopes students will strive for excellence in all clinical activities, but in reality students perform at a higher level when they know they're going to be graded. (An important exception is the student whose usually competent performance deteriorates due to extreme anxiety about the evaluation process.) For example, the instructor might inform students that her observations during the last two to three weeks of the clinical experience will contribute to the final clinical evaluation.

Standards for Evaluation

The instructor's philosophical perspective contributes greatly to the standards selected for evaluation. Careful consideration of "what matters" enables the instructor to clearly articulate the standards that will be used in evaluating students, and helps to promote consistency in conducting the evaluation.

The clinical evaluation instrument is a beginning point for clarifying the standards to be used in the evaluation process. While the clinical evaluation instrument usually is based on course objectives, few guidelines are available for interpreting these objectives within the context of the clinical practice setting. The rating scale that accompanies the instrument may contain only two categories (pass and fail), or it may be a more elaborate scale. Descriptors of each rating are intended to guide and, to some extent, standardize their use among faculty teaching in the clinical area. For example, a three-point rating scale might contain the following descriptors:

    1 = Is unable to meet objective, even with guidance
    2 = Meets objective most of the time; may require guidance
    3 = Consistently meets objective, with minimal guidance

Similar descriptors, specific to the clinical setting in which the instructor is teaching, might be developed by the instructor for each of the objectives on the clinical evaluation instrument. This exercise helps clarify for the instructor what standards of performance will be used in evaluating students.

In addition to the objectives, model of performance, or other standard adopted by the instructor, the instructor must determine whether the evaluation will be *norm-referenced* or *criterion-referenced*. Norm-referenced evaluation ranks students within their group, requiring the instructor to identify the best and poorest performers and then sort the remaining students within these two poles. Norm-referenced evaluation is ill-suited to the clinical setting, where the goal is for every student to achieve the objectives for the course. Criterion-referenced evaluation rates each student against the standards (criteria) for successful performance, without comparisons among students. Use of criterion-referenced evaluation could result in all students passing—or failing—the clinical experience. Criterion-referenced evaluation also serves as a credible defense against complaints of partiality in grading.

Another consideration in relation to standards for evaluation is the stimuli situations in which students are evaluated. Ideally, the patient for whom the student is providing care during the evaluation will represent a typical patient in that clinical setting, and will require interventions previously practiced by the student. This ideal is seldom achieved, and the instructor must factor in the actual circumstances encountered by the student during the evaluation.

Evaluation Methods

Several factors must be considered in planning an approach to evaluation: sources of data, sampling, scheduling, and instrumentation.

Sources of Data.   Gomez et al. (1998) identify the following sources of data contributing to the evaluation of clinical performance: observation, students' written work, students' oral reports, simulations, and self-evaluation. Observations by the instructor are best recorded in an anecdotal note, which attempts to capture the essence of the observed situation in writing close to the time it occurs, with evaluation of the incident occurring later.[1] (Sample anecdotal notes are shown in Appendix D.) In the college laboratory setting, observations may be guided by an observational checklist of steps in various procedures. Videotaped observations, which can be used for either formative or summative evaluation, are best reserved for the college laboratory. Patient confidentiality issues coupled with logistical problems hamper the use of videotaping for clinical performance observations. Students' written work includes nurses notes and other forms of documentation, written care plans prepared to analyze elements of the patient's situation, completion of observation guides, and other reports related to the clinical experience. Students' oral reports include communications with staff concerning patients as well as participation in conferences and formal presentations related to the clinical experience. Simulations, whether written, videotaped, computer-assisted, or involving the use of models, role-play, or standardized nurse-patient interactions, provide a comparable stimulus situation within a controlled environment that provides stability in the evaluation of student performance. This permits more reliable comparisons across students, particularly important when letter or numerical grading is used in the clinical area. Depending on how they are constructed, simulations also can provide insight into the student's intellectual processes as she deals with the stimulus situation. Self-evaluation materials include student logs or journals, but these should be used only for formative evaluation in order to encourage students' honesty and self-revelation. Students usually are asked to complete the clinical evaluation instrument in relation to their perceptions of their own performance. While these evaluations may result in some overstatement of the student's abilities, the completed form can provide the basis for discussions in a

---

[1]Documentation of an incident that places a student at risk for clinical failure is somewhat different, in that it includes both the evaluation of the recorded behavior in terms of actual or potential effects on the patient and/or health care personnel, steps taken by the instructor to communicate with the student concerning the incident, and the student's response.

student-instructor conference, and may contribute to the instructor's insight concerning the meaning of observed student behaviors.

Sampling.   The instructor is unable to observe all students during the entire clinical experience. Instead, episodes of care are observed. The collection of episodes should reveal a pattern of performance that can form the basis of the evaluation. Episodes of care can be recorded in anecdotal notes that describe the patient situation and the actions of the student in relation to patient needs. The sampling process can be guided by identifying a focus for the day's evaluation activities, for example, assessment techniques or documentation practices. It is essential that the instructor sample episodes of care provided by each student that involve a range of patient situations. Similarly, it is essential to sample equivalent numbers of episodes for each student. When a weaker student is observed more frequently than others, she can rightfully claim differential treatment, even though the instructor's intent is to better monitor performance for safety. It is better to ask a staff member to work with the weaker student while the instructor observes others, or to pair the weaker student with a peer. Sampling techniques in the college laboratory practicum involve sampling the skills that were to be mastered during the semester. Slips of paper indicating the skill (draw medication into a syringe) or skill set (calculate the dosage of medication required, draw the medication into a syringe, locate the correct site for the injection) to be performed are placed in a fishbowl or hat, and drawn at random by students.

Scheduling.   Formative evaluation occurs throughout the clinical experience, but the instructor must demarcate the point at which observations will begin to contribute to the final clinical evaluation. Formative evaluation feedback should be provided as close in time to the stimulating incident as possible, so that the student is able to make appropriate connections between her performance and the instructor's comments. Students should be offered the opportunity to review anecdotal notes at regular intervals, to gain a sense of their overall performance, correct errors, or seek guidance from the instructor if they don't understand a comment or disagree with an observation. In conducting the planned summative evaluation, it is essential to build some flexibility into the planned schedule of observations to account for student absences, an inadequate range of patient situations appropriate for student evaluation, or a rapid change in a patient's condition in the midst of the evaluation process. It is wise to plan to observe episodes of care for all students over the course of the two or three weeks allocated for evaluation. This strategy allows for a better estimate of each student's capabilities and accommodates unexpected disruptions of the evaluation process.

Instrumentation.   It is essential to determine—prior to the start of the clinical experience—how various components and sources of evaluation data will be allocated in computing the final clinical grade. Each of the sources of data to be included in the final evaluation must be scrutinized to ensure that data reflect different aspects of clinical performance (that is, are not redundant) and contribute to the objectives established for the experience. This determination should be agreed upon and applied by all clinical faculty teaching the course. A master form can be used to summarize data collected through anecdotal notes, checklists and rating forms, and graded assignments. Such a form provides explanatory support for the final grade, enabling the instructor to respond to student questions about how the grade was computed.

Analyzing Results

Having collected performance data throughout the clinical experience, the instructor must take time to review the assembled data in order to construct a picture of each student's success in meeting course objectives. Contradictory elements of data, usually indicative of a student's uneven performance or an unusual clinical situation, must be reconciled in some manner to determine whether a preponderance of this evidence supports a passing or failing grade. In analyzing results, the instructor must be careful to discriminate between data reflecting incremental learning by students, as with the progressive development of clinical competence, and data suggestive of an uneven performance that does not improve over time. The instructor will also have to reconcile observed behaviors in the clinical area and written reports revealing the intellectual processes used by the student in providing care. Critical thinking is an essential element of clinical performance; a student's ability to make the intellectual connections evidencing critical thinking should weigh heavily in the overall clinical evaluation.

Although it is a time-consuming process, the instructor is well served to write a brief note describing the student's overall performance in relation to each objective for the clinical experience. Examples of behaviors supporting the description further clarify the data upon which the evaluation is based. This synthesis of data crystallizes the instructor's reasoning concerning each student's level of clinical achievement.

Reporting Results and Making Decisions

Analysis of evaluation data provides the instructor with a fairly certain sense of each student's final grade for the clinical experience, but actual grading should wait until the results of the evaluation process have been reviewed with the student. Comparing the student's self-evaluation with the instructor's clinical evaluation is one means of structuring the conference at which this review is done.

If the instructor has kept the student apprised of progress in the clinical experience, the final evaluation conference will contain no surprises. However, a discussion of those areas in which the student's self-evaluation and the instructor's final evaluation differ, including the rationale of each for the rating, provides a chance for the student to correct any misperceptions that might have occurred and for the instructor to reinforce the standard of behavior in relation to the objective that the student should be striving to achieve. The instructor should remain open to the possibility that errors were made in components of the evaluation that might affect the student's final grade. For example, an error in recording a grade on a major written assignment might be missed if not discussed during the conference as an aspect of the evaluation.

Using Results

The aggregate information concerning each student's performance is reduced to a final grade for the clinical experience. This grade is communicated to the lead instructor of the course for inclusion in computing the final course grade. In most nursing programs, a failure in the clinical component of a course results in a failure in the course. This decision is not made lightly, and the instructor should expect to meet with the lead instructor to review the evaluation data and the rationale for the decision to fail the student. The instructor is likely to have sought feedback and guidance on a student with borderline performance during the ongoing process of clinical evaluation, and the final decision should be no surprise to the lead instructor. A thorough discussion with another knowledgeable nurse educator helps to bolster the instructor's confidence with this difficult decision.

Evaluation results contribute to far more than the final grade the student earns in the clinical component of the course. Formative evaluation, occurring throughout the clinical experience, helps to shape and refine the student's performance. Formative evaluation also informs the student of where she stands in relation to the achievement of course objectives and identifies areas for improvement. Beyond these student-centered uses of evaluation results, the clinical instructor should engage in a continuous dialogue with evaluation data as these are collected, seeking to understand what the results are indicating beyond the assessment of student achievement. Evaluation procedures give the instructor insight into each student's level of ability and aptitude to develop at more advanced levels. (Is this student's assignment too basic? Is she ready to care for several patients?) The evaluation process also provides feedback on whether the instructor's expectations for students are realistic or need to be modified. Evaluation data contribute to the evaluation of the clinical setting as an appropriate source of learning experiences. (Does the clinical provide ample opportunities for students to demonstrate achievement of objectives? Are students truly engaged in the clinical, or is there too much downtime?) Results of evaluation also speak to the success of instructional strategies. (Were off-unit experiences beneficial? Were guidelines for these experiences sufficiently detailed to foster learning?) Oral and written assignments may miss the mark not because of student deficits but because the directions for completing them were unclear.

Evaluating the Evaluation Process

Four elements contribute to the assessment of the evaluation process: technical accuracy, effectiveness, efficiency, and ethical considerations.

Technical Accuracy.   There are three components that contribute to the technical accuracy of the evaluation process. *Validity* refers to the degree to which evaluation procedures and instruments measure what they intend to measure. Within the clinical laboratory, rating forms should be reviewed to ensure that the areas identified on the form reflect appropriate expectations for the level of student and the clinical setting in which they are used. Written assignments intended to elicit critical thinking should be reviewed to ensure that they require interpretation, application, and synthesis of information rather than its rote regurgitation. Within the college laboratory, skills checklists should be reviewed to ensure that identified "critical elements" in performing a skill are indeed "critical" and not reflective of one instructor's approach to the skill. All evaluation instruments miss the mark to some extent; critical assessment of these instruments as they are used helps to refine and improve them. *Reliability* refers to the degree to which evaluation processes remain consistent over time and across students. This aspect of technical accuracy is very difficult to achieve in the clinical setting, but is essential to the unbiased evaluation of students. The clinical instructor must apply the same standards of performance for all students, taking into account differences in the clinical assignment where this is appropriate (for example, where the complexity of patient care requires more assistance than usual, or where the instability of a patient hampers prioritizing). Sampling of episodes of care must be equivalent for all students, in length, number, and frequency of observations. *Practicality* concerns how workable the evaluation process is. Does the evaluation process take too much time away from instructional efforts? Is the clinical evaluation form cumbersome and confusing? Difficulties encountered in conducting the evaluation that are attributable to procedures and instruments can confound the results as well as frustrate the evaluator.

Effectiveness.   To be effective, the evaluation process has to achieve its purposes. The process should provide timely and relevant data on performance that inform the learning and instructional processes and contribute to the final grades awarded to students. To assess effectiveness, review the goals of the evaluation process and determine the degree to which results achieve these goals.

Efficiency.   The time, personnel, and materials used to conduct the evaluation contribute to the assessment of the efficiency of the process. Consider the videotaping of skills performed in the college laboratory setting. This approach to evaluation provides excellent data that can be reviewed by both instructor and student. Review of the tape can pinpoint problems and verify the accuracy of observations. However, the approach is time-consuming (each student's performance must be taped and reviewed), involves additional personnel (someone must man the video camera), and is somewhat expensive in terms of materials (tapes, camera, monitor). The superior results achieved with this approach to evaluation in the laboratory setting must be weighed against these costs.

Ethical Considerations.   Two overriding principles must guide all evaluation efforts. First, the evaluation process must respect the learner. Evaluation should be a positive reinforcer of learning rather than a negative experience that diminishes the learner's self-confidence and self-concept. Second, evaluation outcomes must remain confidential. Except when sharing of data with another instructor is essential for decision making concerning grading, the assessment of the student's performance should remain between instructor and student. (O'Connor, 1986, pp. 260–264)

SUMMARY

Novice instructors find evaluation to be a difficult part of their responsibilities because they have little experience with this aspect of the educator role. An awareness of the multiple dimensions and issues embedded in the evaluation process helps the instructor to make decisions concerning her own conduct of evaluation in the clinical setting. Over time, the process becomes easier to manage and the instructor gains confidence in her judgments concerning students' performance.

REFERENCES

Bourke, M.P.; & Ihrke, B.A. (1998). The evaluation process: An overview. (pp. 349–366). In Billings, D.M.; & Halstead, J.A. *Teaching in nursing: A guide for faculty.* Philadelphia: W.B. Saunders.

Gomez, D.A.; Lobodzinski, S.; & Hartwell West, C.D. (1998). Evaluating clinical performance. (pp. 407–422). In Billings, D.M.; & Halstead, J.A. *Teaching in nursing: A guide for faculty.* Philadelphia: W.B. Saunders.

O'Connor, A.B. (1986). *Nursing staff development and continuing education.* Boston: Little, Brown.

CHAPTER 10

EVALUATION STRATEGIES FOR THE LABORATORY AND CLINICAL PRACTICE SETTINGS

Identifying the Goals of Evaluation   178
Clarifying the Standards for Evaluation   181
Selecting and Applying Evaluation Methods   185
     Observations   185
     Written Work   190
     Oral Presentations   192
     Simulations   192
     Self-Evaluations   193
     Testimonials   194
Analyzing Results   194
Reporting Results   195
     Due Process Issues   195
     Confidentiality Issues   197
Making Decisions   198
Using Results   199
Evaluating the Evaluation Process   199
References   199

The clinical practice component of nursing education, which has evolved from the apprenticeship model established by Nightingale, remains ill defined. Efforts to identify how learning proceeds in the clinical practice setting, as a means to developing instructional approaches that enhance such learning, have attempted to differentiate between learning that occurs as a result of students' "contact" with clinical material and the clinical experience as a means to learn (Monahan, 1991). Nursing educators recognize that not all experiences are educative, and that not all learning requires practical experience with its subject matter. But the tradition of clinical nursing instruction

177

persists, and students identify their clinical experiences as a major contributor to their eventual success in the profession (Davidhizar & McBride, 1985).

Two potential outcomes of the learning that occurs in laboratory and clinical practice settings seem to capture the multiple goals for clinical experiences in nursing education programs: the demonstration of accurate clinical nursing judgments and the development of a professional identity (Woolley et al., 1998). These outcomes seem possible to achieve only in the reality-based setting of clinical practice. Benner's (1984) model of skill acquisition suggests that experience is essential for the development of the expertise that leads to accurate clinical nursing judgments. The abstract principles and rules that the student learns in the classroom are challenged by the realities presented in the clinical setting, enabling the student to transform principles into paradigms that eventually guide practice. This "perspective transformation" takes place over time, based on accumulated clinical experiences. The development of a professional identity occurs as the student's self-concept as a nurse is transformed through the mastery of nursing skills (Monahan, 1991).

Given the difficulty in articulating how learning occurs in the clinical practice setting, and the fact that "clinical performance of students in nursing is a complex phenomenon comprised of aptitudes, abilities, cognitions, skills, and affect" (Kirchbaum et al., 1994, p. 397), it is not surprising that the evaluation of clinical learning poses problems for the instructor. These problems include balancing instruction, supervision, and evaluation; differentiating between diagnostic evaluation, intended to assist the learner to develop further, and grading (also termed *formative* and *summative* evaluation, respectively); recognizing the limits of objectivity and the necessity for subjectivity in clinical evaluation; ensuring reliability and validity in measuring performance; managing the unsafe or failing student; providing for due process; and avoiding discriminatory practices. A clear understanding of the evaluation process (see Table 10–1) as it is applied to the evaluation of students' clinical performance can guide the clinical instructor in making sound judgments that meet the procedural standards required in the academic setting. Critical to the use of the evaluation process is clear, timely communication of expectations and feedback on performance.

IDENTIFYING THE GOALS OF EVALUATION

The goals established for clinical learning form the basis of the clinical evaluation of students. These must be clearly articulated to students, along with a description of the progressive steps toward those goals that should occur during the course of the clinical experience. When the instructor communicates the goals for clinical learning, makes these seem feasible, and expresses a desire to facilitate students' success in the clinical experience, students are motivated to achieve, and know what behaviors they are striving toward. This approach empowers students and makes the clinical experience exciting rather than fearsome.

TABLE 10-1   THE EVALUATION PROCESS

- Identify the goals of evaluation.
- Clarify the standards for evaluation.
- Select and apply evaluation methods.
- Analyze results.
- Report results.
- Make decisions.
- Use results.
- Evaluate the evaluation process.

The ultimate goal of evaluation is to determine whether or not the student has attained an acceptable level of achievement in performing expected behaviors, usually articulated through the course objectives. The clinical instructor's goals for clinical learning usually reflect some abbreviated version of these objectives, and may be conceptualized as success in problem solving, demonstrated skill mastery, evidence of behaviors critical to job success, behavior conforming to the standards of practice as an accountable, responsible professional, safety, or some combination of these. Consistency of performance plus growth throughout the clinical experience often serve as touchstones for performance evaluation (Orchard, 1994). The student's goals for learning, while important to her sense of success, are seldom incorporated into the clinical evaluation.

The evaluation of a student's clinical performance necessarily involves both objective and subjective judgments. Certain behaviors are amenable to objective appraisal (whether or not a medication was charted accurately or the performance of the critical steps in a procedure, for example), but most clinical actions require complex goals and strategies and evidence a high level of abstraction. Often, several alternative courses of action are acceptable, placing the focus of evaluation on the student's decision-making process as well as observed behavior (Orchard, 1992). These more complex, intellectual activities—so essential to the development of clinical judgment and to success in clinical nursing situations—can only be evaluated subjectively. Wilhite (1990) asserts that all grading is subjective, because any evaluation is based on what the evaluator thinks is important.

The instructor must provide timely feedback on each student's performance so students can recognize and expeditiously correct their errors during the course. This feedback is the result of a diagnostic, or formative, evaluation process that assesses the student's strengths and weaknesses at a given point in time, and suggests how to improve performance.

Diagnostic evaluation is embedded in the instructional role because it guides the teaching effort. Previous learning is reinforced by the identification of positive behaviors and those requiring improvement. Feedback on skill performance can mold psychomotor skills as the student develops mastery of the technical aspects of practice. When diagnostic evaluation reveals that all students are having similar difficulty with a concept or skill, the instructor learns that a review is necessary and can structure this into a pre- or postconference session.

Diagnostic evaluation also contributes to the instructor's supervisory role. When repeated observations of a student's performance indicate problems, the instructor is alerted to a need for increased supervision or other intervention to support student learning. Brooke (1994) asserts,

> A major responsibility of clinical faculty members is the correct and early detection of students who are clinically unsafe. Once this discovery is made, the faculty member has the duty to supervise this student more closely. This is not harassment or discrimination, but rather sound professional judgment. (p. 252)

Communicating to the student the behaviors that make her practice unsafe, and therefore requiring additional supervision, helps the student to recognize problems and provides the opportunity for remediation. The instructor may seek the assistance of staff or a student-peer in working with the student who requires more than the usual amount of supervision; however, she must periodically reassess the situation to monitor the student's progress (or lack of progress) toward safe practice. Offering the student opportunities to improve performance (the goal of clinical instruction) must be balanced with the need to remove the student from the clinical area if her performance continues to jeopardize patient safety. "The longer a faculty [member] waits to remove an unsafe student from a course, the more difficult it becomes to deny the student the right to progress." (Brooke, 1994, p. 253)

Diagnostic evaluation also is essential to ensuring due process in evaluation practices. Feedback on performance lets the student know where she stands in relation to overall expectations for clinical learning. Providing guidelines for improvement gives the student a chance to overcome deficits. Misperceptions concerning a student's performance can be identified along the way, instead of at the end of the clinical experience during the final evaluation conference.

While feedback is essential, the instructor should avoid labeling a student's performance with an interim grade, unless this is required by nursing program policies at a point midway through the experience. Students' clinical performances fluctuate greatly during the course of the semester, and a satisfactory performance at the start of the clinical experience may deteriorate over time. Similarly, the weaker student may advance dramatically toward the end of the semester. The ability to perform a clinical action and consistently doing it as part of a clinical experience are two different matters; the instructor should avoid implying that a single instance of success (or failure) is all that will be considered in evaluating the student's overall performance. Providing feedback that includes a tentative grade creates an expectation in the student that may not be realized at the end of the course. Instead, feedback should be framed in terms of relative progress toward the goals for learning and should include comment on behaviors the student should seek to further develop or add to her clinical repertoire.

Grading is the final outcome of the evaluation process, and represents the results of summative evaluation. At this point, the student's performance is assessed against the goals for the experience, and a judgment made as to whether the student has or has not succeeded in achieving these. Students must be alerted to the point in time when evaluation procedures take this shift. The pattern of performance observed over the course of the clinical experience, especially the student's consistency in practice and progress toward goal achievement, will figure largely in the final evaluation, but there is a point in time at which goals must be achieved in order for the student to pass the course.

CLARIFYING THE STANDARDS FOR EVALUATION

Clinical instructors must make two professional judgments about student performance: whether the student has met course objectives and whether the student can safely provide care (Orchard, 1994). In making these judgments, the instructor must apply an appropriate set of standards for performance to each critical behavior or learning outcome desired at the end of the clinical experience, and apply these standards consistently across students.

Goals set forth those behaviors expected to be mastered by students as a result of the learning that has occurred during the clinical experience; standards identify the level of performance achieved by the student for each identified goal. Standards describe the hallmarks of an exceptional, average, mediocre, or failing performance. While students cannot expect equivalency of evaluation procedures across clinical areas and with different instructors, they should know the "ground" below which problems occur, as well as what marks a superior level of performance.

A degree of objectivity in applying standards to the evaluation of students' clinical performance can be achieved by creating a "snapshot" of the superior, adequate, and failing student. Written descriptions that depict each level of potential student performance further support the instructor's efforts to apply standards consistently. Care must be taken not to set performance standards based on the actions that would be taken by a nurse with several years' experience, or what the instructor would do. Rather, standards must be geared to the progressive development of skillful performance appropriate to the student's level in the program; that is, they must be valid for the level of student being evaluated as well as the clinical setting in which learning experiences take place.

Reliability in the application of standards is facilitated by the use of rating scales. Rating scales describe various aspects (e.g., consistency of behavior, amount of guidance needed, time required to complete tasks) of each objective or learning outcome selected for evaluation. Definitions of the components of each performance standard help in the use of the rating scale. Table 10–2 provides an example of standards established for various levels of performance in clinical experiences at the University of Minnesota School of Nursing (Krichbaum et al., 1994). A midlevel performance ("assisted" in this typology) may be acceptable for a beginning student, but inadequate for a senior student in a clinical practicum experience. Such terms as "assisted" and "supervised" must be distinguished from the student's appropriate request for guidance, which should be encouraged. If little or no supervision is the criterion that distinguishes superior performance, students may fail to seek guidance when it is needed, jeopardizing patient safety. Similarly, if the instructor has identified a student's need for supervision, the student might claim that she could have functioned more independently if only the instructor had given her the opportunity to do so. In using the rating scale in conjunction with course objectives, the instructor must determine how ratings are to be used in making grading decisions. For example, will a "provisional" or "dependent" performance for any one of the objectives result in a failure in the clinical component of the course, or must a majority of objectives be rated at a low level to justify a clinical failure. The use of ratings in determining final grades should be agreed upon by all faculty teaching in the course.

Certain elements critical to minimally safe practice may be identified as overriders. These are elements that must be present whenever a skill is performed. Table 10–3 defines the behaviors involved in the overriders selected by faculty at the School of Nursing at Miami-Dade Community College (Woolley

---

TABLE 10–2   LEVELS OF STUDENT PERFORMANCE IN CLINICAL PRACTICE

Independent
- Performs safely and accurately each time behavior is observed without supportive cues from the preceptor/instructor.
- Demonstrates dexterity.
- Spends minimal time on task. .
- Appears relaxed and confident during performance of task.
- Applies theoretical knowledge accurately each time.
- Focuses on client while giving care.

Supervised
- Performs safely and accurately each time behavior is observed.
- Requires a supportive or directive cue occasionally during performance of task.

TABLE 10–2 CONTINUED
<hr>

- Demonstrates coordination, but uses some unnecessary energy to complete behavior/activity.
- Spends reasonable time on task.
- Appears generally relaxed and confident; occasional anxiety may be noticeable.
- Applies theoretical knowledge accurately with occasional cues.
- Focuses on client initially; as complexity increases, focuses on task.

Assisted
- Performs safely and accurately each time observed.
- Requires frequent supportive and occasional directive cues.
- Demonstrates partial lack of skill and/or dexterity in part of activity; awkward.
- Takes longer time to complete task; occasionally late.
- Appears to waste energy due to poor planning.
- Identifies principles, but needs direction to identify application.
- Focuses primarily on task or own behavior, not on client.

Provisional
- Performs safely under supervision, not always accurate.
- Requires continuous supportive and directive cues.
- Demonstrates lack of skill; uncoordinated in majority of behavior.
- Performs tasks with considerable delay; activities are disrupted or omitted.
- Wastes energy due to incompetence.
- Identifies fragments of principles; applies principles inappropriately.
- Focuses entirely on task or own behavior.

Dependent
- Performs in an unsafe manner; unable to demonstrate behavior.
- Requires continuous supportive and directive cues.
- Performs in an unskilled manner; lacks organization.
- Appears frozen, unable to move, nonproductive.
- Unable to identify principles or apply them.
- Attempts activity or behavior, yet is unable to complete.
- Focuses entirely on task or own behavior.

<hr>

Source: Krichbaum, K.; Rowan, M.; Duckett, L.; Ryden, M.B.; & Savik, K. (1994). The clinical evaluation tool: A measure of the quality of clinical performance of baccalaureate nursing students. *Journal of Nursing Education, 33*, 399. Used with permission.

TABLE 10–3   DEFINITION OF TERMS RELATED TO OVERRIDERS

Overriders: The specific nursing competencies inherent in the safe performance of all skills. Overriders must be demonstrated in all aspects of nursing care.

Asepsis

- Washes hands in the presence of the examiner before and after each client situation and each skill.
- Follows universal precautions.
- Protects self and others from contamination by microorganisms.
- Uses a sterile field when necessary.
- Disposes of contaminated articles in designated containers.

Communication

- Verifies written orders.
- Checks clients' name bands.
- Provides privacy.
- Explains procedure(s) to clients.
- Reports changes in clients' conditions.
- Documents findings.
- Uses verbal and nonverbal communication that demonstrates respect, understanding, and caring.
- Avoids abusive, threatening, patronizing, or familiar communication patterns.

Safety

- Demonstrates principles of body mechanics.
- Raises side rails when beds are in an elevated position or clients are in need of protection.
- Keeps environment free of potentially harmful elements (e.g., cleans up spills, avoids electrical hazards).
- Protects clients from temperature extremes.
- Provides care consistent with knowledge gained from previous courses.
- Uses universal precautions.

Source: Based on Wooley, G.R.; Bryan, M.S.; & Davis, J.W. (1998). A comprehensive approach to clinical evaluation. *Journal of Nursing Education*, 37, 362. Used with permission.

et al., 1998). It might be assumed that failure to demonstrate safe practice in relation to these overriders would result in a failure on the objective being rated, but faculty in the course must agree on how many instances of unsafe practice will result in a failure in the course. Providing opportunities for remediation is essential to ensure the due process rights of students. Consequently, some breaches of minimal safety requirements must be tolerated in the earlier phases of the clinical experience.

SELECTING AND APPLYING EVALUATION METHODS

Because the goals for clinical learning include higher-level cognitive, psychomotor, and affective objectives, and combinations of these, it is logical that multiple methods of evaluation be used to assess student achievement. Each source of information used in the final evaluation should contribute in some way to the assessment of student achievement of one or more course objectives, with all objectives represented in the final set of measures selected.

In identifying assignments, the instructor must be clear as to whether the work is intended to foster student development, in which case evaluation of the assignment will be formative in nature, or will contribute to the final grade. In some instances, assignments designed to guide instruction also may provide evidence of the student's progressive development. For example, clinical logs or journals that record the student's thought processes as she reflects on the care she has provided may reveal refinement of critical thinking skills. Note, however, that grading of logs and journals can hinder students' free expression of their reactions to clinical situations, which is the goal of such assignments. Use of such materials in the final evaluation should be limited to evidence of progress in the process of critical thinking or reflective practice rather than the content of the writing. When assignments serve such a dual function (both formative and summative evaluation), students should be alerted to this at the onset of the clinical experience. Written guidelines should include all of the elements that will contribute to the final evaluation, including their proportional weight in determining the final grade.

Sources of information that may contribute to student evaluation include observations, students' written work, students' oral reports, simulations, and self-evaluations (Gomez et al., 1998). When the instructor systematically rates and records the information derived from these sources, they become evaluation instruments, and should be assessed for validity and reliability. (Validity refers to the degree to which an instrument measures what it is intended to measure. In this context, validity refers to the degree to which an observation or assignment contributes to the assessment of student achievement of one or more course objectives. Reliability refers to the degree to which the instrument measures what it measures consistently, across students. Reliability is best assured by developing grading criteria for each assignment and then using these criteria—and only these—in evaluating student work.)

Observations

The instructor's observation of students as they carry out clinical assignments probably contributes most to the overall evaluation of students' clinical performance. Observations consider the contextual aspects of the situation in which the student is operating (e.g., relative complexity of care being provided, interruptions that interfere with timely completion of the assignment), allowing the instructor to make appropriate adjustments in her assessment of the student. The degree of caring exhibited by the student in interactions with the patient, the patient's comfort level while the student administers treatments, the accuracy of the student's assessments concerning the patient's responses to his illness and its treatment, and the processes used by the student in discharge teaching are some examples of clinical performance that are most amenable to assessment through observation.

Anecdotal Notes.   Anecdotal notes are the means by which data obtained through observations are recorded for later evaluation. (Sample anecdotal notes are shown in Appendix D.) An anecdotal note should capture the following data:

- student who is the subject of the evaluation;
- patient or patients for whom the student is providing care during the observation (using patients' first names or initials to preserve confidentiality);
- pertinent elements of the patient's condition, such as medical diagnosis, current status, treatment requirements, nursing diagnoses;
- brief description of what care the patient required during the observation;
- description of what the student did or failed to do in providing necessary care (e.g., Alma gathered the necessary supplies for the dressing change prior to entering the patient's room. She explained the procedure to the patient and provided for privacy. The dressing change was completed without a breach in technique. Alma accurately recorded the status of the wound in the patient's chart.); and
- description of any contextual variables that contributed to the observed situation (e.g., Bella's attempts to provide morning care for the patient were interrupted by visits from the house staff, the patient's attending physician, and a technician taking a portable x-ray).

Not all observations need to involve student-patient interactions. For example, the instructor may elicit from the student her plan of approach to the day's activities or a verbal report about what is going on with a patient in the student's care. Evidence of the student's preparation, critical thinking, or decision-making processes might then become the material for an anecdotal note (e.g., Although she had received report from the primary nurse, and had visited with the patient, Clara was unaware that the patient had developed a spontaneous pneumothorax the previous evening, requiring the insertion of a chest tube).

While observations are subjective in nature, the anecdotal note should be free of value judgments. Instead, the note should record what occurred, including any observed omissions (e.g., Despite a verbal reminder by the primary nurse to check the patient's IV site and the intravenous drip rate, Dora

did not do so during the observed interaction with the patient, requiring a reminder from the instructor).

An equivalent number of observations should be recorded for each student, both to adequately assess each student's performance and to counter
charges of discrimination in evaluation practices. Ideally, a note on every student in the group should be made every clinical session; however, the realities of the clinical environment, and the need for the instructor to balance
evaluation with instruction and supervision, make this virtually impossible.
Both positive and negative observations should be recorded, even for the
borderline student. When these are observed in a single situation, both positive and negative observations may appear in the same note. If the observed
performance is atypical for the student, a note to this effect might be made,
although the instructor should follow-up with the student to determine what
other factors might be operating in the situation.

Having made the note, the instructor should provide verbal feedback to
the student, commenting on the positive aspects of the care and correcting
any errors or omissions that were observed. Students also should have periodic access to the anecdotal notes themselves, as a means of tracking their
own progress in the clinical experience.

To supplement the observations recorded in anecdotal notes, the instructor should keep notes on each student's assignment for each clinical session.
These notes should briefly capture core elements of the care each assignment
required, along with a note as to why this assignment was selected for this student. While this "history" of clinical assignments is useful in balancing assignments among students and ensuring that each has the opportunity to achieve
course objectives and master required skills, the clinical assignments data are
also useful in determining whether students consistently met the challenges
presented in the assignments or whether some assignments had to be modified for less capable students. The record of clinical assignments also can help
to defend the instructor's decision to fail a student, who then claims that she
was given the most difficult assignments.

Incident Reports.   Anecdotal notes should not be used to report incidents
of unsafe performance, although incident reports will form part of the student's overall evaluation record. Incident reports should include the data
gathered for anecdotal notes, but also note the actual or potential effect of the
student's actions or omissions on patient safety, any intervention done to protect the patient (e.g., the instructor completed the procedure for the student;
the student was removed from the clinical area and responsibility for the patient's care returned to the primary nurse), and the plan for meeting with the
student to provide feedback and, where appropriate, develop a plan for remediation. While immediate feedback on the problematic behavior must be
communicated to the student, any lengthy discussion should occur after the
clinical day is concluded. Selecting a time and place apart from the clinical
setting diffuses the situation for both the instructor and the student, prevents

the discussion from being overheard by others in the clinical area, and frees the instructor to continue to work with the other students in the group.

At the earliest possible time following the incident, the student and instructor should meet to review the incident report. Both the instructor and the student should sign the report to confirm that the meeting took place. If the student disputes the report, she should be encouraged to write down her own evaluation of the situation. This evaluation should be filed with the original incident report. A plan for remediation or enhanced supervision should be developed with the student if this will contribute to improved performance. For example, the student might be counseled to practice changing a sterile dressing in the college laboratory, and contact the instructor to demonstrate her technique before the next clinical session. Enhanced supervision might involve a requirement that the student have the instructor present when she next attempts a sterile dressing change. A record of the conference, along with the signed evaluation plan, should be filed with the incident report.

The recording of an incident and the counseling that follows such an event protect the due process rights of the student. If no further incidents occur following counseling and remediation, the incident report can be ignored in the final evaluation of the student's performance. It is the accumulation of incidents, without improvement by the student, that support a decision to fail a student or remove her from the clinical area. If identification of the problem and supportive intervention achieve their goals, the student should not be penalized for errors that accompany learning.

Rating Scales.   Rating scales provide a summary of accumulated observations of students' clinical performance. These scales usually comprise the course objectives accompanied by standards of performance (such as those outlined in Table 10–2) or a three- to five-point ranking system (such as unmet, partially met, fully met) which the instructor uses to rate performance. If the scale does not provide descriptors of the types of behaviors that constitute each level of performance in relation to each objective, the instructor should attempt to construct such descriptors to ensure the validity of the instrument for the clinical setting in which she is teaching and the reliability of her use of the scale across students.

Instructors with limited experience in using the clinical rating scale adopted for the course should fill out the form periodically for each student based on observations in the clinical area and/or anecdotal notes collected thus far. Reflection on the intellectual processes used in completing the scale (and, sometimes, gut-level reactions to the results) can alert the instructor to potential problems in using the scale to evaluate students. This awareness may prompt a more thorough consideration of what behaviors and level of ability the instructor expects for students in the clinical group.

External Raters.   Because evaluation processes can interfere with the instructional and supervisory responsibilities of the instructor (and cloud the evaluation), some programs seek the input of others into the observation of student performance. Anderson and Knuteson (1990) report on a program used at Alverno College, in which two practicing nurses observe students in the clinical area at the end of the junior and senior year, providing evaluations of each student's ability to use the nursing process, to interact effectively with others, and actions reflecting respect for the dignity of others. This evaluation is then factored into the total evaluation of the student's clinical performance.

A more conventional approach to using others in evaluating students' clinical performance seeks "another look" at a student by a clinical instructor teaching in the same course who has not worked with the student previously. This process usually is reserved for the borderline or failing student whose clinical failure would result in dismissal from the nursing program, or when the clinical instructor is concerned that the student's performance to date may be biasing the instructor's ability to provide a fair evaluation. The student joins the second faculty member's clinical group and is given a regular assignment. Expectations for the student's performance are established in advance in a conference with the student. Two to three clinical days may be required to conduct an adequate second evaluation; consequently, the evaluation should occur before the end of the semester. A final decision on performance is made by the lead instructor of the course, in consultation with both clinical instructors.

Skills Checklists.   Skills checklists have their primary use in the college laboratory. Such lists detail the sequential steps to be executed when performing a technical skill. Certain steps are labeled as "critical" to the safe or effective performance of the skill. Failure to perform these steps results in a failure on the skill. Because they provide clear instructions on how a skill is to be performed, skills checklists can serve as a teaching device for students learning a skill as well as an evaluation device for verifying that the student has at least beginning ability in performing the skill. The drawback of skills checklists is that they do not allow for variations in technique, but the beginning student is best introduced to one approach to the skill rather than confused with alternatives. The identification of critical steps signals aspects of the skill that are essential regardless of technique and those that might be modified.

Observation of the student as she performs a skill is recorded on the checklist. There are several approaches to this observation. The instructor can observe each student as she performs each skill to be mastered for the course. Alternatively, a skills examination can be set up to randomly assign skills under the assumption that the student who is prepared to perform one skill is likely to be prepared to perform others.

Peer instruction is an approach that saves the instructor considerable time in both teaching skills and in evaluating students. Students are taught each skill, either by the instructor or through mediated instruction (films, videotapes, computer instruction), and practice the skill in the college laboratory. When a student feels ready to be examined on the skill, the instructor observes her and verifies performance using the skills checklist. The student is then identified as a peer instructor, who both assists other students in learning the skill and then verifies their performance using the checklist. As each student "passes" the skill, she becomes a peer instructor to the other students who are still struggling to master the technique. In addition to freeing the instructor to assist students who are having particular difficulty with the skill, the peer instructional approach acknowledges prior skills learning by students who work as nursing assistants or licensed practical nurses as well as the differences in technical aptitude among students. Students may be more relaxed in learning from their peers, and the act of instruction reinforces and clarifies the technique for the peer instructor. Periodic checks by the instructor can assure that technique has not lapsed as the chain of peer instructors lengthens.

Still another approach involves videotaping the student's skill performance, and then rating the tape against the skills checklist. This alternative allows the instructor to rate performances at a time apart from the laboratory session, and also provides a review for the student, who can watch her own performance and identify breaks in technique.

Written Work.   Students' written work reveals the intellectual processes that guide students' clinical performance. While students often feel burdened by multiple written assignments, their use reinforces the notion that nursing is as much about thinking as about doing. These assignments also may prevent the development of habitual, rote practice that is disengaged with its subject matter—the patient. Of course, some students fail to integrate the written work with the clinical assignment. This usually is revealed when the student is asked to talk about what she is doing. Written work is, at the same time, a teaching strategy and an evaluation strategy. Thoughtful feedback on written assignments provides formative evaluation that can further the student's insights regarding practice. If a record of ungraded assignments is maintained by the instructor, the cumulative performance of the student on these assignments can contribute to summative evaluation as an indicator of the development of critical thinking ability as well as professional accountability. A simple recording device might be developed by the instructor with reference to such assignments. For example, a satisfactory rating (S) might be recorded for work that is complete, accurate, and submitted on time. A pass rating (P) might be recorded for work that meets basic requirements or is improved after guidance from the instructor. An unsatisfactory rating (U) might be recorded for work that is incomplete, inaccurate, is uncorrected even after guidance is provided, or that is submitted late. Some portion of the overall clinical grade should be attributed to such assignments, as an indication of their value in the process of clinical learning. Written assignments intended to integrate theory and practice, such as a major nursing care plan, usually must be completed by all students in a course and carry a grade that contributes to either the course grade or the clinical grade. Detailed grading criteria should be developed collaboratively by all faculty teaching in the course, so that similar standards are applied to all students.

Observation Guides.   Guidelines for observing an off-unit experience are intended to focus the student's attention on aspects of the experience related to course objectives. (Samples of such guides appear in Appendix G.) For example, a student assigned to attend a class on how to stop smoking might be guided to observe and comment on the role of the instructor, the group process, and the teaching-learning process. A student observing a surgical procedure might be guided to observe and comment on the role of the nurse in the operative setting, and aspects of the surgical experience that suggest nursing measures to be taken postoperatively. Another form of observation guides focus students' attention on some aspect of patient care. For example, assessment guides stimulate the student to perform a physical assessment, nutritional assessment, or family assessment.

Process Recordings.   Process recordings capture interpersonal interactions between the student and another person, usually a patient. Their purpose is to focus the student's attention on the communication processes used in the interaction as a means to fine-tune the student's communication skills. Often the clinical instructor can pick up nuances in the interaction that the student has missed. Pointing these out helps to develop the student's sensitivity to verbal and nonverbal cues from the communication partner, as well as her own behaviors as they affect the interaction.

Nursing Care Plans.   Two forms of nursing care plans are used in clinical teaching. Brief nursing care plans focus on one or two nursing diagnoses that the student has identified for emphasis during the clinical day. Assessment factors contributing to the diagnosis; objectives and goals for the patient; planned interventions, including a rationale for each activity; and evaluation approaches are detailed by the student. The plan may be derived from the student's previous work with the patient, or from the patient's record and the nursing care plan developed by staff. Students should not be required to reinvent the care plan. They should be required to understand the rationale for the plan elements, so that they can independently assess the accuracy of the nursing diagnoses, the suitability of nursing interventions, and the patient's progress toward identified goals.

Most nursing programs use a standardized format for the nursing care plan, which cues the student to the elements of the nursing process. The form usually includes space for evaluation of the plan following implementation, as well as evaluation of patient progress toward goals. In using brief nursing care plans as a device for student preparation for the clinical experience, the instructor may elect to focus on some element of the nursing process, such as assessment factors contributing to nursing diagnoses, rather than the entire plan. The instructor also may modify the focus of the plan, for example, by having students complete a nursing care plan pertinent to the medications the patient is receiving.

The major nursing care plan details the application of the nursing process for all nursing diagnoses identified for a selected patient. Here, students are expected to provide greater detail in their elaboration of rationales, as well as support from the literature for their assertions and conclusions. The purpose of this assignment, to demonstrate the student's ability to integrate theory and practice, is defeated when students rely entirely on published standardized care plans. While such plans may serve as a base for the student's work, the emphasis should be on individualizing the plan for the patient.

Documentation.   Students' documentation practices must be monitored by the instructor to ensure their accuracy and completeness, the appropriate use of abbreviations, notation, and technical language, and timeliness. For beginning students, drafts of nurses notes can be reviewed by the instructor prior to their entry into the patient's record. Alternatively, notes can be developed for submission to the primary nurse, who remains responsible for documentation. A student's failure to document usually is brought to the instructor's attention after the clinical session has ended. The instructor must follow-up with the student to emphasize the importance of documentation to the patient's safety and continuity of care.

Oral Presentations
Oral presentations include communication with staff and with the instructor, active participation in pre- and postconferences, and formal presentations. Except for formal presentations, which can be graded in accordance with written evaluation criteria, it is difficult to objectively measure and record the caliber of students' oral reports and comments. Indeed, it is rare for these to be formally considered in the evaluation process, despite the centrality of communication skills to nursing practice and the effect that a student's communication style has on the instructor's subjective evaluation of her performance. When it is evaluated, assessment of the communication component of a student's practice often is confined to interactions with patients. However, effective communication with staff is essential to the nurse's advocacy role, and active involvement in conferences provides evidence of participation in the group process. In both types of interactions—those with other health care providers and those with student peers—effective communication is central to the demonstration of leadership in the clinical setting. Anecdotal notes that capture the quality of students' oral communication with staff and periodic analysis of the group process as it occurs in the conference that follows the clinical experience can yield data on students' communication skills as a reflection of the achievement of objectives related to advocacy, group process, and leadership.

Simulations
Simulations present students with a clinical situation to which they must respond. The use of simulations as part of the evaluation process standardizes the stimuli to which students are exposed, providing stability that contributes to reliability and objectivity in evaluating performance. Simulations may be

written, videotaped, computer-assisted, or involve the use of models and mannequins or live actors.

An example of a written simulation is the case study, which presents clinical data for the student to analyze. Questions are posed concerning the data and appropriate nursing actions to be taken in response to the data. The student's verbal or written response is evaluated for accuracy. Videotaped simulations provide similar data in a video format, permitting the inclusion of data elements that test the students' observation skills. Again, a verbal or written response to questions concerning the depicted situation is the basis for evaluation. Computer-assisted simulations utilizing an interactive format present basic clinical situations. The student must ask for additional data to reveal further aspects of the case and respond appropriately to data indicating a need for nursing action. In addition to assessing the student's knowledge base, computer-assisted simulations can provide data concerning the student's decision-making processes.

The use of models and/or mannequins to create simulated situations is a common approach to evaluation in the college laboratory. Typical of such simulations is testing skills in cardiopulmonary resuscitation (CPR) using Resusci-Annie. Sophisticated mannequins are available that provide variable data in response to students' actions. Observations of students as they perform skills with models or mannequins usually are recorded in a checklist format.

The use of actors to present stimuli to students is the form of simulation most closely aligned with clinical practice, lending validity to the evaluation process along with reliability in presenting similar stimuli to all students. The student is required to assess the "patient" and identify appropriate nursing diagnoses in response to elicited data. A "chart" containing laboratory and other test results may be available if the student requests these. The student also may be asked to develop a plan of care in collaboration with the "patient," or do health teaching suggested by the data. The interaction may be videotaped for later analysis, or an observer may rate the interaction as it occurs. Any written component of the simulation (for example, the care plan or nurses note recording results of a physical examination) is evaluated in accord with preestablished criteria.

Self-Evaluations

Students' self-evaluations of their performance can provide valuable insights for the instructor. Students often are asked to complete the clinical evaluation form at midway through the clinical experience, as a self-assessment device. Discussions with students concerning their ratings and their perceptions of their performance in the clinical setting provide an opportunity for the instructor to structure feedback and identify areas in which the student might enhance her performance.

More than a picture of how the student rates herself in relation to course objectives (the most common approach to self-evaluation), the student's expression of her thoughts about the clinical experience can reveal problem-solving and decision-making skills, critical thinking abilities, areas of practice that pose problems the student would like to overcome, and experiences the student would like to have in the clinical setting. These expressions are best elicited in a clinical log or journal that is maintained on an ongoing basis by the student. By posing general questions to consider in writing an entry, the instructor can guide the content of the log or journal so that it represents more than a factual accounting of the day's experiences. The instructor should collect the logs regularly, and provide written feedback on their contents. This feedback should strive to create a dialogue with each student that supports the expression of thoughts and the posing of questions. When students reveal their decision-making processes, the instructor gains insight into what she has observed in the clinical setting. When students ask questions about aspects of the clinical experience or ask for a more or less challenging assignment, the instructor can better shape the learning experiences to meet student needs.

Testimonials

Frequently, the clinical instructor will be approached by patients, their families, staff members, other students, and students' significant others to provide information related to a student's clinical performance. Except for information provided by staff members, these testimonials have little to contribute to the evaluation process. Patients and their families can be encouraged to write a brief note concerning the student to the department chair, and be assured that the note will be placed in the student's file. Students should be discouraged from commenting on other student's performance unless an immediate safety concern arises. Family members and friends of students also should be politely discouraged from contributing comments concerning a student's performance.

Staff members often have important insights concerning student performance, and can be a safety check for the harried instructor. In considering staff comments on student performance, the instructor should accept the input and then validate the observation for herself. Staff members have a different set of expectations for student performance than the instructor does, as well as a different frame of reference for evaluating performance. Their input alerts the instructor to potential problems, but should not color her own evaluation of the student's clinical competence.

ANALYZING RESULTS

After assembling the data collected throughout the clinical experience, the instructor must consider whether, taken together, the evaluation data indicate that the student has progressed toward meeting the course objectives and has demonstrated achievement of these objectives by the final clinical session. Data might be grouped based on these objectives, enabling the instructor to rate the student's performance in relation to each objective. The instructor also will analyze the data to derive a more general sense of the student's clinical performance. For example, has the student demonstrated at least a minimal level of competence in meeting course objectives? Has the student demonstrated growth and development of knowledge, skills, competence, and confidence throughout the experience? Has the student demonstrated the knowledge and skills necessary to move forward to the next program level? Is the student's practice safe?

REPORTING RESULTS

In addition to completing the clinical evaluation form in accordance with the rating criteria, the instructor should take the time to write a description of each student's performance as a whole and in relation to each objective.

The act of writing descriptive statements requires the instructor to reflect on the accumulated data and crystallize her impressions of each student's performance. The written evaluation also provides feedback to students that is more useful than a simple rating. Students naturally will be relieved to learn they passed the clinical portion of the course, but they want and need more information on how well they are developing toward their goal of entering the profession as competent nurses.

Written descriptive evaluations provide valuable information to instructors who will have the student in subsequent clinical experiences. They also provide input for faculty who are later asked to write letters of recommendation about a student's clinical skills. Such descriptions also contribute to the program's self-evaluation by tracking students' growth and development through successive courses and clinical experiences. This is particularly important in relation to data describing the progressive development of students' critical thinking skills, because this is a major area assessed during program accreditation reviews despite the fact that there are few—if any—valid and reliable instruments to measure this.

Due Process Issues

With respect to academic performance, due process concerns the right of students to know what they must do to successfully complete a course (the faculty responsibility is to communicate these expectations); to receive timely feedback on their performance, especially if it fails to meet expectations; and to be told the consequences of their continued failure to meet expectations (Halstead, 1998). Providing the opportunity for the student to remediate, or improve, performance often is identified as a component of due process, as is informing students of their rights under any established grade review or appeal procedures. Guidelines for providing academic due process for students are shown in Table 10–4. The clinical instructor must be familiar with the program's provisions for due process and procedures for grade appeal, as well as

TABLE 10–4   GUIDELINES FOR PROVIDING ACADEMIC DUE PROCESS
FOR STUDENTS

- Clearly communicate student and faculty rights in student and faculty handbooks.
- Systematically review catalogs, handbooks, and so on to determine whether they are up-to-date with current policies and procedures.
- Course requirements and expectations should be clearly established at the beginning of the course.
- Maintain all tests and written work in files until the student has successfully fulfilled program or course requirements.
- Students should have the opportunity to view all evaluation data that are placed in their student file.
- When the potential for course failure or dismissal exists, students should receive notification of their academic deficiencies.

Source: From Halstead, J.A. (1998). The academic performance of students; Legal and ethical issues. (pp. 39–41). In Billings, D.M.; & Halstead, J.A. *Teaching in nursing: A guide for faculty*. Philadelphia: W.B. Saunders. Used with permission.

policies concerning grading practices, progression in the program, graduation, and dismissal from the program.

As soon as problems in clinical performance are detected, inform the student verbally and in writing of the observed behaviors. Provide detailed information concerning the episode, including an explanation of how the behavior failed to meet the standards of practice or jeopardized patient safety. Have the student sign a copy of the written evaluation, and give her a copy to review. Place the signed copy of the evaluation in the student's file along with a notation of the date on which the meeting reviewing the evaluation occurred. Avoid any speculation as to the student's intellectual ability, aptitude for nursing, attitude or commitment to studies, or overinvolvement in social, work, or family activities to prepare adequately for clinical. Instead, focus on the student's deficiencies in relation to academic standards (Graveley & Stanley, 1993). Any underlying reasons for these deficiencies are for the student to recognize and correct.

When making clinical assignments, provide the student with opportunities to demonstrate improved performance. If the student remedies the problematic behavior, make a note of this for the file, and provide feedback to the student. Continue to observe the student, however, because faulty performance may recur.

If the student is unable to correct performance promptly, schedule a meeting to develop a plan to remedy identified deficiencies. The plan should be developed collaboratively with the student, and then put in writing. The plan should identify the student's deficiencies and the strategies that would improve performance. The plan should note that it is the continuous improve-

·ment in performance and safety in patient care activities that will be evaluated, not isolated instances of improved or deficient performance, and that the student's ultimate success in the clinical component of the course will be rated in relation to the objectives for the course rather than the remediation plan (Graveley & Stanley, 1993). It is at this point that the student must be informed of the consequences of failure to improve performance: removal from the clinical area if patient safety is being compromised or potential failure in the course if performance is inadequate but still safe. The safe student must be given the opportunity to finish the clinical experience even if it is improbable that she will achieve course objectives. The final evaluation cannot be done until the course is completed. Giving such a student a midsemester "failure," however, communicates the potential consequences of the problematic situation more clearly than does a notation of "marginal" on the clinical evaluation form. The unsafe student is another matter. The remediation plan for this student should involve activities outside the clinical area, such as in the college laboratory, with a requirement that a safe level of practice be attained before the student will be permitted to return to the clinical setting. A dated, signed memo summarizing the content of the meeting should be placed in the student's file, along with a copy of the remediation plan.

In developing the remediation plan, it is important for the instructor to give consideration to the effects of implementing the plan on her ability to provide adequate instruction and supervision to other members of the group. Due process does not require that the instructor abandon all other responsibilities to provide instructional support for the failing student. Similarly, the instructor's obligation to ensure that patients' safety, comfort, and care needs are met when students are assigned to provide care must be considered in developing and implementing the remediation plan.

It is likely that the student will be very upset to learn that she is in danger of failing the clinical component of the course. The instructor should avoid impulses to comfort the student; rather, a referral should be made to available counseling services. The student also can be referred to support services that provide sessions on stress reduction and study skills.

As the clinical experience progresses, the instructor should make note of teaching strategies and other approaches, such as enhanced supervision using staff or a student peer, she has implemented in support of the remediation plan, as well as providing frequent feedback to the student on her progress.

Confidentiality Issues

All evaluative data—both verbal feedback and written evaluations—should be shared only with the involved student. The instructor must take care to provide corrective feedback that identifies student deficiencies away from the bedside, staff, and other students. Comments on another student's performance—whether excellent or marginal—should be avoided. Instead, frame references to other students' activities in terms of the challenge that was presented that might enhance the learning of others in the group.

Parents of a student who is in danger of failing the clinical component of a course often will demand to discuss the student's performance or to review the evaluation data. The instructor should decline this request, and refer the parents to the department chairperson, who can make a determination of the appropriateness of such an action. Parents are not professionally competent to analyze these data, even if they have a health care background. Evaluation is the responsibility of the instructor who supervises students in the clinical area, who is best able to determine whether or not the student has achieved course objectives or is practicing in a safe manner. The student has a right to privacy concerning academic evaluations, regardless of who is paying for the education. The student may waive her right to privacy and request that the data be provided to her parent, but such a waiver may be coerced. In any event, the matter is best referred to the appropriate academic authority.

MAKING DECISIONS

The final decision on grading clinical performance should be made after students have had the opportunity to review results. If upon this review the instructor decides that a failing grade must be entered for the student, the student should be promptly informed of this and given information on the grade appeal process in place at the college.

In general, the academic judgments of faculty are upheld in internal and external review processes, because faculty are considered to be the best judges of academic standards and student performance in relation to these. Consequently, grade appeal processes focus on two issues: were the student's due process rights preserved and was the decision to fail the student academically made in a discriminatory manner. Discrimination involves the situation in which the student was held to a different standard of performance than other students in the group.

To counter potential charges of discriminatory practices, the instructor must keep scrupulous records on all evaluation practices. Anecdotal notes reflecting observations of both positive and deficient performances by all students demonstrate that the failing student was not subject to special scrutiny. Where extra supervision of the failing student was required because of problems with performance, the decision to do this—and notification of the student—explain the differential treatment in terms of patient safety. The record of assignments made for all students in the clinical group helps to support the instructor's assertion that the assignments given to the failing student were no different than those of her peers and were designed to permit the student to demonstrate her ability to achieve course objectives.

USING RESULTS

The ongoing review of evaluation data provides excellent feedback to the instructor on her own performance teaching in the clinical setting. Novice instructors often expect too much or too little of students. Actual student performance can challenge the instructor's initial assumptions and guide the creation of an experience that is more appropriate to the students and the clinical setting. Student comments, as on observation guides, reaction papers, and journals or logs, help to shape assignments and instructional methods. By remaining open to these comments, the instructor can grow in her role and develop an instructional style and approach that enables students to achieve goals.

EVALUATING THE EVALUATION PROCESS

Many of the instruments used for the evaluation of clinical performance have been created by others, and the clinical instructor may find these difficult to apply in the clinical setting in which she teaches. In many instances, modifications can be made within the framework of the established form, for example, by developing written descriptors reflecting various levels of performance in relation to course objectives. This permits the intelligent use of the instrument while complying with a requirement to use the form. When established instruments are inadequate to the task of eliciting evaluation data on an important component of clinical performance, the instructor can supplement the form with additional data recorded in a suitable format. Where students in all clinical groups will be completing a similar assignment, such as a major nursing care plan or case presentation, the instructor should become involved in establishing the criteria to be used in evaluating these assignments, or at the very least, discuss the criteria with other instructors to gain insight into what should be expected of students.

At the end of the clinical experience, providing feedback on experiences with the evaluation procedures in place for the course to the lead instructor and other faculty members teaching in the course can help to shape the future approach to clinical evaluation, which is, after all, an imprecise process.

REFERENCES

Anderson, E.; & Knuteson, C. (1990). Co-assessment as a unique approach to measuring students' clinical abilities. *Journal of Nursing Education, 29,* 42–43.

Benner, P. (1984). *From novice to expert: Excellence and power in clinical nursing practice.* Menlo Park, CA: Addison-Wesley.

Brooke, P.S. (1994). Comment on Orchard's "Clinical evaluation procedures." *Journal of Nursing Education, 33,* 252–253.

Davidhizar, R.E.; & McBride, A. (1985). How nursing students explain their success and failure experiences. *Journal of Nursing Education, 24*, 284–290.

Gomez, D.A.; Lobodzinski, S.; & Hartwell West, C.D. (1998). Evaluating clinical performance. (pp. 407–422). In Billings, D.M.; & Halstead, J.A. *Teaching in nursing*: A *guide for faculty*. Philadelphia: W.B. Saunders.

Graveley, E.A.; & Stanley, M. (1993). A clinical failure: What the courts tell us. *Journal of Nursing Education, 32*, 135–137.

Halstead, J.A. (1998). The academic performance of students; Legal and ethical issues. (pp. 37–50). In Billings, D.M.; & Halstead, J.A. *Teaching in nursing*: A *guide for faculty*. Philadelphia: W.B. Saunders.

Krichbaum, K.; Rowan, M.; Duckett, L.; Ryden, M.B.; & Savik, K. (1994). The clinical evaluation tool: A measure of the quality of clinical performance of baccalaureate nursing students. *Journal of Nursing Education, 33*, 395–404.

Monahan, R.S. (1991). Potential outcomes of clinical experience. *Journal of Nursing Education, 30*, 176–181.

Orchard, C. (1992). Factors that interfere with clinical judgments of students' performance. *Journal of Nursing Education, 31*, 309–313.

Orchard, C. (1994). The nurse educator and the nursing student: A review of the issue of clinical evaluation procedures. *Journal of Nursing Education, 33*, 245–251.

Wilhite, M.J. (1990). Diagnostic evaluation and grading in nursing laboratory courses. *Journal of Nursing Education, 29*, 39–40.

Woolley, G.R.; Bryan, M.S.; & Davis, J.W. (1998). A comprehensive approach to clinical evaluation. *Journal of Nursing Education, 37*, 361–366.

CHAPTER 11

INTERPERSONAL ISSUES IN CLINICAL NURSING EDUCATION

The Instructional Role 202
    The Clinical Instructor as Teacher 203
    The Clinical Instructor as Supervisor 204
    The Clinical Instructor as Evaluator 206
    The Clinical Instructor as Nurse 206
Communicating Caring 207
Conveying Enthusiasm 209
Communication Strategies 210
    Setting Goals 210
    Communicating Values 211
    Motivating Performance 212
    Praising 212
    Providing Corrective Feedback 212
    Preventing Unsafe Practice 212
    Describing Performance Deficits 214
    Disciplining a Student 215
    Failing a Student 215
    Removing a Student from the Clinical Area 215
Responding to Student Stress 216
Helping Students to Cope with ... 218
    ... Death and Dying 219
    ... Disfigurement, Deformities, Wounds, and Other Alterations in Body
        Integrity 220
    ... A Patient's Sexuality 221
    ... Racist or Sexist Remarks by Patients 222
    ... Staff or Physician Harassment 222
Strategies for Working with the ... 223
    ... Reluctant Learner 223

... Reticent Learner   223
... Monopolizer   224
... Distractor   225
... Student Who Lies   225
... Student Who Plagiarizes   226
... Student Who Exhibits Inappropriate Behavior   227
... Student Who Is Defiant   228
... Student Who Is Poorly Groomed   228
... Student Who Is a Family Member or Friend   228
... Older Student   228
... Male Student   229
... Student Who Is Repeating the Course   229
... Student Who Is Licensed as an LPN or RN   229
... Student for Whom English Is a Second Language   230
Maintaining Relationships with Staff   230
Controlling Emotions   231
Summary   232
References   232

As in nursing, interpersonal relationships are at the heart of the clinical instructional role. Many aspects of interpersonal interactions that are seemingly peripheral to the actual act of teaching are, in fact, critical to success. This chapter explores a variety of interpersonal issues and strategies for managing interpersonal relationships in the clinical setting.

THE INSTRUCTIONAL ROLE

The role of the clinical nursing instructor is multifaceted, requiring shifts in the nature of interactions with learners as the instructor recognizes and responds to learners' needs in the various situations that evolve both in the clinical setting and in encounters outside that setting. The instructional role can best be described as involving a continuum of interactions that begin with a student-teacher relationship in which the learning situation is largely teacher-controlled and move toward a collegial relationship in which learning involves a mutual encounter between two nurses. As students progress in a nursing program, their confidence in their knowledge and skills and in their mastery of the intricacies of the nursing role grows. The instructor seeks to shift the student-teacher relationship along the continuum, encouraging independence in learning while providing a supportive presence that enhances learners' growing confidence in their ability to function independently in the professional nursing role.

Three principles guide the evolving instructional relationship with students. First, the instructor must maintain boundaries while fostering trust and communicating caring. Boundary maintenance in this context involves avoiding social friendships with students. The instructor may like and enjoy students as people, but she must maintain the student-teacher relationship in order to avoid role conflict and confusion. Because friendships naturally develop among nursing colleagues, the neophyte instructor easily can find herself slipping across the boundary that marks the instructional relationship and moving into a friendship relationship with one or more students. An awareness of this potential hazard helps the instructor to structure the student-teacher relationship in more appropriate ways. Second, the instructor must immerse herself in the instructional role, developing her ability to move across and function in its various components with ease, "being in" the role rather than "playing" the role. Playing the role occurs when the instructor adopts attitudes and behaviors that seem to "fit" with an external conceptualization of the role, shedding her authenticity in the process. Playing the role almost always results in a distancing from students, placing the instructor in an authoritarian relationship with them. This, in turn, interferes with the development of mutual respect and collaboration between instructor and students, necessary elements of collegiality. Although at first glance these two principles may seem contradictory, they enable the instructor to find a "center place" in her relationships with students that allows her to function effectively as a clinical instructor while remaining an authentic, caring human being. The third principle, continual performance as a role model of professional nursing, helps the instructor to maintain her "center place." The relationship of teacher to student parallels in many ways the relationship between nurse and patient: both respect the uniqueness of the individual; both structure interactions to evidence a humanistic concern for the other; both strive to enable the recipient to achieve goals; and both require that boundaries be placed on the nature of the relationship.

The Clinical Instructor as Teacher

Initially, the teacher provides a great deal of structure and focus for students, deliberately guiding their activities. The teacher designs learning experiences to meet the identified learning needs of students within the context of program goals, course objectives, and the possibilities presented by the college laboratory and/or clinical settings. She presents relevant content, demonstrates skills, describes processes of care, and discusses alternative approaches necessary to negotiate the experience, either with the clinical group as a whole or with individual students. Throughout the learning experience, the teacher monitors the situation to ensure that it continues to provide an appropriate context for learning.

As students gain a modicum of confidence and competence, the teacher's role shifts to that of *coach*. In this role, the teacher continues to design the learning experience, but allows the students freedom in functioning within the overall plan, including improvising as needed. As coach, the teacher continues to monitor the unfolding situation, making adjustments in assignments as needed or calling a student aside to explain a new procedure or make a suggestion about an approach to care. When the student is hesitant in performing an aspect of care with which she has had previous experience, the teacher as coach refrains from reteaching, but provides cues to get the student started in the appropriate direction. Above all, the teacher as coach expresses her belief in the capacity of the students to succeed, and instills in them an expectation of their own success.

Further along the continuum, the teacher may assume the role of *preceptor*. She still designs the learning experience through the assignments she makes, but her role involves more "watchful listening" (Rittman & Osburn, 1995), with teacher-initiated interventions confined to preventing unsafe practices. The student has more control of the learning experience, coming to the instructor with questions or when she needs guidance in performing some aspect of care.

At the far end of the teaching continuum, the teacher and student *collaborate* in the learning process. They cooperatively design learning experiences, mutually seek answers to problems arising in the clinical setting, discuss alternatives and make suggestions as equal partners, and together evaluate the results of interventions.

Because each clinical experience will present students with new content and skills to be mastered and applied in the care of patients, the instructor can expect to move back and forth across the teaching continuum, even with more advanced students. Recognizing what is needed in each situation and responding appropriately constitutes part of the art of teaching.

The Clinical Instructor as Supervisor

Much of the clinical instructor's time is spent supervising students as they carry out assignments. Akin to the managerial style of "walking around," clinical supervision keeps the instructor alert to each student's progress in the clinical area, both in executing the assignment and in demonstrating competence and skill in performing nursing functions with patients. The instructor's supervisory presence can be interpreted in various ways by students, depending on the approach to supervision adopted by the instructor. The instructor who lurks unannounced behind the curtain as a student performs care activities creates in students a sense of distrust and apprehension. In contrast, the instructor who enters the room, warmly greeting the patient and asking the student how things are going, offers the student the opportunity to ask a question or request the instructor's guidance in performing a task.

The instructor as supervisor must function as a *safety officer* during the clinical experience, and part of "walking around" is done to detect student practices that might affect patient safety. In this aspect of the supervisory role, the instructor may decide to select a specific location for supervisory activities.

For example, when students are learning to administer medications, the instructor may situate herself near the medication room so that she can readily check students as they prepare medications for their patients. At the end of the clinical day, the instructor may stay at the nursing station, to listen to students as they report to staff. As with general supervision, the instructor's vigilance as a safety officer can be variously interpreted by students. The instructor who is open about the potential for errors and her role in monitoring the situation to prevent these from happening is seen by students as supporting them in their role as learners, and freeing them to focus on their activities rather than on the fear of making mistakes. The instructor who insists on being with each student as they perform certain activities not only blocks the flow of clinical activities, but communicates distrust of the students' ability to provide care.

As a supervisor, the instructor may be required to take the role of *disciplinarian* in discussing unacceptable behavior with a student or pointing out errors and their consequences. In performing the disciplinarian function, the instructor must act in ways that protect the patient and maintain the dignity of the student. When the student's behavior is unacceptable, for example, when the student is chronically late or unprepared for the clinical experience, the instructor should ask this student to wait in a private location while the instructor completes her involvement with other students. When a student is observed performing in an unsafe manner, the instructor must first intervene to complete the procedure safely without alarming the patient. For example, the instructor might say, "Let me show you another approach to doing this," or "Let me help you finish this task." Such a statement should signal the student to step aside and observe rather than continue with her activities. When the patient situation is stabilized, the instructor can then ask the student to come with her to a private location to discuss why the student's actions required the instructor's intervention. Students might be alerted beforehand to verbal cues the instructor will use in the patient's presence. For example, "May I . . ." might signal the instructor's offer to assist, which the student should feel free to accept or reject. "Let me . . ." might signal the need for the instructor to intervene.

All student discipline should occur where the interaction cannot be overheard by patients, staff, or other students. The discipline should focus on the observed behavior and the reasons it was unacceptable or unsafe. The instructor should avoid generalizing about the student's behavior (for example, "You're never prepared for clinical"), which, in effect, places a final judgment on it. Instead, the conversation should center on the specific behavior that is the focus of the discipline and its consequences for patient care. If the behavior is a repetition of behavior that has been commented upon previously, the instructor should identify the commonalties between this and past episodes and the conceptual link (e.g., unreliability, problems with priority setting) that joins the episodes, because the student is unlikely to be able to make these connections herself.

While no student enjoys being disciplined, the instructor's actions to maintain the dignity of the student while protecting the legitimate interests of patients and the other students create an impression of fairness and respect. Knowing that inappropriate or unsafe practices will be disciplined reconfirms the importance of the activities that surround the clinical experience and the value attached to these by the instructor.

The Clinical Instructor as Evaluator

As the instructor assesses student performance against expectations established for the course, she functions as an evaluator in two important and distinct ways. The ongoing evaluation of student progress enables the instructor to shape the experience to best meet the needs of the student group and of individual learners. In this respect, evaluation is not unlike that which occurs in the clinical setting as the nurse implements a plan of care, continuously evaluating its suitability for the patient's current situation and its success in achieving the goals of patient care. In addition to providing feedback to the instructor on the design of the clinical learning experience, this formative evaluation provides feedback to students on how well they are progressing in meeting course objectives and how they can improve their performance as the experience continues. Students who get continuous feedback on their performance as well as guidance and support in improving that performance come to view evaluation as a positive means of growth and development, and a natural corollary of the learning process. Students who lack such feedback tend to feel insecure and hesitant to try out new experiences. Formative evaluation requires a lot of openness and interaction between instructor and students as each communicates their observations and experiences in the clinical setting.

Summative evaluation is the process of applying judgments to evaluative data to determine the grade each student will receive in the clinical component of the course. Summative evaluation encompasses all course objectives, and provides a determination of the success of the student in achieving these by the end of the course. This evaluation cannot be avoided by the clinical instructor, who must communicate a final grade for each student at the end of the experience regardless of the nature or extent of the evaluation processes she has used during the semester. The instructor who has used formative evaluation throughout the clinical experience will find summative evaluation relatively easy to accomplish; students who have gotten continuous feedback on performance are unlikely to be surprised by their final grades.

The Clinical Instructor as Nurse

Despite her clear communication that she is functioning in an instructional role, the clinical instructor is likely to be perceived as a nurse by both staff and patients. Indeed, it is important that the instructor maintain this role as an aspect of the instructional role. Staff members' recognition of the instructor as nurse facilitates communication concerning practices and protocols unique to the unit, patient needs, student performance, and so forth. For the patient, the presence of the instructor who presents herself as a skilled nurse supports the student as she functions in the nursing role.

As a role model, the instructor is able to demonstrate aspects of the nursing role that are difficult to articulate to students, such as a way of touching a patient or of using nonverbal approaches to communicating concern and caring. When working with a student who is focused on a task, the instructor can model those aspects of the nursing role that have not yet been incorporated into the student's delivery of care but are an important aspect of technique—for example, explaining the procedure to the patient before proceeding with it. This action complements the student's care, meeting patient needs while also demonstrating the fuller approach to care that should be the student's goal.

As a nurse, the instructor is also a future colleague of the students she teaches. In relating to students as future colleagues, the instructor should strive to communicate her enthusiasm for nursing and the joyful aspects of this professional career. The instructor who expresses her relief to be off the unit and away from patients communicates disdain for the profession that is quickly picked up by students. The instructor who expresses a delight in her teaching role that is tempered by her urge to return to patient care communicates the richness of the profession that also is picked up by students.

As a nurse with experience in the profession, the instructor may elect to become a mentor for one or more students. Despite some mistaken references to the term, which confuse mentoring with teaching, coaching, and other aspects of the instructional role, mentoring is an activity undertaken by a more experienced person on behalf of someone she believes has the potential and drive to succeed. Mentoring is the process of guiding that individual as she makes career decisions, and opening doors of opportunity for further growth. The clinical instructor should avoid entering a mentoring relationship with students in her clinical group, as this might be viewed as favoritism of one student over others.

COMMUNICATING CARING

The centrality of caring to the act of nursing has been rediscovered by numerous nurse theorists and is the focus of a growing body of research. One component of that research has explored students' experiences of being cared for by faculty, and whether being treated in a caring manner is a contributing factor in students' development of caring approaches to patients in their practice of nursing. Knowledge and experience are assumed to contribute to learning nursing (else there would be no need for clinical experience in nursing programs), so it is easy to infer that students' interactions with their instructors might also contribute to learning.

Building on work that has described caring as involving authentic presence and connectedness with the other, characterized by active patterns of helping and enabling, Hanson and Smith (1996) analyzed interviews in which baccalaureate nursing students described caring and not-so-caring interactions with a faculty member. Their findings confirm those of other researchers. They report that "[t]he essence of the caring interaction between faculty and student in this study was recognition, connection and affirmation/confirmation" (p. 109). *Recognition* involved attending (really listening to the student without being distracted by other events in the environment); initiating (acknowledging the presence of the student, reaching out to the student); and responding (recognizing the student's need for help and providing it). *Connection* involved connecting (permitting an authentic interpersonal relationship to develop between student and teacher) and empathizing (recognizing and responding to student's questions or concerns; acknowledging that the teacher makes mistakes too). *Confirmation* involved affirming (providing positive reinforcement and encouragement; expressing sincere concern that the student succeed) and motivating (the teacher's caring about the student's success makes the student want to do the best she can) (p. 109). The structural description of a caring teacher–student interaction that resulted from the data contains an excellent picture of the instructor who cares:

> The experience of being cared-for by nursing faculty may be initiated by the teacher or it may be the teacher's response to noticing, observing, or listening to a student. While it occasionally lasts over a significant period of time, it more often is quite brief. Sometimes it involves specific actions or words on the part of the faculty, but just as often it is a moment in which a connection is made between two persons with minimal regard to status or roles. The student is recognized as an individual and a special person. At times the teacher listens without judgment and conveys a sense of acceptance. The teacher acknowledges the student's whole life, not just the student role. The teacher conveys an attitude of flexibility, fairness, warmth, and genuineness. The specific action or words are sometimes directive and sometimes supportive and accepting. The caring teacher not only is skilled in interpersonal relationships, but is skilled in teaching. The competent, well-prepared teacher gives information, offers suggestions, helps problem-solve, and works hard to ensure a good [clinical] experience. For the student, the result of this caring connection is a feeling of comfort, confidence, competence, and motivation to keep on, to strive more, to study harder. The student is affirmed in having chosen nursing as a profession. In seeing the teacher care, the student learns to care (p. 108).

Instructors' acts of caring enhance students' self-esteem and positive feelings about themselves as human beings. This humanistic response, in which the carer facilitates and promotes the growth of the person cared for toward self actualization, has been proposed as an alternative to the behaviorist approach to curriculum design and teaching in nursing programs (Bevis, 1988). By behaving in caring ways toward their students, instructors role model caring acts that can be transferred to interactions with patients. When students witness the instructor in caring interactions with patients and with other students, they learn what it means to care or to be caring in addition to feeling cared-for.

Caring acts with students are inherently motivating because they affirm the worth and potential of the individual. Such acts convey the instructor's belief that the student can succeed, that she is worthy of the instructor's efforts and able to benefit from the learning experience. The vast majority of students in nursing programs are there because they want to become nurses, good nurses, successful nurses. Receiving the instructor's confirmation that this is a goal that can be achieved by each of them—and is worthy of their own investment in their learning—causes them to work harder to achieve that goal.

Caring acts also affirm the student's choice of nursing as a professional career. Most students enter the field to take care of others. The experience of being cared-for themselves broadens the possibilities inherent in caring acts with patients. It feels good to be cared-for and to be part of a profession that values caring.

Three ingredients contribute to the clinical nursing instructor's success in communicating caring to students. The first, described above, involves "being in" the instructional role rather than "playing" the role. The instructor need not be a perfect teacher (indeed, acknowledging imperfections frees students to be themselves—imperfect as well); she does need to be an authentic one. Second, knowing the content (that is, feeling confident and comfortable in the clinical setting) frees the instructor to know the learners as people. Third, the instructor needs to value people. If the instructor has not developed the capacity to express caring with patients, she is unlikely to readily develop this capacity with students.

CONVEYING ENTHUSIASM

The clinical instructor sets the tone not only for the clinical experience, but also for students' perceptions of nursing as a career. In this regard, the clinical instructor's enthusiasm—or apathy—about nursing and about teaching and learning can be contagious. It is the instructor's leadership skills that enable her to motivate and inspire students as they engage in learning.

People follow leaders who articulate and are committed to worthy and achievable goals. Commitment is demonstrated in enthusiasm for both the tasks and processes involved in goal achievement. Leadership is accomplished through the instructor's *power* as a clinical expert, her *authority* as the person responsible for learning activities in the clinical setting, and her *influence* as a role model (Claus & Bailey, 1977).

The clinical competence of the instructor is demonstrated not only in her skillful performance of nursing activities but also in her work ethic. Because the work of nursing is meaningful and important, it is essential that nurses take responsibility for performing that work to the best of their ability. Setting high standards and attaching accountability to assignments communicates to students the significance of the nursing endeavor. The instructor's engagement in the work of nursing by becoming involved with students as they provide direct patient care demonstrates the instructor's continued commitment to and involvement with nursing practice.

In establishing the day's activities, the instructor can communicate her enthusiasm by highlighting the unique possibilities contained in the students' assignments. For example, the instructor might suggest to students that they take time to observe an icteric patient to develop a better sense of skin color in this condition. Most students arrive in the clinical setting excited about engaging in clinical learning activities, but their expression of this excitement may be tempered by normative standards of peers, which may view enthusiasm about learning as "not cool." The instructor's own enthusiasm counterbalances this, and permits students to embrace the potentials inherent in the clinical learning environment.

The instructor's sense of passion about nursing—and about teaching nursing to others—encourages and inspires students to emulate her high standards. The clinical instructor who feels and expresses satisfaction and fulfillment in her choice of a nursing career confirms students' own choice of nursing, and motivates them to engage fully in the clinical learning process.

Finally, the instructor's sense of humor goes a long way to alleviate the stress that naturally accompanies clinical learning. Nursing can be a source of great delight and fun, and students should be encouraged to recognize the humor in many of the situations they encounter. Enjoying the work of nursing and learning nursing contributes to emotional health, uplifts staff, and can be a source of comfort and reassurance to patients.

COMMUNICATION STRATEGIES

Communication with students must be focused and structured to achieve its purposes. Many of the communication skills and strategies that the instructor has developed as a clinical practitioner can be applied in clinical teaching. Planning general approaches for interactions likely to be encountered while teaching in the clinical setting further expands the instructor's communication abilities.

Setting Goals

It is essential to articulate the goals of the clinical experience as a whole and for each clinical session. These goals establish the instructor's expectations for student performance. The focus of goal setting should address both goals for patient care and goals for student learning.

A general set of goals with respect to patient care is necessary to address such issues as safety and confidentiality. More specific goals for individual patients need to be clarified for students, especially early in the educational program. Although each patient's nursing care plan should identify goals for care (outcomes and associated objectives in relation to each nursing diagnosis), these may be difficult for students to relate to, or, possibly, missing from the patient's record. Helping students to identify appropriate, achievable goals for their work with patients provides some structure for the clinical experience. This is particularly important when continuity of the nurse-patient relationship is impossible due to shortened patient lengths of stay coupled with the student's presence on the clinical unit for only one day per week.

Goals for student learning are likewise both general and specific. General goals are related to the objectives for the clinical experience. More specific goals may be developed in relation to past performance or experience. For example, the instructor may identify assessing the safety of the patient's home environment as a goal for all students in the group, or improved priority setting as a goal for an individual student. Students' own goals for the clinical experience also should be solicited and built into the instructional plan.

In addition to establishing goals for the clinical experience, students need concrete directions as to how those goals can be achieved as well as endpoints that signal goal achievement. By providing interim milestones that can serve as markers for students to assess their own progress toward goals, the instructor clarifies the assignment and how it might be accomplished.

Because each student's progress in the clinical area is influenced by the nature of the patient assignment and the vagaries of learning, particularly psychomotor skills, which take time to develop, it is useful to set both short-term and long-term goals for clinical learning. The student's sense of progress toward goals is an important facet of motivation, and contributes to continued engagement in clinical learning at the high level necessary for mastery to occur.

Communicating Values

As with many other aspects of nursing practice, students benefit when the instructor explains the impact of her values in providing patient care. Once a value has been incorporated into one's practice, it is seldom articulated; the action in accord with the value speaks for itself. But students are not yet able to identify the values that underlie many nursing actions, and are assisted in examining and reflecting upon value-based practice when the instructor explains both the value and its corresponding rationale. For example, the instructor might say, "I believe it is important to take some time to talk with the patient before planning the day's activities, so that I can incorporate his preferences and current situation into my planning." Such a statement expresses the instructor's valuing of individualization of care, how she operationalizes the value, and why she believes this is important. The statement also expresses the instructor's ownership of the value, rather than imposing it on students.

Motivating Performance

Students do not intuit the rationale for many of the assignments and activities undertaken in the course of nursing education. Their enthusiastic engagement in these activities can be promoted by an explanation as to why the activity is important and how it contributes to future nursing practice. For example, observations of preschool children become salient for students when they are guided to reflect on the behavior of well children as a basis for assessing the child who is ill and understanding the impact of hospitalization or immobilization on usual levels of child activity.

Praising

While positive feedback on performance is an important component of formative evaluation and contributes to the student's motivation, it is important not to praise prematurely. As with discipline, recognize successful performance by focusing on the observed behavior and its effects on patient care. This helps to mitigate the roller-coaster effect of being praised one day and corrected the next. Passing along positive comments of staff, patients, and families is an important reinforcer of success.

Providing Corrective Feedback

Acquisition of psychomotor skills is a gradual process, as students refine these skills with repeated performances that come closer and closer to the smooth, well-coordinated action that signals mastery. Similarly, students' ability to attend to multiple facets of a patient's condition—and respond appropriately to each—is acquired gradually. Formative evaluation needs to acknowledge approximations of successful performance, so the student knows she is on the right track. Such feedback reinforces not only the behavior, but also the body and intellectual senses that accompany the behavior. As the student becomes more "tuned in" to the elements that comprise success, she is able to refine the performance.

When providing corrective feedback, focus on the behavior and its effects. Describe what is wrong, why it is wrong, and how it can be corrected (or what is right, why it is right, and how it can be improved). When they receive corrective feedback from the instructor, students assume that the whole process they have engaged in is flawed. Be certain to point out the aspects that were satisfactory, for example, "Up until this point, everything went well. Then, you contaminated the sterile field by reaching across it."

Preventing Unsafe Practice

No student wants to commit an error in the clinical setting. Fear of making mistakes was cited as one of the highest sources of anxiety by junior and senior baccalaureate students in a study by Kleehammer et al. (1990). Anticipatory guidance in the prevention of errors is an important factor in alleviating stress and focusing students' attention on situations that could result in error or jeopardize patient safety. For example, alert students to the problems that might be encountered with the confused patient, and how these might be prevented, as with keeping the side rails up and frequently checking on the patient's status during the course of the day.

War stories are an excellent way to identify potential sources of error and alert students to red flags that should signal a need to double-check before proceeding. As an example, I share three stories with students in relation to administering medication. The first concerns my roommate shortly following our graduation from nursing school, who came home one evening and asked whether quinine and quinidine were the same drug. Lesson: Just because drug names sound similar does not mean they are similar. The second concerns my own error in giving a double dose of an antibiotic to a patient who insisted that she usually received only one tablet. Lesson: Listen to your patient. The third concerns a student who was preparing to give 10 capsules of procainamide to a cardiac patient. Lesson: If the dose requires more than 2 pills, check it out.

War stories accomplish several goals. First, they acknowledge that errors are possible—for anyone. Second, they provide graphic examples of the types of errors that can be made. Third, they provide "rules of thumb" for preventing errors that are applicable in a variety of situations, demonstrating the learning that can occur as a result of errors. For example, the situation involving a potential drug overdose can be extended to rechecking dose calculations when an intramuscular injection requires more than 2½ cc of fluid.

The instructor also can help to alleviate anxiety (including her own) over potential problems by monitoring situations that might give rise to errors or accidents. Her supervision of a situation that already has been identified as potentially problematic reinforces the need for extra care by the student, and provides a welcome backup for the student.

Rittman and Osburn (1995) identify signals that should raise the instructor's concern about a student's safety:

- The student can't be depended upon to seek appropriate backup or assistance in patient care.
- The student enters the clinical area more anxious than others.
- The student arrives late for the experience.
- The student approaches patients in a tentative, uncertain manner.

They further identify hallmarks of danger that indicate a need for close monitoring and for redesigning the experience to create possibilities for success while safeguarding patient safety:

- The student does not know when care is complete; cannot recognize gaps in care.
- The student has difficulty in setting priorities and organizing care activities.

- The student's performance is inconsistent, even after having made progress.
- The student cannot be counted on to report important observations or occurrences.
- The student does not know when to ask for backup or help.
- The student does not recognize or acknowledge errors.

Describing Performance Deficits

There is a significant difference between performance deficits that are a natural part of the learning process, and those that signal that the student is not making progress in clinical learning. Repeatedly deficient performance requires counseling to get the student back on track or to begin the process of documentation necessary to support a failing clinical grade. Discussions with the student who is not meeting expectations should occur away from the clinical area, in a conference designed specifically for this purpose.

Prepare for the conference by categorizing deficient behaviors under broad conceptual headings that relate to course objectives. Group such behaviors logically, eliminating redundancies by indicating the number of times such a behavior has occurred, with an example reflecting the latest observed episode. Prioritize the deficient behaviors, with the most significant deficit listed first. Focus on patterns of behavior rather than on isolated episodes, and on the behavior and its consequences rather than on the student and her inadequacies. Organize any anecdotal notes documenting episodes of deficient performance for the student's review during the conference.

In the meeting with the student, review the accumulated data. Do not ask the student "why" she has behaved in the observed manner; instead, ask "what's going on" that might be interfering with her practice. Seek some evidence of whether the student is aware of or oblivious to deficits. Determine whether the student has any insight into what might be behind her actions or inactions.

If the student is able to communicate a problem that is interfering with her performance, help her to identify an appropriate means to deal with this, such as getting counseling or "stopping out" of the program until a major life issue is resolved. If there is no significant external issue to be dealt with, develop a plan with the student to help her to improve performance. This may involve a less demanding or complex assignment, pairing with a more skilled peer, or reviewing the day's activities with the instructor before beginning. Clarify that these measures are intended to move the student in a more positive direction in terms of her clinical performance, but that overall performance will be evaluated on the basis of established course objectives. It is important to communicate the potential for the student's success if this is at all evident, as well as the instructor's commitment to facilitating the student's achievement of clinical objectives.

Meet with the student at a predetermined interval after the conference, to follow-up on the plan and communicate any observed change in performance.

Disciplining a Student

When it is necessary to discipline a student, do so immediately after removing her to an isolated area to provide privacy. Identify the problematic behavior in a matter-of-fact manner. Cite any prior instances of the same or similar behavior (e.g., dependability). Outline the consequences of continued episodes of similar behavior and the rationale for these. For example, the student who has been late for clinical on two occasions might be charged with a clinical absence when she is late again, with accumulated "absences" reflected in a clinical failure.

It is important that similar behavior among students be disciplined similarly. It is unfair to allow one student to come to clinical late while chastising another for the same behavior unless something else distinguishes the two cases; for example, the first student may have called the unit to alert the staff and instructor to her delay.

On occasion, it may be necessary to discipline the whole clinical group for a pattern of behavior that is unacceptable. It is important to identify the overarching problem as well as the instances of behavior that illustrate this. Such discipline should take place early in the clinical experience to underline the instructor's expectations and the high standards of performance to which all students will be held.

Failing a Student

A clinical failure should not be a surprise to the student if appropriate feedback and counseling have been provided during the clinical experience. Communicate the failure in a matter-of-fact, straightforward fashion, in private, and provide time for the student to collect herself before she leaves the meeting. Offer to review the accumulated record with the student, or to meet with her on another occasion to do so. Outline the steps available to the student to dispute the grade if she wishes to pursue this option.

Removing a Student from the Clinical Area

Occasionally, the student's behavior poses a potential hazard to patients, the student herself, or others in the clinical setting. The student who arrives in the clinical area unwell, under the influence of drugs or alcohol, or emotionally unstable poses such a potential risk. The student who is totally unprepared for the clinical experience poses a different problem. In the first instance, the instructor must quickly evaluate the situation in terms of the possible hazards it presents and the potential to resolve the issue quickly and effectively without removing the student from the setting. In the second instance, the student who is unprepared is better sent to the library for an hour to do the necessary preparation than sent home for the day, which does not address the underlying issue of preparation.

When the hazard presented by a student's behavior cannot be dealt with by the instructor, the student may be required to leave the clinical area.

However, the instructor must take steps to safeguard the student and patients if this is necessary. For example, the belligerent student may require escort off the premises by agency security personnel. The student who is under the influence of drugs or alcohol will need to be driven home or to treatment. The emotionally disturbed student should be guided to call a family member or counselor before leaving the agency.

When a student must be removed from the clinical area, notify staff that the student is leaving and make plans to cover her assignment, either by returning the assignment to staff or arranging for other students to complete it. Determine what, if anything, has been done by the student before leaving, and report this to staff. Reassure the patient if the student's behavior has been upsetting to him, and identify who will be providing the remainder of his care that day.

As soon as possible, report the incident to the school contact, briefly explaining the incident and the steps taken to protect those affected by it. Acknowledge to others in the clinical group that the student has left for the day, but avoid discussion of the reasons. A simple "Sarah is unable to attend clinical today" should suffice.

After the clinical experience is over, attempt to determine what happened after the student left clinical. Did she arrive home safely? Is she under appropriate care? Discuss with the program coordinator and department chairperson the consequences of the student's behavior for her continuation in the program. For example, substance abuse or dependency may be a cause for suspension or dismissal from the program until the student has evidenced rehabilitation.

RESPONDING TO STUDENT STRESS

The clinical environment is inherently stressful because of the existence of "uncertainties and unique situations which cannot be taught in the classroom alone or through readings and other assignments completed by students" (Oermann, 1998, p. 197). Oermann describes the stress that students feel at the start of the clinical experience as "anticipatory anxiety," which is nonspecific and nonfocused. As they proceed through the program, students' stress increases (p. 199), reaching a peak in the semester just prior to graduation. Consequently, the clinical instructor must anticipate and respond to student stress at all stages of the educational program.

Stress is a broad term that encompasses experiences that are perceived as challenging, with the potential for mastery, growth, or gain, and those that are experienced as threatening, with the potential for harm (Pagana, 1990). A challenge is accompanied by a feeling of excitement. A threat causes worry.

People who respond to new experiences as challenges tend to value change and unpredictability. They have a high tolerance for risk, and are able to identify the potential for gain despite the existence of difficult odds. In the clinical learning situation, however, risk-taking is not necessarily an entirely positive characteristic. One approach to helping students cope with the stressors encountered in the clinical learning experience—without encouraging them to dash headlong into a potentially risky encounter—is to encourage them to reconceptualize a perceived threat as a challenge that is within their ability to meet successfully.

Regardless of its source, stress tends to present as a diffuse feeling of unease. A beginning point for reconceptualizing stress is to articulate the source of anxiety to make it more finite and hence more manageable. Once both instructor and student are clear about the source and nature of the stress, they can work on the steps necessary to identify the challenges inherent in the situation so as to achieve a successful outcome. For example, Pagana (1990) identifies as a source of student stress the feeling of uncertainty in the clinical environment and the fear that something will happen that the student will be unable to handle. By exploring with the student the potential "somethings" that can go wrong, and brainstorming responses to each, the instructor places coping with stress into a problem-solving framework that can be applied by the student in other situations. Reassuring the student that the instructor is there to back her up should she be unable to handle a problem is a major means by which perceived threats can dissolve and challenges emerge.

Admi's (1997) research concerning the stress experienced by nursing students prior to, during, and following the initial clinical experience explored six categories of stressors derived from beginning nursing students' descriptions of stressful situations they had encountered in their initial clinical experience. These categories were: "(1) inadequate knowledge and training; (2) averse and embarrassing sights; (3) instructor's close supervision; (4) insufficient hospital resources; (5) causing pain and suffering; and (6) education-reality conflict" (pp. 324–325). Study results indicated that students' mean stress levels in all but one category—reality conflict—were higher prior to the start of the clinical experience than during or at the end of the experience. While Admi places on nurse educators the responsibility for helping students to develop more realistic expectations of the clinical setting as a means to control stress, she fails to note that the major preexperience stressor for students *is* the instructor. This finding is confirmed by Oermann (1998), who found the clinical instructor to be the predominant stressor for associate degree students and second only to the demands associated with patient care for baccalaureate students, despite the instructor being identified as "the primary facilitator of learning" (p. 200).

How, then, can the clinical instructor help students cope with stress when she herself may be a cause of that stress? Oermann (1998) identifies "[d]isplaying caring behaviors and empathy, providing immediate feedback, being available to answer students' questions and assist them, and demonstrating enthusiasm" (p. 200) as approaches to facilitating learning by mitigating stress. Kleehammer et al. (1990) identify the creation of a nonthreatening atmosphere, through the use of humor, respect, and enthusiasm, as important in reducing student stress. Providing time for students in the clinical group to share their apprehensions about and responses to the clinical experience may serve as an effective means of helping students cope with stress. Pagana (1990) speculated that the sources of social support students have used to alleviate stress in the past may be unavailable because of the "unique and intensely personal aspect of the clinical experience" (p. 259). Encouraging students to use the instructor and the clinical group as a support system provides an alternative source of social support that often persists throughout the program. Students often have developed ways to cope with stress, but fail to apply these in the stressful situations encountered in the clinical setting. Students can be encouraged to share the approaches they use to manage stress in other settings, and to adapt these for use in the clinical setting.

The clinical instructor should remain aware of the potentially disabling effects of stress, and encourage students to take "time out" when they appear to be overwhelmed. Suggesting to the student that she slow down and think things through before proceeding is another approach to relieving stress. In the midst of a crisis, it is important to remember that anxiety interferes with information processing. Do not assume that students hear and absorb what is being said. Get feedback.

Disabling stress may arise in response to events occurring in the clinical area either because they reactivate a student's response to a previous traumatic life experience (Posttraumatic Stress Disorder, or PTSD) or are reminiscent of a traumatic event experienced by another. Shearer and Davidhizar (1998) offer the following guidelines for faculty intervention when such stress immobilizes a student:

1. Recognize that unhealed psychological scars can cause pain.
2. Assess students who seem to be experiencing psychological stress.
3. Encourage the expression of feelings and thoughts.
4. Debrief students after they have engaged in stressful clinical situations.
5. Encourage students to take "breaks" if care experiences are stressful.
6. Encourage students to engage in stress-releasing activities.
7. Refer students who evidence greater than usual levels of stress for professional counseling.

These guidelines are also useful in helping students cope with more normal sources and levels of stress. However, the instructor must refrain from entering the role of nurse or therapist to students and, instead, refer those for whom stress is a persistent problem to appropriate sources of guidance and counseling.

HELPING STUDENTS TO COPE WITH . . .

In a powerful discussion of the "hidden" work of nursing, Wolf (1989) describes as "largely undisclosed to the public and shielded from professional outsiders" (p. 463) those aspects of providing nursing care that involve patients' pain, fears, physical persons, sexuality, excreta, dying, death, and so forth. Is it any wonder, then, that students entering the profession from the "outside" often experience difficulty in coping with "the unseen work and the dirty work" (Wolf, p. 467) required of nurses?

To the extent possible, students need to be forewarned about unpleasant experiences before they encounter them and provided with a framework for functioning effectively with patients whose condition or behavior may present problems for the neophyte. To work effectively with students in this regard, the instructor must reflect on her own approaches to managing distasteful aspects of nursing practice. Three concepts that provide a useful beginning point for such a discussion are empathy, boundary maintenance, and intellectualization. *Empathy* involves the capacity to participate in another's feelings. By imagining oneself in the other's situation, the nurse is able to recognize what needs to be done to promote the comfort and well-being of the other. The danger of the empathic response is that the nurse may become overwhelmed by the patient's plight, and rendered ineffective in providing care. *Boundary maintenance* is one means of protecting against being overwhelmed by an empathic response to the patient, and involves recognizing the unique role the nurse plays in meeting patient needs—a role that cannot be performed by anyone else. To remain effective as a care provider, the nurse must maintain an awareness of the differentiation between herself and her patient. *Intellectualization* is an effective defense mechanism that supports boundary maintenance. A conceptual understanding of the nature of and reasons for the feelings the patient, family, and nurse might be experiencing helps to distance the nurse emotionally from difficult situations without disengaging entirely from them.

In addition to such a discussion, the instructor must provide a supportive presence to the student until she feels able to deal with the situation on her own.

. . . Death and Dying

Most students are troubled by their initial work with the dying patient, which raises significant existential issues for the student that she may have not yet contemplated and resolved. Few students will have had a personal experience with death; if they have, it is often the death of a grandparent, which, while sad, was likely to have been expected. Traumatic deaths of people their own age, for example, in automobile accidents, are quite different than the lingering death of the young mother with cancer or the prolonged dying of the man with degenerative neurological disease. While the theoretical grounding provided by a knowledge of Kübler-Ross's stages of dying (1969) enables the student to understand the responses of the patient and his family to impending death, this knowledge doesn't provide any clues as to how the student ought to behave in providing care for the patient. Helping the student to explore what she would want for her family members, friends, or herself in a similar situation, supplemented by the instructor's sharing of her own experiences with the dying, assists the student to uncover effective approaches to care. For example, enabling the dying person to retain control of his care to the extent possible, maintaining dignity, relieving pain, providing uninterrupted time for interaction with loved ones, and offering an upbeat, caring presence are goals for care that the student can embrace and work to attain.

While it is unusual that the student will be present when a patient dies, this does occur. The first experience of a patient's death is a milestone for any nurse. Thoughtful reflection on the event and her responses to it is an essential element of integrating the finality of death into the nurse's work with the dying. The student's initial response to the death may be a concern that she did something to cause or hasten the death. This is rarely the case, but presents a serious concern for the student that must be discussed and resolved. The necessary physical work of caring for the dead body—for example, cleansing and wrapping—can be made easier by helping the student to recognize such care as an extension of the dignity she tried to promote while the patient was alive, and as a shift in focus to the family members who may want to view the body. More frequently, students learn of the death of a patient for whom they have provided care in the past, and need time to mourn this passing. By gathering any details concerning events surrounding the death, the instructor can help students to meaningfully integrate this experience into their nursing practice.

. . . Disfigurement, Deformities, Wounds, and Other Alterations in Body Integrity

Anticipatory guidance is essential in preparing students to work with patients who have experienced disfiguring surgery or disease processes or whose wounds are unusually large or grossly infected. The sights and odors that accompany certain illnesses make it difficult for most care providers to remain unperturbed, but their reactions to the patient have a profound effect on his self-image. Students need help to overcome their fear and, perhaps, horror, in entering the patient's room and in working with him, as well as ways to control nonverbal expressions of aversion.

Provide the student with a focus—for example, the patient's eyes—so that she is not mesmerized by the disfigurement. Encourage her to enter into dialogue with the patient prior to beginning care activities. This humanizes the patient for the student, converting him from a potential monster into a person in need of compassionate nursing care. Before the student enters the room, describe the wound or disfigurement in precise, graphic terms so that the student is not shocked by what she sees. Telling the student that a patient has a third-degree pressure ulcer does not prepare her for the sight of muscle and bone when the dressing is removed.

The most useful support the instructor can provide is to offer her presence to the student when she first provides physical care involving a significant alteration in body integrity. Prepare the student for the vagomimetic response that many people have to particularly gruesome sights, as well as the warning signs of an impending fainting spell so that the student can leave the room to recover physically. Provide a means for the student to signal that she must leave the room if she feels she must—for example, to get more supplies—and allow that this may happen. If the student does need to leave the room, continue the care of the patient, and encourage the student to reenter the room as soon as she is ready to do so. It is vital that the student not abandon the patient, even if she has not been able to complete an aspect of care, both for the patient's sake and for the student's self-confidence. If possible, enable the student to work with the patient on another occasion, to overcome her initial response and discover that she can cope with the unthinkable.

. . . A Patient's Sexuality

Sexuality is a profoundly personal subject for most people. Social taboos discourage conversations about sexuality with casual acquaintances, although this is changing, particularly in relation to the advertising media addressing erectile dysfunction (ED), which may offer a smooth entry point for initiating a discussion with students concerning patients' needs in relation to their sexuality. As with so many other aspects of nursing, this taboo often is suspended in interactions between patients and nurses as patients struggle to frame questions concerning their own capacity for sexual expression in light of a disease condition or its treatment. While many students today are sexually active, most will have had limited experience in responding to others' sexuality outside an intimate relationship. When a disturbance in sexual functioning is an actual or potential problem for a patient, the student will need help in structuring her communications with the patient to elicit concerns and provide the information the patient is seeking.

A second aspect of sexuality involves providing intimate personal care to patients. It is unreasonable to expect that the patient who is unable to wash his face will be able to effectively wash his genitals, and it is not necessary that a person of the same sex insert or care for a urinary catheter. Providing such care in a matter-of-fact manner, maintaining a professional demeanor, is the appropriate approach, but students need to be reminded of this. When male students are in the clinical group, the instructor should recognize the potential for a female patient to object to his providing personal care for her. The instructor can mediate this reaction by reassuring the patient of the student's professionalism, but offering to be present in the room while intimate care is being provided.

A third aspect of sexuality involves the patient's sexual orientation, which may be difficult for the student to accept. This issue is likely to arise in relation to HIV and AIDS, which, because of the association of the HIV virus with promiscuous male homosexuality, raises in the student immediate concerns for safety. A good approach to this issue is to review the conceptual basis of Universal Precautions, which assumes that anyone can be infected with HIV or other blood-borne disease. This can lead to a discussion about the intrinsic worth of human beings, regardless of their lifestyle choices, and the nurse's professional obligation to provide care to those who need it.

A final aspect of sexuality concerns a patient's overt sexual advances to a student.[1] The student is likely to be either bewildered or outraged by such behavior. She may feel somehow responsible for the patient's response, may feel that ignoring or laughing off the advance is the best approach to dealing with it, or avoid further contact with the patient. Because this sort of patient behavior is unlikely to be confined to an interaction with one student, the instructor may be aware of the potential for such actions and should warn the student. This offers the opportunity to guide the student in dealing with such behavior by telling the patient that it is inappropriate and unwanted. The instructor's presence during such a discussion reinforces the message and provides support for the student. If the behavior persists, the instructor must evaluate its effect on the student's learning, and alter the assignment if necessary.

. . . Racist or Sexist Remarks by Patients

Patient's hurtful remarks (or their nonverbal equivalents) also are likely to result in a student feeling bewildered or outraged. The student who is the victim of such a verbal assault needs to be supported in the appropriateness of her response of outrage, but counseled concerning her professional responsibility not to retaliate in kind. The instructor must advocate for the student and confirm her worth and dignity as a human being. Although a reassignment, which serves to reinforce the bigotry, would unlikely occur with staff nurses, it is important for the instructor to assess the effect of the patient's harassment on the student's learning, and alter the assignment if necessary. Allow the student to express her feelings in response to the event, and provide time for the student to "regroup" emotionally before expecting her to proceed with clinical activities.

. . . Staff or Physician Harassment

Students are often the brunt of staff or physician frustrations. Because they feel like the "low man on the totem pole," subordinate even to nursing assistants and housekeepers, students are likely to absorb abusive behavior by those they perceive to be superior to them. The instructor's relationships with staff and physicians can go a long way in preventing such harassment, but it may still occur.

If nurses are providing care for patients, it is likely to be because that is the patient's primary need. This notion must be reinforced for students, who need

---

[1]Nurses have also violated the sexual boundary that should exist between patient and nurse, either on their own initiative or in response to a patient's advances. This possibility also needs to be explored with students in the context of boundary maintenance.

to be reminded of their importance to the patient and their right—and duty—to be involved in his care. The instructor's advocacy and role modeling in this regard—for example, asking a physician to wait to examine a patient until a treatment has been completed—provide students with the tools of assertive interaction with other health care providers.

STRATEGIES FOR WORKING WITH THE . . .

Every clinical group contains at least one student who presents a challenge to the instructor. Although this section is far from exhaustive, it does offer suggestions for working effectively with a variety of problematic situations that may arise with students while teaching in the college laboratory or clinical setting.

. . . Reluctant Learner

The reluctant learner is the one who hangs back. She seldom volunteers to try something new and tends to distance herself from patients, staff, and other learners. She completes her assignment quickly, and then sits somewhere seemingly absorbed in patient charts or textbooks rather than becoming involved in other unit activities. Working with the reluctant learner requires a diagnosis of the underlying problem. She may be shy, insecure, bored, or she may not want to be there in the first place.

Encourage the reluctant learner to become involved by pointing out an activity she can perform or a procedure she can observe that will expand her knowledge and skill base while reengaging her in clinical activities. If she persistently completes assignments ahead of others, check out the completeness of her work with the patient, including nonphysical aspects of care, such as interpersonal or teaching needs. If the reluctant learner's nursing care is satisfactory, explore the possibility of increasing the complexity of her assignment. This discussion is likely to bring to light the reasons she isn't actively engaged in learning.

. . . Reticent Learner

The reticent learner is actively engaged in clinical activities, but contributes little to discussions during pre- and postconferences. When called upon to comment on some aspect of care provided during the day, her answers are brief, and usually conveyed in a nearly inaudible voice. Most reticent learners would prefer to be left alone, and will claim that they are intellectually engaged in conference activities but, because they agree with what has been said, have little to add to other students' comments. Because the ability to speak assertively and authoritatively on behalf of patients is such an essential component of the nursing role, it is important for the instructor to diagnose the underlying problem (usually shyness or insecurity) in order to help the student to become more active in this aspect of learning.

A discussion with the student might communicate the instructor's observations and create opportunities for the reticent learner to actively contribute during conference. For example, the instructor might comment on the student's ability to clearly articulate the rationale for nursing care activities in one-to-one conversations with the instructor, and her plan to ask the student to share this rationale with students during the postconference. By authenticating the student's ability and providing a fair warning that she will be called upon to present information in conference, the instructor is addressing one possible reason for reticence (insecurity) while facilitating the student's active participation in conference. The student's manner of presentation will enable the instructor to evaluate the alternative reason for reticence (shyness), based on whether the student speaks very softly and rushes the presentation. Continue to encourage the reticent learner's participation in conference discussions, asking open-ended questions that do not put the student "on the spot," but do elicit comment. Over time, the reticent learner will begin to contribute on her own, although probably not at the level of other students.

. . . Monopolizer

The opposite of both the reluctant learner and the reticent learner, the monopolizer pushes to the front, volunteers for everything, and always has something to say. The monopolizer is distinguished from the simply enthusiastic learner by her insensitivity to the effects of her actions on other members of the clinical group. Often the monopolizer has little competition among her peers, who initially are quite willing to let her take the risks involved in volunteering. Group members soon tire of her constant contributions, however, as they begin to recognize that their own learning needs are in danger of being co-opted by her behavior.

Once again, the instructor needs to determine what might be causing the monopolizer's behavior. Two possible reasons are competitiveness and camouflage. The student who continuously vies for the instructor's attention may be seeking recognition as a star performer, and attempting to ensure a high clinical grade. The monopolizer who is motivated by a desire to camouflage lack of knowledge or skill speaks up when she is confident of an answer to avoid being called upon at other times. She often touts her knowledge and ability to distract the instructor's attention from her. She also knows that her behavior will eventually wear out her audience, who will tune out—and so be less critical of—what she is saying.

In working with the monopolizer, the instructor needs to provide reassurance that she is aware of the student's competence (if this is the case), with a comment on the need for others to have opportunities to demonstrate their own level of performance. If the instructor suspects that camouflage may be operating, she will need to double-check on the student's work rather than accept her verbal assurances that her care is accurate and complete. As a skilled leader of the group process, the instructor must structure group interactions to permit all students to participate equally. The monopolizer often needs a firm directive, such as, "Let's hear from someone else, Monica. Judy, what was going on with Mr. A this morning?" Similarly, the instructor should select "volunteers" from among all group members when demonstrating procedures or encouraging students to try out new activities. Care must be taken, however, not to discourage the monopolizer; providing periodic opportunities to contribute at a level similar to other group members prevents a perception that the monopolizer is being punished for her enthusiasm.

. . . Distractor

Whether intentionally or inadvertently, the distractor disrupts the teaching-learning process. She arrives late—and loudly—to conferences, or rushes off before they have ended. She engages other students in side conversations. She tells jokes or giggles inappropriately. She interrupts the flow of a discussion with unrelated questions or comments.

The distractor may be seeking attention through her behavior, or she may have not yet associated the college laboratory and clinical setting with a need for a more professional level of behavior. Regardless of the reason for her behavior, it is important for the instructor to put a quick end to it by identifying it for what it is: unacceptable. Because it is possible that the distractor is still "stuck" in the classroom, where such behavior is better tolerated, the instructor should let the student know in a private conversation that her behavior is inappropriate and will not be tolerated. If the behavior persists, the instructor should deal with it firmly, by asking the student to stop it immediately or to leave. If the instructor fails to address such behavior early in the clinical learning experience, she runs the risk of losing control of the learning environment as other students join the distractor in testing boundaries.

. . . Student Who Lies

While most students are in the nursing program to learn, and steadfastly abide by rules governing integrity in the learning process, a few will resort to dishonesty in order to "get by" a learning or testing experience. In the clinical area, the student may lie about having attended a required off-unit activity or she may lie about the care provided to a patient or she may lie about the patient's vital signs. While the instructor would be justified in failing a student for violating the professional principle of integrity and accountability, it is wise to explore with the student the reasons she felt it necessary to lie in order to determine whether the situation can be salvaged.

Students may lie to cover up their inadequacies. Instead of acknowledging difficulty in performing some activity or reporting an error she has made, the student may attempt to bluff her way through the situation, hoping no one will notice. If the instructor has established a climate for learning that allows for the possibility of error when this is counterbalanced by the protections afforded by openness and honesty, and if learners feel that they will be treated respectfully if they admit they do not know how to do something, then lying is less likely to occur. Students may lie because accumulated stress in both their personal and educational lives causes them to devalue certain learning activities, especially if they believe that no one will be the wiser.

It is essential that the instructor confront the student who lies, identifying the nature of the lie, how the instructor uncovered the lie, how the lie affects patient safety if this was compromised, and asking the student to explain why she felt it necessary to lie. Before doing so, however, the instructor must be certain of her claim. If she is unable to determine whether the problem is an honest error or a lie, she should explore this openly with the student. For example, the instructor might say, "This blood pressure reading on Mr. B is consistent with previous readings but not with his current condition. I'm concerned that you may not have recorded it accurately. Are you certain this is the reading you got? Let's recheck his blood pressure together, to be sure it is correct." This approach enables the instructor to determine whether the student's technique is at fault, and also clears the way for a discussion of the importance of accuracy. Or, "You reported to the primary nurse that you had changed Mr. C's dressing, but it is still dated with yesterday's date. Can you explain this to me?" If the student insists that she was just about to do the change, reinforce the importance of timely and accurate reports. In these two instances, the instructor's alertness to potential lies—and willingness to confront the student with the possibility—discourages the student who might have lied from doing so in the future.

When the student is caught in a lie, the instructor must create some consequences for the student as a result of the behavior. There should be an extremely low tolerance for lies involving patient care. The student who lies in this regard should be warned both verbally and in writing that she will automatically fail the clinical portion of the course should she lie again. Written documentation of the incident and the consequences of a second episode of dishonesty, signed by both the student and the clinical instructor, should be placed in the student's file. When a student confesses to a lie before the instructor has uncovered it or confronted the student, the instructor may wish to be more lenient, particularly if the situation does not involve patient care activities. One instructor had such a student describe the episode in writing to reinforce the importance placed on honesty. This documentation remained in the student's file until the course was completed.

. . . Student Who Plagiarizes

Akin to the student who lies, the student who plagiarizes commits academic dishonesty by adopting another's work as her own. Plagiarism most often involves written work, and so is evident in term papers and nursing care plans, but may also arise in connection with formal oral presentations. It is easy to spot, since the work usually is at an intellectual level much higher than that demonstrated by the student during the semester, and involves language usage (sentence construction, spelling, etc.) far better than in other samples of the student's work, such as nurse's notes or journal entries.

Students may claim ignorance of their plagiarism, indicating that they were relying on accepted sources in preparing their work. Therefore, it is wise to review the rules pertaining to attribution of sources in conjunction with discussions about written assignments. Then students are forewarned about the standards that will be applied in terms of their use of sources when the instructor evaluates their written work. The instructor is well advised to determine the college's policies about academic dishonesty in advance of such a discussion, so as to incorporate the appropriate language into her comments concerning the consequences of plagiarism.

A simple way to deal with the assignment that obviously has been plagiarized is to return it to the student ungraded with a note that indicates that the paper is unacceptable because it follows too closely the work of another (citing that source and providing a copy of the "lifted" area documents the plagiarism) and inviting the student to resubmit a more original version the paper. Where there is a suspicion but no proof of plagiarism, the instructor is better advised to ask the student to meet with her to explore the sources used in preparing the assignment. (Indeed, asking the student to bring those sources to the conference may be one way to confirm the plagiarism.) Quizzing the student on aspects of the paper that go beyond those sources may uncover the plagiarism.

. . . Student Who Exhibits Inappropriate Behavior

The student who engages in behavior that is inappropriate to the clinical setting is likely to be unaware that she is violating standards of professionalism. Such behavior may involve alarming the patient with inaccurate or unfounded information concerning his condition or its treatment, discussing the student's personal problems with the patient, violating patient confidentiality in conversations in public areas, engaging in noncare communications with patients and their families (evangelizing, distributing political information, selling Girl Scout cookies or Tupperware), using access to medical records to determine the health status of people other than the assigned patient, bringing contraband (cigarettes, drugs, alcohol) to a patient, and any number of other, clearly inappropriate activities.

The student's poor judgment coupled with a lack of awareness that the behavior is inappropriate should send a strong signal to the instructor that problems are likely to recur in the future. As a first step, the instructor will need to meet with the student to discuss the behavior and why it is inappropriate. An opportunity should be given to the student to explain her reasons for behaving in the way she did. This gives the instructor some sense of the degree of insight the student has regarding the impropriety of her acts. Documentation of the episode and of the conference should be placed in the student's folder. If the behavior is so out-of-line as to raise questions about the student's continued presence in the clinical area, a joint conference with the program coordinator or department chairperson should be arranged to review the situation and make a final determination as to the student's continued status in the program.

. . . Student Who Is Defiant

Occasionally a student will defiantly disregard the ground rules the instructor has set for the clinical experience. Even after being reminded of those rules—and provided with a rationale for them—the student may continue to ignore them. It is essential that the instructor act quickly and decisively to persuade the student to change her behavior. Depending on the nature of the defiant act, this can be done with a degree of good humor as long as the student gets the message. For example, the student who continues to refuse to remove an engagement ring can be told to have it off her finger in 10 minutes or leave the unit. The instructor must then follow through on her warning and require the student to leave if she does not comply.

. . . Student Who Is Poorly Groomed

Some students feel that they must make a fashion statement in the clinical area. They alter uniform hems and make them too short, wear kneesocks instead of stockings, wear too much makeup, reek of perfume, and so forth. Alternatively, some students fail to attend to personal hygiene, and come to clinical areas with noticeable body odor, dirty fingernails, and scraggly hair.

Explore with the student in a private setting the problems that may underlie the grooming problem, and then work with the student on ways to correct these, providing a patient-related rationale for standards of dress and grooming. Keep in mind that the student whose uniform is too tight or too short may be borrowing a classmate's uniform because she cannot afford her own. Another may be unaware of body odor, or have a physical condition that is contributing to the problem.

. . . Student Who Is a Family Member or Friend

It is difficult to remain objective when a student in the clinical group is a family member or friend, and it is wisest to avoid this problem entirely. Speak with the program coordinator before the experience begins, and ask that this student be placed in another clinical group.

. . . Older Student

More and more nontraditional (26 years of age or older) students are entering nursing programs after having raised families or in search of a second career. These students bring to the learning enterprise a wealth of practical knowledge coupled with maturity that can add new dimensions to everyone's experience. Unfortunately, it is easy to assume that the older student is more skilled and knowledgeable with regard to nursing practice than are more traditionally aged students. This is rarely the case, and it is important to recognize that older students share the same fears and concerns, and often the same learning curve, as their classmates. In working with the older student, provide assignments and experiences that are equivalent to those of other students, while capitalizing on their special strengths.

. . . Male Student

Male nurses still make up only 5–10% of the overall nursing population, and this is reflected in the composition of students in nursing programs. As with the older student, the male student should be treated identically to other students in the group. It is particularly important to guard against the male student being subjected to the jokes and jibes that would be labeled "sexist" if directed toward the female student, and to avoid asking for this student's physical assistance with difficult tasks if this will draw him away from learning activities.

. . . Student Who Is Repeating the Course

The expectations for the student who is repeating the course, either because she was forced to withdraw due to illness or other personal problem or because she failed either the classroom or clinical portion of the course (or both) during her previous registration, must be the same as those of other students. While the instructor cannot assume that the student has forgotten everything that was learned in the course previously, neither can it be assumed that the student should demonstrate greater comfort and ease—as well as greater knowledge and skill—than other students in the group.

It is helpful to meet with the student in advance of the first clinical session to develop a plan that will enable the student to succeed in both the classroom and clinical components of the course. For example, if the student failed the clinical component, try to pinpoint the problems the student encountered and create opportunities for the student to overcome identified deficits. If clinical performance was satisfactory but academic performance problematic, it may be best to focus on assisting the student to make the theoretical connections that might enhance academic performance. Regardless of the planned approach, the student must be confident that she is not being "set up" for failure, but being guided toward success.

. . . Student Who Is Licensed as an LPN or RN

The student who already holds licensure as a licensed practical or registered nurse requires a clinical learning experience akin to the enriched special education that is provided for a gifted child. Such an experience covers the same general content and objectives as those identified for other students, but with greater depth and breadth. Nurses who are returning to school for a higher degree often have developed skilled technical performance but need more work on assessment, diagnosis, analysis, and making the theoretical connections expected of the nurse with more advanced education. Calling upon these students to provide assistance to others helps to reinforce their strengths while challenging them to think through the rationale for activities and their approaches to patient care.

The LPN may avoid revealing her status to program instructors, for fear of being required to do more or being judged in a manner different than other students, and it is important to guard against this possibility.

. . . Student for Whom English Is a Second Language

Most students for whom English is a second language will have sufficient facility with the English language, if only by virtue of having negotiated the prerequisite courses in the arts and sciences that are a prelude to clinical nursing courses. On occasion, however, a student may demonstrate a great deal of difficulty in communicating with peers, staff, and patients as a result of an inadequate command of English. This student should be encouraged to use available supportive devices, such as a bilingual medical dictionary, to gather and interpret information. In the final analysis, the ability to communicate clearly and accurately is an essential skill in nursing practice, and the student must be held to a communication standard similar to that maintained for other students. If problems with language persist, the instructor should seek guidance from the program coordinator or department chairperson to identify appropriate resources for the student and to avoid actions that may result in a claim of discriminatory practices.

MAINTAINING RELATIONSHIPS WITH STAFF

The instructor sets the tone for relationships with staff, and paves the way for students to function comfortably in the clinical agency. The instructor's clinical expertise is her strongest asset in her relationships with staff members, for if staff members trust that the instructor knows what she is doing, they have less concern about the accuracy and completeness of care being provided by students under the instructor's direction. The instructor's reciprocal respect for the expertise of staff members opens the door to more effective communication concerning events that occur on the unit. For example, staff may alert the instructor to a change in the condition of one or another patient so that she can adjust the students' assignments accordingly, or staff may make learning opportunities available to students, by encouraging them to observe or participate in clinical activities that are not part of the regular assignment.

The instructor should encourage staff to let her know about any problems that arise with students in the course of providing patient care. If she is alerted quickly to difficulties, the instructor is able to work with the student to ensure patient safety and effective care. When she has addressed the problem, the instructor should report back to the staff member who alerted her to the situation so that staff know that the instructor cares about quality of care and is responsive to their concerns.

Despite her clinical expertise, the clinical instructor must guard against being co-opted as an extra staff member. The instructor can—and should—pitch in on an ad hoc basis, but gently refuse to become responsible for a patient assignment or to accede to a request to cover the floor during a staff meeting. A simple explanation that the instructor will need to be in a patient's room while Susie demonstrates her ability to do a complete physical examination (or some other teaching or supervisory obligation) lets staff know that the primary focus of the instructor's activities is the students and the learning activities with which they are engaged.

CONTROLLING EMOTIONS

The clinical instructor's role is an inherently stressful one. She faces demands from students, patients, and staff. She needs to communicate with staff to identify changes in patient status or interventions. She must be well versed in the nursing needs of each patient for whom students are providing care, as well as prepared to intervene to complete care activities when necessary. She must be constantly alert to potential problems while remaining free to provide necessary instruction to students. She must be visible without being intrusive. She must present a picture of coolheaded professionalism, even as one patient's status deteriorates, another is discharged prematurely, and a student is stuck with a needle.

It is essential that the instructor keep any anxiety she may be feeling well in check. Anxiety is contagious, and students will quickly sense when their instructor is uneasy, and be concerned that they, too, will be unable to cope with the clinical situation. The instructor must also avoid expressions of anger and exasperation, because students will fear disruption of their working relationships with staff and spillover of anger onto the students.

To control emotions, the instructor must develop the habit of reflecting before reacting. The proven technique of counting to ten before saying or doing anything works well. While she reflects, the instructor should attempt to determine what is going on in the larger situation beyond the stimulus that triggered her anxiety or anger. Making sense of the situation tends to diminish its immediate effects on the instructor as an individual. When the instructor finds herself frequently distressed in the clinical setting, she should try to pinpoint triggers for this emotional response, and determine why she is responding as she is. As the clinical instructor settles into her new role, she should expect to be surprised and, perhaps, confounded by the various demands placed on her as well as the emotional responses they elicit. As in any new work situation, the instructor must find her own path to a comfortable way of operating in the clinical setting.

SUMMARY

Transmitting of knowledge and skill, which is at the heart of the teaching act, relies heavily on the interpersonal effectiveness of the instructor. Her ability to interact and communicate effectively with students, staff, and patients is an essential component of her success. Mindful of her effect on others, as well as their effect on her, the instructor tailors her interactions to meet the multiple demands of the situations in which students are learning nursing. At bottom, however, she strives to maintain her authenticity as a person, and as a nurse.

REFERENCES

Admi, H. (1997). Nursing students' stress during the initial clinical experience. *Journal of Nursing Education*, 36, 323–327.

Bevis, E.O. (1988). New directions for a new age. In National League for Nursing, *Curriculum revolution: Mandate for change*. New York: NLN.

Claus, K.E.; & Bailey, J.T. (1977). *Power and influence in health care*. St. Louis: C.V. Mosby.

Hanson, L.E.; & Smith, M.J. (1996). Nursing students' perspectives: Experiences of caring and not-so-caring interactions with faculty. *Journal of Nursing Education*, 35, 105–112.

Kleehammer, K.; Hart, A.L.; & Keck, J.F. (1990). Nursing students' perceptions of anxiety-producing situations in the clinical setting. *Journal of Nursing Education*, 29, 183–187.

Kübler-Ross, E. (1969). *On death and dying*. New York: Macmillan.

Oermann, M.H. (1998). Differences in clinical experiences of ADN and BSN students. *Journal of Nursing Education*, 37, 197–201.

Pagana, K.D. (1990). The relationship of hardiness and social support to student appraisal of stress in an initial clinical nursing situation. *Journal of Nursing Education*, 29, 255–261.

Rittman, M.R.; & Osburn, J. (1995). An interpretive analysis of precepting an unsafe student. *Journal of Nursing Education*, 34, 217–221.

Shearer, R.A.; & Davidhizar, R.E. (1998). Recognizing a post-traumatic stress disorder in a nursing student. *Journal of Nursing Education*, 37, 222–224.

Wolf, Z.R. (1989). Uncovering the hidden work of nursing. *Nursing & Health Care*, 10, 463–467.

CHAPTER 12

ETHICAL AND LEGAL ISSUES IN NURSING EDUCATION

Ethical Issues in Nursing Education   234
    Ethical Systems and Analytical Tools   234
    Approaches to Guiding Students through Ethical Dilemmas
    in Practice   235
    Ethical Issues Related to the Instructional Role   239
Legal Issues in Nursing Education   242
    Licensure Issues   243
    Due Process Issues   246
    The Student with a Disability   247
    Contractual Issues   248
Summary   249
References   249

Ethics describe standards of conduct by which people choose to act based on conceptions of what is good and what is bad; the obligations and duties people have in relation to good and bad acts and their outcomes; and the principles underlying decisions to conform to one or another standard of conduct. Laws are socially accepted rules of conduct, devised to protect society. Rooted in the values held by the majority of people in a given society, laws attempt to create order in people's dealings with one another through the application of the principles of fairness and justice, so that the rights of individuals and of society are protected.

Ethics and law both guide conduct. The special circumstances of nursing practice, which places nurses in intimate relationships with patients, demands attention to those ethical guidelines and legal requirements that govern the conduct of the professional nurse. The clinical instructor carries much of the responsibility for guiding students' ethical decision making as they encounter ethical dilemmas in the course of providing nursing care. The clinical instructor must also identify and articulate for students the legal parameters within which nursing practice takes place.

Beyond practice-related issues, the clinical instructor also must consider additional ethical and legal issues specific to nursing education as she works with students in the clinical setting.

ETHICAL ISSUES IN NURSING EDUCATION

Aiken (1994) defines ethics as "systems of valued behaviors and beliefs" (p. 22) that provide a framework for decision making in seeking to secure values or ideals. Ethical dilemmas occur when an action to secure individual rights will violate the rights of others; when an obligation to an individual will result in failure to meet an obligation to others; when one value must be given a higher priority than another, equally compelling value; when no one good solution can be secured; or when the system of ethical decision making adopted by the individual offers no guidance for selecting an action.

In her work with students, the clinical instructor will be challenged by students' responses to the ethical dilemmas they encounter. The instructor usually has successfully resolved many of these same issues in the course of her practice experience, and is likely to apply a framework for ethical decision making without having articulated its basis. Students' questions often evoke a response from the instructor that reflects her own framework rather than a response that initiates a discussion of alternative ways of analyzing the dilemma. This latter approach helps students to develop their own approach to ethical issues.

Ethical Systems and Analytical Tools

The ethical decisions required in the situations nurses encounter are called normative decisions, because they require a choice as to what action the nurse will take when faced with an ethical dilemma. Three frameworks or ethical systems describe the major approaches to these day-to-day ethical issues.

Egoism entails decision making that centers on what the moral agent (the person making the choice) thinks is right, rather than the effects of the decision on the comfort of others. A nurse who operates from this framework would choose to initiate cardiopulmonary resuscitation—despite a DNR order or the patient's express wishes not to be resuscitated—because it makes her more comfortable to do so.

Deontology entails actions taken on the basis of the inherent moral significance of the standard to be used in selecting an action. In *act-deontology*, the moral values of the agent (what the agent believes to be right) are of major significance in determining how to resolve an ethical dilemma; in *rule-deontology*, external rules become the standard for response. A nurse who operates within an act-deontological framework will very consistently apply her own value system in resolving ethical dilemmas, for example, by giving the minimum amount of narcotic prescribed for a patient regardless of source or level of pain, age of the patient, or imminent death. A nurse who operates within a rule-deontological framework will consistently apply rules in resolving such dilemmas, for example, by taking vital signs at the intervals ordered without regard to the patient's need for rest.

Utilitarianism entails decision making that attempts to balance predicted outcomes of various decision options so that the action selected is the one that will yield the greatest good (or the least harm) for the most people. The nurse who operates within a utilitarian framework would choose to restrain the patient who is wandering so that she is able to attend to other patients in her care.

These three systems of ethical decision making are not mutually exclusive, and a moral agent may operate from different systems or a mix of systems when faced with different ethical dilemmas. An understanding of these basic approaches to ethical decision making enables the clinical instructor to elicit from students their reasoning in response to the moral issues they encounter in practice and to work within that existing framework to assist students to consider alternative perspectives.

Many nursing students have not yet completed their own moral development. The issues they encounter during their clinical learning experiences raise profound questions of right and wrong and of how the nurse ought to respond, particularly to the pain and suffering of those she cares for, creating a fertile field for further moral growth. Kohlberg's (1981) cognitive-developmental framework attempts to outline the sequence of moral development in children, which parallels the ethical systems described above. In his research with young boys, Kohlberg identified three levels of moral development, each with two stages. Gilligan's (1982) work with young girls identified a similar schema. At the *preconventional* level, the child distinguishes right from wrong on the basis of consequences rather than internalized rules. Initially, the child seeks to do right to avoid punishment. Later, the child's own interests determine what is right, with those interests including a desire to obey. At the *conventional* level, the child begins to understand and internalize rules for behavior. Initially, the child's behavior is in response to other's expectations. Later, the child begins to develop a social conscience and a sense of duty that operates even when authoritative others are not present. At the *postconventional* level, the child's behavior in relation to right and wrong is self-chosen, on the basis of social utility versus individual rights or based on universal ethical principles. Kohlberg asserts that many children reach adulthood without attaining the postconventional level of moral development.

Approaches to Guiding Students through Ethical Dilemmas in Practice

Ethical dilemmas in nursing practice tend to arise in relation to fundamental perceived rights—

- the right to live;
- the right to die;
- the right to health;

- quality of life;
- societal needs; and
- competition for resources

—as well as fundamental perceived obligations of the health care system and the providers of health care—

- to do good;
- to do no harm;
- to provide equal treatment to all, in particular the disenfranchised and marginalized persons in society; and
- to maintain an acceptable level of competence in performing the responsibilities inherent in the work of health care.

A first step in helping students to work through the ethical dilemmas that emerge in their clinical learning experiences involves guiding them in identifying the standard or principle involved. Identifying the core value or values represented in the dilemma is facilitated by reference to the American Nurses Association's Code for Nurses (see Box 12–1) or by relating the dilemma to one or more ethical principles (see Table 12–1). Either of these can provide a beginning point for discussion. For example, a question involving a patient's right to refuse care can be explored in relation to the first statement in the Code for Nurses (concerning human dignity and the uniqueness of the patient) or the ethical principle of autonomy.

Second, students need help in identifying the source of their moral discomfort in a given situation. Because they often are groping with the moral imperatives raised by their own developmental issues and, in the process, developing a personal moral code, students tend not to acknowledge—let alone honor—the legitimacy of another's belief system or moral perspective. This egocentric stance creates a conflict of value systems, which is the true source of the ethical dilemma. Shall the student honor her own lust for life, or support the patient's decision to forego additional treatment for a terminal condition? Students also tend to respond to the most immediate and predominant characteristics of the dilemma rather than exploring its deeper levels to consider the consequences of alternative decisions. Emergency triage exemplifies this source of ethical dilemmas: the need to prioritize values that are equally compelling. The same tendency to attend to the immediate situation also causes students to explore the first presenting issue that they encounter rather than recognizing that other ethical standards or principles are involved that present conflicting stimuli for response. Should the student undertake to inform the patient of a terminal prognosis, abiding by the principle of veracity, or work instead to rally the patient's support system to provide the comfort and counsel he will need when he learns the prognosis from his physician, abiding by the principle of nonmaleficence? Third, students lack sufficient knowledge and experience to fully grasp many of the ethical issues they encounter in practice. They recognize that something is wrong in the situation

Box 12–1   American Nurses Association Code for Nurses

1. The nurse provides services with respect for human dignity and the uniqueness of the client unrestricted by considerations of social or economic status, personal attributes, or the nature of health problems.
2. The nurse safeguards the client's right to privacy by judiciously protecting information of a confidential nature.
3. The nurse acts to safeguard the client and the public when health care and safety are affected by the incompetent, unethical, or illegal practice of any person.
4. The nurse assumes responsibility and accountability for individual nursing judgments and actions.
5. The nurse maintains competence in nursing.
6. The nurse exercises informed judgment and uses individual competence and qualifications as criteria in seeking consultation, accepting responsibilities, and delegating nursing activities to others.
7. The nurse participates in activities that contribute to the ongoing development of the profession's body of knowledge.
8. The nurse participates in the profession's efforts to implement and improve standards of nursing.
9. The nurse participates in the profession's efforts to establish and maintain conditions of employment conducive to high quality nursing care.
10. The nurse participates in the profession's effort to protect the public from misinformation and misrepresentation and to maintain the integrity of nursing.
11. The nurse collaborates with members of the health professions and other citizens in promoting community and national efforts to meet the health needs of the public.

Source: Reprinted with permission from *Code for Nurses with Interpretive Statements*, © 1985. American Nurses Publishing, American Nurses Foundation/American Nurses Association, Washington, DC.

that calls for a response, but need more information to understand the ethical principles involved and the nature of potential outcomes of alternative decisions. For example, the student observing a normal delivery that turns into an emergency delivery does not know what—if anything—can be done to preserve the mother's life while salvaging the fetus. She recognizes that an ethical decision-making process is occurring, but not its basis.

Fourth, students need to know that there are constraints on the ability of any individual to act in accordance with his or her values. Having analyzed

---

TABLE 12–1   PRINCIPLES UNDERLYING ETHICAL DILEMMAS

- **Autonomy**—the right of self-determination, independence, and freedom.
- **Justice**—the obligation to be fair to all people; often called distributive justice.
- **Fidelity**—the obligation to be faithful to commitments made.
- **Beneficence**—doing good.
- **Nonmaleficence**—doing no harm; protecting others from harm.
- **Veracity**—truthfulness.
- **Standard of Best Interest**—what others decide is best for a person who cannot express a choice; based on the principle of beneficence (but raising the problem of paternalism).
- **Obligations**—demands to fulfill and honor the rights of others; may be moral or legal in nature.
- **Rights**—claims or entitlements; may be legal, in relation to a claim to some good or benefit; may be moral; may be option rights, involving freedom of choice within a prescribed set of boundaries.

Source: Based on Aiken, T.D. (1994). *Legal, ethical, and political issues in nursing.* (pp. 23–26). Philadelphia: F.A. Davis.

---

an ethical dilemma in terms of the ethical principles involved and the source of the dilemma, can the student act on her decision concerning the right thing to do in the situation? Three constraints on action need to be considered. *Impotence* involves the lack of means, power, or the right to act. A student may determine that her best action in a situation would be to stay with the patient through the night, but she is prevented from doing this because of her role as a student. *Organizational barriers* to action, such as policy considerations or obligations as an employee, present other constraints on nurses' ability to act in accordance with the ethical decisions they have made. This reality cannot be ignored in discussing ethical dilemmas with students, who are often frustrated with the "system" and its seeming inhumanity. A discussion of ways that nurses can act to change the system and foster better care provides an outlet for frustration while confirming the appropriateness of an ethical response. Finally, *legal constraints*—in particular, liability issues—impact the nurse's ability to act in accordance with an ethical decision, and must be included in discussions with students concerning ethical dilemmas.

The educational approach to ethical decision making in the clinical practice setting is one of exploring the parameters of the presenting dilemma and the alternatives, consequences, and constraints that exist and impact the nurse's moral agency. Such an approach seeks to initiate a process of analysis rather than to provide answers. Coupled with the following "rules of thumb" governing value selection, this analysis equips students for the myriad dilemmas they will encounter throughout their educational experiences and subsequent practice, and provides an excellent foundation for their development as moral agents.

1. Intrinsic (good in themselves) values are preferred to extrinsic (means to attain other goals) values.
2. Productive, relatively permanent values are preferred over those that are less enduring.
3. Value selection should be based on self-chosen ends or ideals that are internally consistent and related to one's own life as lived.
4. Of competing positive values, the preference is for the most positive; of competing negative values, the preference is for the least negative.

Ethical Issues Related to the Instructional Role

The same principles that underlie the ANA Code for Nurses can serve as guidelines for considering ethical issues likely to arise in the course of clinical teaching. While students are not patients, they *are* clients of the educational system, and share many of the vulnerabilities that give rise to ethical issues in providing direct nursing care.

Student-Teacher Relationships. Students, like patients, are unique persons of worth and dignity and deserving of respect. The clinical instructor must develop core behaviors evidencing mutual respect for and collaboration with those she teaches. Interpersonal sensitivity and humanistic caring are the means by which the "respect for the human dignity and the uniqueness of the [student as] client" are preserved in the clinical, instructional setting.

The clinical instructor holds a position of power and control over the students she teaches. Abuse of this power and control is unethical. Inappropriate behaviors include sarcasm and belittling; threatening; criticizing the student in front of others; acting in a superior fashion; showing favoritism to one student over another; refusing to answer student's legitimate questions; rudeness; and authoritarianism. It is interesting to note that often it is the instructor who feels least in control and least competent in the role of instructor that abuses the power and control inherent in the role as a means of bolstering her own self-confidence.

There is often a fine line between student-teacher interactions intended to stimulate student thinking or provide corrective guidance and those that are dismissive and rude. The student who arrives on the clinical unit unprepared for the day's activities needs to be directed to prepare for the assignment before beginning work with the patient, rather than given the necessary information by the instructor. In the same vein, the student whose question concerns material previously covered needs guidance in retrieving the information and applying it in the present situation. A few stimulus questions by the instructor to initiate the student's thought processes are more useful than simply providing the answer, because discovering her own answers increases the student's confidence in her ability to apply theory to practice. In contrast to these examples, the instructor who tells a student "to look it up" when she asks a question is communicating disdain for the student and for the educational process. Students rightly resent such nonresponsiveness in their instructors, who are, after all, the experts to whom they should look for guidance in their learning and also the persons responsible for teaching.

In her efforts to demonstrate humanistic caring and concern for students and maintain a collaborative approach to teaching and learning, the instructor must be careful not to cross the boundary that should exist between student and teacher. Being warm and friendly does not require being "one of the girls," which creates confusion for students, who need someone to be in charge of their learning rather than in competition for their friendship.

Although less frequently a problem in nursing than in some other academic disciplines, the instructor must guard against interactions with students that constitute inappropriate sexual behavior. The same guidelines used with patients apply to student-teacher situations. The instructor's position of control and authority precludes intimate relationships with any student.

Privacy.   The Family Education Rights and Privacy Act of 1974 seeks to protect student confidentiality by prohibiting the disclosure of student grades, class standing, and other similar information to other students, the student's parents, or any other persons. Such common practices as posting course, exam, or paper grades—even with codes substituting for names of students—allowing one student to deliver another student's paper, and placing papers in a common place for pickup are all prohibited under the law. This creates a special burden for the part-time clinical instructor, who may see students only during clinical laboratory hours and so must devise creative strategies for the timely return of papers within the restrictions of the law.

The provisions of this Act also suggest the breadth of the ethical demands for privacy with respect to student performance, underlining the need to conduct disciplining of students in private, away from the earshot of others. Great care must be taken in discussing one student's clinical experiences with others in the group. While such discussions are not proscribed, the instructor must refrain from making evaluative comments concerning an individual student's performance during such conferences.

The clinical instructor also needs to guard patient confidentiality in activities that take place away from the clinical unit. Conferences held in the dining room over a student meal may be time efficient, but run the risk of jeopardizing patient confidentiality. Particular care must be taken to ensure that the patient cannot be identified by the casual observer, who may be a family member or neighbor. Using a first name and unit number is hardly sufficient to guard against this hazard. Conferences held on campus also must be conducted in such a way as to protect confidentiality. The clinical instructor also needs to safeguard written materials, such as student assignments and student papers, from the scrutiny of others.

Dealing with Academic Dishonesty.   The clinical instructor must consider carefully the consequences of such dishonest practices of students as plagiarism, cheating, submission of papers prepared by others (such as completed nursing care plans), and "fudging" documentation in the clinical setting in light of the ethical standard that requires the nurse "to safeguard the client and the public when health care and safety are affected by the incompetent, unethical, or illegal practice of any person." Care must be taken not to falsely accuse a student of academic dishonesty, but there should be a clear message of zero tolerance for such behavior. Cutting corners and attempting to get away with less than adequate provision of patient care, lying about what has been done or not done, and other behaviors that fail to meet the standards of nursing practice tend to persist after the student who has engaged in these during the nursing program has graduated and is in active practice. The clinical instructor needs to reflect on whether such a person should be allowed to continue in the program and express her concerns to the program coordinator or department chairperson.

Meeting Work-Related Responsibilities.   The instructional role is multifaceted, complex, and at times overwhelming. Assuming "responsibility and accountability for individual nursing judgments and actions" in the context of clinical teaching requires that the instructor meet the demands of the job she has undertaken to perform.

The clinical instructor must be prepared for each college or clinical laboratory experience and any associated conferences. College laboratory activities need to be planned to provide for active learning rather than merely being an extension of classroom lectures. A plan must be devised for each day in the clinical area, so that student learning is maximized and proceeds toward the achievement of established objectives. Preparation may require that the instructor visit the unit the day before the clinical experience or, in this era of shortened lengths of stay in most institutional settings, hours before the experience is scheduled to begin. The instructor must have a firm grasp of what she hopes to accomplish with students on any given clinical day, what is possible given the situation as she finds it, and how goals might be achieved. She must also have a firm understanding of the histories, treatments, and nursing care needs of the patients she has selected for students to work with. Conferences must be focused on salient issues that reflect classroom learning. An open-ended discussion of what went on in the clinical area during the experience does not provide sufficient structure to permit integration of theory and practice, a major goal of clinical learning. Preparation places the instructor in control of the learning experience (to the extent that this is possible in the fluid clinical arena) and endows students with a sense of confidence in the instructor and the instructional process.

The clinical instructor must remain visible and available to students on the unit for guidance and assistance. Students should know where to find the instructor if she will be occupied with another student for any length of time, and should be aware of her watchful presence on the unit as the students carry out assigned activities. In the home care setting, contact by telephone or pager is essential, and students should have a general idea of where the instructor will be at various times during the day.

The clinical instructor must provide timely feedback on individual student performance, whether through anecdotal notes describing the student's actions in the clinical area or in response to written work. These written vehicles for communicating with the student, coupled with face-to-face encounters during the course of the clinical experience, provide an opportunity for a dialogue between student and teacher that enhances learning through individualization. Timeliness is critical to learning.

The clinical instructor must "show up," by being available during office hours, attending scheduled meetings, and so forth. At times, her attendance may seem inconsequential, especially when no one comes for office hours or the instructor has nothing to contribute to a meeting. But her availability signals her commitment, and students are comforted by knowing her whereabouts.

By the same token, the clinical instructor should maintain visibility by attending those "ceremonial functions" that are significant to students. Although the new or part-time instructor may feel like an outsider at such functions as pinning ceremonies and honor society inductions, she is not perceived as such by the students she has taught in the clinical laboratory. The clinical instructor's role looms large in students' perceptions of the nursing education experience, for it is in their clinical laboratory that the real work of learning nursing occurs. As the person who has guided and facilitated that learning, the clinical instructor holds a special place for students. Attendance at these functions communicates the instructor's pride in the progress of the students she has taught.

Finally, the clinical instructor must respond to requests from students, particularly for letters of recommendation as they seek employment during the summer or upon graduation. As the person who has observed the student "in action," the clinical instructor has valuable insight into the student's potential as a nurse. Recognizing this, students often seek the endorsement of their clinical instructor when they apply for jobs. When the instructor enthusiastically agrees to send a letter of recommendation to a potential employer or graduate school, she is also welcoming the student into the profession's ranks. If for some reason the instructor believes she cannot write a supportive letter for the student, she should let her know this and guide her to seek such a letter from someone else on faculty rather than allow the request to linger on her desk, possibly jeopardizing the student's employment opportunity.

LEGAL ISSUES IN NURSING EDUCATION

The practice of nursing is governed by each state's nurse practice act. Nurse practice acts typically define nursing and its scope of practice; elaborate the educational and examination requirements to be licensed as a registered nurse; restrict the use of the RN title to those who have met those requirements; identify persons who are permitted to perform nursing acts even if unlicensed, including nursing students; identify conduct which could lead to sanction or revocation of a nurse's license; and establish a board of nursing comprised of professional and lay members to oversee professional issues. Table 12–2 provides excerpts from Connecticut's Nurse Practice Act, which is similar to the nurse practice acts enacted in other states. "Meat" is put on the bare "bones" of the nurse practice act through the board of nursing's promulgation of regulations (for example, those that govern the length and content of nursing education programs) and issuance of declaratory rulings (for example, those that clarify the scope of nursing practice in relation to new technologies). Legal proceedings under the nurse practice act fall in the realm of administrative law.

Nursing practice also is subject to civil law proceedings (those involving malpractice issues, for example) and criminal law proceedings (as when a nurse steals narcotics from her employer). Constitutional law is invoked in situations involving such issues as due process rights and discriminatory practices, which are of particular concern to nursing educators.

Licensure Issues

Clinical nursing instructors are justifiably concerned about the impact on their own licensure status of acts performed by students. The commonly held belief that students "practice on the instructor's license" is not entirely true. Students are responsible for their own acts, and are held to the same standard of care required for the occupation for which they are preparing. Problems arise when the instructor fails to assess the readiness of the student to engage in the assigned activity, fails to provide adequate instruction and/or supervision for the activity, or insists that the student perform an activity that is illegal or beyond the scope of nursing practice. These are the same principles that are applied to an analysis of delegating nursing assignments in the clinical setting. Consequently, a student's act can be attributed to the instructor, and so create a potential action against the instructor's license, only if it can be demonstrated that the instructor's own negligence in overseeing the student's activities contributed to the alleged damage. In our litigious society, the search for the "deepest pockets" (most money) will result in all potential defendants being named in a suit arising from alleged negligence or malpractice. Consequently, the clinical instructor is wise to carry malpractice liability insurance to cover the costs of defending herself, even if the nursing program provides such coverage for its instructors. The instructor also should thoroughly document in writing any guidelines and ground rules she has provided for students, and retain these if an incident that might lead to legal action has occurred. Further, the instructor should record in detail any events that might give rise to legal action, including her own response to a student's actions. These contemporaneous notes, which should be dated and signed, can be

TABLE 12–2   Selected Provisions of the Connecticut State
Nurse Practice Act

Sec. 20-87a. Definition of "nursing," "advanced nursing practice," and "practical nursing". (a) The practice of nursing by a registered nurse is defined as the process of diagnosing human responses to actual or potential health problems, providing supportive and restorative care, health counseling and teaching, case finding and referral, collaborating in the implementation of the total health care regimen and executing the medical regimen under the direction of a licensed physician or dentist.

Sec. 20-99. Improper professional conduct. (b) Conduct which fails to conform to the accepted standards of the nursing profession includes, but is not limited to, the following: (1) Fraud or material deception in procuring or attempting to procure a license to practice nursing; (2) illegal conduct, incompetence or negligence in carrying out usual nursing functions; (3) physical illness or loss of motor skill, including but not limited to deterioration through the aging process; (4) emotional disorder or mental illness; (5) abuse or excessive use of drugs, including alcohol, narcotics, or chemicals; (6) fraud or material deception in the course of professional services or activities; (7) willful falsification of entries in any hospital, patient, or other record pertaining to drugs, the results of which are detrimental to the health of a patient and (8) conviction of the violation of any of the provisions of this chapter by any court or criminal jurisdiction. The Commissioner of Public Health may order a license holder to submit to a reasonable physical or mental examination if his physical or mental capacity to practice safely is the subject of an investigation.

Sec. 20-101. Construction of chapter. Permitted practices. Temporary practice. No provision of this chapter shall confer any authority to practice medicine or surgery nor shall this chapter prohibit any person from the domestic administration of family remedies or the furnishing of assistance in the case of an emergency; nor shall it be construed as prohibiting persons employed in state hospitals and state sanatoriums and subsidiary workers in general hospitals from assisting in the nursing care of patients if adequate medical and nursing supervision is provided; nor shall it be construed as prohibiting students who are enrolled in schools of nursing approved pursuant to section 20–90, and students who are enrolled in school for licensed practical nurses approved pursuant to section 20–90, from performing such work as is incidental to their respective courses of study; nor shall it prohibit graduates of schools of nursing approved pursuant to section 20–90, from nursing the sick pending the results of the first examination for licensure scheduled following their graduation, provided such graduate nurses are working in hospitals or organizations where adequate supervision is provided.

Source: Connecticut General Statutes. Chapter 378. Nursing.

used to refresh the instructor's memory of the incident should litigation be brought in the future.

The ultimate purpose of nurse practice acts is to protect the public from harm by unqualified or incompetent practitioners. The section of the nurse practice act detailing improper professional conduct provides guidance to the instructor as she attempts to balance patient safety concerns with her instructional responsibilities. The behaviors listed in this section are those that would be grounds for the suspension or revocation of a nurse's license. The same behaviors may warrant a student's removal from the clinical setting or a failure in the clinical component of the course. Reviewing the provisions of this section of the act with students alerts them to the seriousness of such behaviors and the potential consequences that may follow.

Illegal conduct (pilfering hospital supplies, for example), incompetence (inability to perform tasks, whether intellectual or physical, even with maximum guidance and supervision), and malpractice (practice that consistently fails to conform to the standard expected of students at the same educational level, even after remediation) are all grounds for failure or, at the very least, removal from the clinical area until further remediation can be provided. However, the due process rights of the student, discussed below, must be preserved in taking such an action.

Physical illness, loss of motor skill, emotional disorders, or mental illness that interferes with the student's ability to perform normal nursing functions and cannot be accommodated in some way also are grounds for removing the student from the clinical area. The issue is not the illness per se, but its effect or potential effect on patient safety and well-being. Once a nurse has been licensed, a chronic disability that interferes with her ability to function in one or more settings may lead to a restriction being placed on her license, limiting her to work in areas in which she is able to function safely. Within the nursing program, however, students are expected to accomplish a broad range of activities in the course of their nursing education, some of which may be beyond the ability of the disabled or chronically ill student. In such circumstances, care must be taken not to violate the student's rights under the Americans with Disabilities Act (ADA) while still conforming to the standards established for program completion.

Abuse or excessive use of drugs, alcohol, or other substances is another ground for removal of a student from the clinical area. The student who arrives hung over or under the influence of alcohol or drugs (even prescribed medications, such as analgesics) must be sent home. The student whose substance abuse or addiction does not interfere with clinical practice activities presents a different issue. The policies and procedures of the nursing program and college with respect to this problem must be adhered to in order to protect the student's rights under the ADA and to conform to due process procedures.

Fraud, deception regarding clinical activities, and falsification of records pertaining to drug administration are clearly proscribed by the nurse practice act, and merit a similar response (removal from the clinical area or failure in the course) by the clinical instructor. In responding to a student's fraudulent behaviors, the clinical instructor, once again, must take care to preserve the student's due process rights.

Conviction of a criminal act or a finding against a nurse as a defendant in a civil action (for example, a malpractice suit) that arises from the nurse's clinical activities may constitute grounds for revocation of the nurse's license. The court's decision carries over into any administrative proceedings against the nurse involving the same matter. A criminal conviction may render a nursing student ineligible for licensure upon graduation from the nursing program. The clinical instructor must be guided by established policies and procedures.

Due Process Issues

A student's due process rights are implicated whenever the actions of the instructor will have a negative impact on the student's status in the nursing program. Due process safeguards are intended to ensure that the student's voice is heard, as well as to ensure that the instructor has taken all reasonable and necessary steps to enable the student to succeed. The procedures for appeal of an instructor's decision should be written and contained in the college's handbook as well as in nursing department documents. It is essential that both the instructor and students know—in advance of any problems—what recourse they have if a dispute arises.

Due process procedures usually follow a stepwise pattern as the student seeks review of the instructor's decision by a higher authority empowered to amend or overturn that decision. The person or persons to whom the appeal is taken do not review the basis for the instructor's decision, but instead review the process used to reach that decision to determine whether the student has been treated differently than others in her clinical group or whether a palpable injustice has occurred. An example of discriminatory treatment that would provide grounds for appeal might be failing a student clinically for chronic lateness while tolerating the identical behavior in other students. An example of palpable injustice that would provide grounds for appeal might be accusing a student of deliberately falsifying a patient's record when the student had made an innocent mistake. Because clinical instruction is a learning process, where the student should be able to make mistakes, it is essential that the instructor discriminate between errors committed in the course of learning and lapses that are more likely to be attributable to incompetence or academic dishonesty.

To avoid due process issues the instructor should incorporate the following strategies in all her clinical teaching:

1. At the start of the clinical experience, review with students the program's policies with respect to appeals in the event of a dispute between the instructor and a student.
2. Clearly communicate, both orally and in writing, expectations for students' performance and behavior in relation to the clinical

experience and retain a dated file copy of these for future reference. Such expectations should include student behaviors that are unacceptable, and the consequences for the student should she breach the rules governing conduct in the clinical area.

3. Structure assignments in such a way that all students have equivalent opportunities to achieve clinical objectives and so demonstrate competent practice.

4. Provide timely feedback, both orally and in writing, on each student's conduct—including any instances of problematic behavior—again preserving a dated file copy. Make detailed notes concerning student practices that are unsafe or fail to meet the standards expected of .other students.

5. Inform the student (again, in writing) of the grounds for removing her from the clinical area (such as illness or substance abuse) if this becomes necessary, and the steps the student must take to reenter the clinical area. Make every effort to provide the student who is legitimately ill with an opportunity to complete an alternate assignment so that she can keep pace with the group.

6. Develop a written remediation plan—dated and signed by both the instructor and student—for the unsafe or incompetent student, outlining performance expectations and detailing approaches and strategies for meeting these expectations.

7. Insist that all students conform to the ground rules detailing acceptable and unacceptable behaviors in the clinical area. Maintain performance standards at a comparable level for all students. Standards should not be lowered for the unsafe or incompetent student.

The Student with a Disability

The Americans with Disabilities Act prohibits discrimination against persons with physical and mental disabilities. This means that otherwise qualified candidates must be admitted to nursing programs and, once they are admitted, provided with reasonable accommodations to overcome their limitations. Creativity and flexibility are key to successful adaptation of the learning environment to accommodate the disabled student. Obviously, the clinical experience presents the most challenges in this regard.

As Magilvy and Mitchell (1995) note, "A functional limitation does not necessarily result in disability, but in the context of a society in which that limitation is not accommodated, disability can occur" (35). A student's limitation may be visible, as with vision and hearing deficits, mobility problems, or the physical or functional loss of one or more limbs, or it may be invisible, as with chronic illness, learning disabilities, and mental disorders. It is essential for the instructor to have prior knowledge of the type and degree of limitation that is present, and the kinds of accommodations that have worked in the past. While the student's file is likely to contain notations in this regard, the best source of information is the student herself. Having progressed this far in her education, the student is likely to have discovered many approaches to accommodating her limitations and is an excellent resource to the instructor as she plans clinical learning experiences. The instructor also can turn to the college office that manages issues related to disabled students.

The goal of accommodation is to create an even playing field for the disabled student by providing a means for her to compensate for her disability so that she can fully participate in the learning experience. In addition to identifying those adaptations, whether technological or otherwise, that will support the student's functioning in the clinical area, the instructor must carefully analyze planned learning activities to determine which are essential to meet course objectives. When considering the needs of the disabled student, there is a tendency to focus on the physical tasks and demands of nursing practice, despite the fact that much of the real work of nursing is mental. Is it most important that the student reposition a patient, or that she recognizes the need for repositioning and can direct a nursing assistant to accomplish the task safely? This type of analysis presents the real challenge in working with the disabled student to identify activities and approaches to clinical learning that will accomplish the goals of the experience.

Once appropriate accommodations have been made, the disabled student must be evaluated using the same criteria as are applied to other students. Not all problems with learning can be attributed to the disability. A marginal student may remain marginal despite the accommodation provided for a physical or mental limitation.

Contractual Issues

The nursing program's affiliation with a clinical agency usually is formalized in a written agreement or contract in which the parties agree to the conditions under which the agency will accept nursing students. Under the terms of the contract, the agency generally reserves control over the care of patients in its facility and the school retains control over the educational curriculum. Both students and instructors must meet specified health requirements (recent physical examination, PPD, immunizations) and hold current CPR certification. The contract often specifies the maximum number of students who can be supervised by one instructor, and requires that the full names of all students and instructors be submitted to the agency prior to the start of the clinical experience. Any restrictions on student activities, such as administering medications, are stipulated in the contract. Liability issues and insurance coverage for students and instructors may be detailed.

Although the instructor is not a party to the affiliation agreement, she is responsible for abiding by its terms. Therefore, it is wise to ask the program coordinator or department chairperson for a copy of the agreement with the agency in which the instructor will be supervising students to ensure that she knows the terms under which the affiliation is proceeding. A sample of such an agreement is reproduced in Appendix E.

The instructor also needs to understand the employment contract under which she is working, in particular the dates on which employment begins and ends, any provision for sick days or holidays, and any fringe benefits. The rate of compensation should be clearly identified in the employment contract, but the instructor should inquire as to when payment can be expected. A benefit package that includes health care, disability and life insurance, and so forth, usually is not available to part-time employees, but there may be some non-monetary perquisites, such as free or reduced tuition at the college, that the instructor should be aware of.

SUMMARY

Ethical and legal issues surround nursing practice and nursing education. Because students have had limited experience with ethical decision making, the clinical instructor must help students to recognize ethical dilemmas as they occur in their practice with patients as well as approaches to resolving those dilemmas. Students also have little exposure to the legal parameters of practice; the clinical setting is an ideal place in which to introduce and reinforce the behaviors expected of the professional nurse.

At the same time, the new clinical instructor must deal with ethical and legal issues that are embedded in the educational experience to ensure that she is meeting the highest standards in this new role.

REFERENCES

Aiken, T.D. (1994). *Legal, ethical, and political issues in nursing*. Philadelphia: F.A. Davis.

American Nurses Association. (1985). *Code for nurses with interpretive statements*. Washington, D.C.: The Association.

Gilligan, C. (1982). *In a different voice; Psychological theory and women's development*. Cambridge, MA: Harvard University Press.

Kohlberg, L. (1981). *The philosophy of moral development*. New York: Harper & Row.

Magilvy, J.K., & Mitchell, A.C. (1995). Education of nursing students with special needs. *Journal of Nursing Education, 34*, 31–36.

SAMPLE PROGRAM, LEVEL, AND RELATED COURSE OBJECTIVES FOR A BACCALAUREATE NURSING PROGRAM

The program and level objectives for this baccalaureate nursing program, which reflect program outcomes and the plan for the sequential development of the knowledge and competencies necessary to achieve those outcomes, all address the same core competencies, but at different levels of sophistication and with different populations. The related course objectives mirror the program and level objectives, but express how the objective is achieved within the content and related clinical experiences students cover in the course.

PROGRAM OBJECTIVES

1. Synthesize knowledge from the arts, sciences, and humanities with nursing theory as the basis for making nursing practice decisions.
2. Exercise critical thinking in using the nursing process to assess, diagnose, plan, implement, and evaluate the care provided to individuals, families, and communities.
3. Apply the nursing process to design, implement, and evaluate therapeutic nursing interventions to provide preventive, curative, supportive, and restorative care for individuals, families, and communities in both structured and unstructured settings, using a variety of technologies.
4. Use a variety of communication techniques, including written documentation, in the process of assessment, counseling, and therapeutic intervention with individual clients, families, groups, and communities.

Source: Department of Nursing, Western Connecticut State University, Danbury, CT.

5. Develop and implement a variety of teaching-learning strategies in providing health teaching for individuals, families, and groups in a variety of settings.
6. Use the process of scientific inquiry and research findings to improve nursing care delivery.
7. Manage information, human resources, and material resources to achieve optimum client outcomes in a cost-effective manner.
8. Use leadership, management, and collaborative skills as a member of a multidisciplinary team within the health care delivery system to develop, implement, and evaluate health care provided to clients.
9. Exercise independent judgment and ethical decision making, and act as an advocate for consumers of health care services.
10. Demonstrate accountability in learning and in nursing actions, based on accepted standards of nursing care and in accordance with standards of professional nursing practice.

LEVEL OBJECTIVES

First-Level Nursing

At this level, which comprises courses in the first semester of the second year of a four-year program of study, students are introduced to the conceptual threads used to organize the nursing curriculum, learn some basic therapeutic nursing interventions, and are expected to integrate and synthesis knowledge obtained in foundational disciplines. Objectives for this level are

1. Transfer and apply knowledge from the arts, sciences, and humanities with nursing theory as the basis for making nursing practice decisions.
2. Develop beginning skill in using the nursing process to assess, diagnose, plan, implement, and evaluate the care provided to individuals.
3. Describe the nurse's role in providing preventive, curative, supportive, and restorative care for individuals, families, and communities.
4. Develop beginning skill in using a variety of communication techniques, including written documentation, in the process of assessment and therapeutic intervention with individuals and families.
5. Apply teaching-learning principles in planning and implementing health teaching for individuals in structured settings.
6. Identify the scientific support for assessments and therapeutic nursing interventions.
7. Identify sources of information, human resources, and material resources used to achieve optimum client outcomes in a cost-effective manner.
8. Participate in the group process.

9. Identify legal and ethical issues that affect the ability of consumers of health care services to meet their health care needs.
10. Demonstrate accepted standards of academic integrity, nursing care, and professional nursing practice.

Second-Level Nursing

At this level, which spans the second semester of the second year of study as well as the first semester of the third year of study, students are expected to apply nursing concepts in clinical settings, develop skill in both the design and implementation of nursing interventions, shift from a consideration of single health problems seen in isolation to a consideration of the nursing care needs of patients with multiple, interacting problems, and develop awareness and skill in utilizing resources to achieve outcomes of care. Objectives for this level are

1. Analyze knowledge from the arts, sciences, and humanities as it is used with nursing theory in making nursing practice decisions.
2. Apply critical thinking skills in using the nursing process to assess, diagnose, plan, implement, and evaluate the care provided to individuals, families, and groups.
3. Apply the nursing process to design, implement, and evaluate therapeutic nursing interventions to provide preventive, curative, supportive, and restorative care for individuals, families, and groups in structured settings, using a variety of technologies.
4. Demonstrate competence in using a variety of communication techniques, including written documentation, in the process of assessment, counseling, and therapeutic intervention with individual clients, families, and groups.
5. Adapt teaching–learning strategies to meet specific needs for health teaching for individuals, families, and groups.
6. Critically analyze and evaluate nursing research and other scientific studies.
7. Identify and begin to use sources of information, human resources, and material resources to achieve optimum client outcomes in a cost-effective manner.
8. Apply the principles of planned change and group process skills as a member of a multidisciplinary team within the health care delivery system to develop, implement, and evaluate health care provided to clients.
9. Articulate principles involved in advocating for consumers of health care services, taking into account pertinent ethical and legal issues.
10. Demonstrate accountability for learning and for nursing actions, based on accepted standards of nursing care and in accordance with standards of professional nursing practice.

Third-Level Nursing

At this level, which spans the second semester of the third year of study as well as the first semester of the final year of study, students are expected to continue to apply increasingly complex nursing concepts in community-based settings, increased skill in the design and modification of nursing interventions, shift from practice within the structured institutional setting to relatively unstructured community, and development of leadership skills in delegation, change initiatives, and resource utilization. Objectives for this level are

1. Synthesize knowledge from the arts, sciences, and humanities with nursing theory as the basis for making nursing practice decisions.
2. Critically evaluate situations through the use of the nursing process to assess, diagnose, plan, implement, and evaluate the care provided to individuals, families, and communities.
3. Apply the nursing process to design, implement, and evaluate therapeutic nursing interventions to provide preventive, curative, supportive, and restorative care for individuals, families, and communities in both structured and unstructured settings, using a variety of technologies.
4. Selectively apply appropriate communication techniques, including written documentation, in the process of assessment, counseling, and therapeutic intervention with individual clients, families, groups, and communities.
5. Selectively apply appropriate teaching-learning strategies in providing health teaching for individuals, families, and community groups.
6. Use the process of scientific inquiry and research findings to design and critically evaluate nursing interventions.
7. Manage information, apply delegation techniques, and utilize material resources to achieve optimum client outcomes in a cost-effective manner.
8. Apply principles of leadership, management, and collaboration in acting as a member of a multidisciplinary team within the health care delivery system to develop, implement, and evaluate health care provided to clients.
9. Demonstrate independent judgment, ethical decision making, and. advocacy in providing care for consumers of health care services.
10. Demonstrate accountability in learning and in nursing actions, based on accepted standards of nursing care and in accordance with standards of professional nursing practice.

Fourth-Level Nursing

This level of the program comprises the clinical practicum taken in the final semester of study. Fourth-level objectives are identical to the program objectives.

RELATED COURSE OBJECTIVES

Course Objectives for a Second-Level Nursing Course, Clinical Nursing Practice I

1. Transfer and apply knowledge from the arts, sciences, and humanities as it is used with nursing theory in making nursing practice decisions.
2. Develop critical thinking skills in using the nursing process to assess, diagnose, plan, implement, and evaluate the care provided to individuals.
3. Apply the nursing process to design, implement, and evaluate therapeutic nursing interventions to provide preventive, curative, supportive, and restorative care for individuals in structured settings, using a variety of technologies.
4. Demonstrate competence in using a variety of communication techniques, including written documentation, in the process of assessment and therapeutic intervention with individuals.
5. Adapt teaching-learning strategies to meet specific needs for health teaching for individuals.
6. Identify the scientific support for assessments and therapeutic nursing interventions.
7. Identify and begin to use sources of information, human resources, and material resources to achieve optimum client outcomes in a cost-effective manner.
8. Apply group process skills as a member of a multidisciplinary team within the health care delivery system to develop, implement, and evaluate health care provided to clients.
9. Articulate principles involved in advocating for consumers of health care services, including pertinent ethical and legal issues.
10. Demonstrate accountability for learning and for nursing actions, based on accepted standards of nursing care and in accordance with standards of professional nursing practice.

Course Objectives for a Third-Level Nursing Course, Clinical Nursing Practice II

1. Synthesize knowledge from the arts, sciences and humanities with nursing theory as the basis for making nursing practice decisions for individuals experiencing complex illnesses.
2. Critically evaluate situations through the use of the nursing process to assess, diagnose, plan, implement, and evaluate the care provided to individuals experiencing complex illnesses.

3. Apply the nursing process to design, implement, and evaluate therapeutic nursing interventions to provide preventive, curative, supportive, and restorative care for individuals experiencing complex illnesses.

4. Selectively apply appropriate communication techniques, including written documentation, in the process of assessment, counseling, and therapeutic intervention with individuals experiencing complex illnesses.

5. Selectively apply appropriate teaching-learning strategies in providing health teaching for individuals experiencing complex illnesses.

6. Use the process of scientific inquiry and research findings to design and critically evaluate nursing interventions with individuals experiencing complex illnesses.

7. Manage information and utilize material resources to achieve optimum outcomes in a cost-effective manner when caring for individuals experiencing complex illnesses.

8. Apply principles of leadership, management of patient care, and collaboration in acting as a member of the health care team to develop, implement, and evaluate care provided to individuals experiencing complex illnesses.

9. Demonstrate independent judgment, ethical decision making, and advocacy in providing care for individuals experiencing complex illnesses.

10. Demonstrate accountability in learning and in nursing actions, based on accepted standards of nursing care and in accordance with standards of professional nursing practice.

APPENDIX B

SAMPLE COURSE OUTLINE FOR A NURSING COURSE WITH A CLINICAL COMPONENT

NUR 235 CLINICAL NURSING PRACTICE I

5 credits (3 hrs class; 6 hrs clinical/college laboratory)

Description
Use of the nursing process in applying foundational concepts and skills in planning and providing nursing care for individuals. Considers human responses to commonly encountered illnesses, including pathophysiological processes and treatment approaches. Laboratory experiences provide opportunities to apply theory and develop skills in the care of individuals in structured clinical settings.

Pre- and Corequisites
Prerequisites: NUR 201, Introduction to Physical Assessment;
NUR 205, Fundamentals of Nursing; BIO 215,
Microbiology

Corequisites: NUR 225, Pharmacotherapeutics and Diagnostics in
Nursing Practice; NUR 230, Principles of Community
Health; HSC 205, Nutrition and Health

Source: Department of Nursing, Western Connecticut State University, Danbury, CT. Note that the content outline reflects the conceptual framework of this baccalaureate nursing program, which organizes content based on the five need categories of food, air, and water; proper use and care of the body; ego preservation and enhancement; control of excessive forces; and control of pathogens.

Objectives

1. Transfer and apply knowledge from the arts, sciences, and humanities as it is used with nursing theory in making nursing practice decisions.
2. Develop critical thinking skills in using the nursing process to assess, diagnose, plan, implement, and evaluate the care provided to individuals.
3. Apply the nursing process to design, implement, and evaluate therapeutic nursing interventions to provide preventive, curative, supportive, and restorative care for individuals in structured settings, using a variety of technologies.
4. Demonstrate competence in using a variety of communication techniques, including written documentation, in the process of assessment and therapeutic intervention with individuals.
5. Adapt teaching-learning strategies to meet specific needs for health teaching for individuals.
6. Identify the scientific support for assessments and therapeutic nursing interventions.
7. Identify and begin to use sources of information, human resources, and material resources to achieve optimum client outcomes in a cost-effective manner.
8. Apply group process skills as a member of a multidisciplinary team within the health care delivery system to develop, implement, and evaluate health care provided to clients.
9. Articulate principles involved in advocating for consumers of health care services, including pertinent ethical and legal issues.
10. Demonstrate accountability for learning and for nursing actions, based on accepted standards of nursing care and in accord with standards of professional nursing practice.

Content Outline

I. Application of the Nursing Process with Patients with Commonly Encountered Illnesses
   A. Assessments
      1. Obtaining objective and subjective data
      2. Identifying underlying pathophysiology
      3. Identifying psychosocial responses to illness and/or its treatment
   B. Diagnostic processes
      1. Analyzing and interpreting data
      2. Searching for additional information
      3. Formulating hypotheses
      4. Testing hypotheses
   C. Care planning and implementation
      1. Collaborative planning
      2. Establishing objectives

        3. Continuity of care
        4. Discharge planning
        5. Delegation principles
    D. Evaluation
        1. Outcomes
        2. Processes
II. Communication Processes among Professionals
    A. Privacy, confidentiality
    B. Timeliness, salience, completeness
    C. Documentation
    D. Delegation
III. Developmental Changes Related to the Aging Process
    A. Physiological changes
    B. Psychosocial considerations
    C. Cognitive changes
    D. Functional impairment
        1. Sensory deficits
        2. Motor deficits
        3. Bowel and bladder function
IV. Ego Preservation and Enhancement
    A. Illness experience
        1. Meaning of illness
        2. Meaning of hospitalization/institutionalization
    B. Stress
        1. General and local adaptation syndromes
        2. Assessment of response to stress
        3. Coping strategies
            a. acute illness
            b. chronic illness
        4. Nursing interventions
V. Control of Excessive Forces
    A. Pain
        1. Nursing assessments
        2. Nursing interventions
        3. Pharmacological interventions
        4. Nonpharmacological interventions
    B. Hazards of immobility
        1. Nursing assessments
        2. Nursing interventions
        3. Pharmacological interventions
        4. Nonpharmacological interventions
VI. Control of Pathogens
    A. Impairment of skin integrity
        1. Inflammatory processes
        2. Wound healing

    B. Urinary tract infections

    C. Gastrointestinal infections

    D. Pulmonary infections

    E. Nursing considerations

       1. Physiological principles

       2. Psychosocial responses

       3. Nursing diagnoses

       4. Nursing interventions

       5. Pharmacological interventions

       6. Nonpharmacological interventions

VII. Principles of Rehabilitation

    A. Continuum of care

    B. Multidisciplinary team planning

    C. Teaching-learning processes

    D. Monitoring progress toward outcomes

VIII. Commonly Occurring Problems Related to the Need for Food, Air, and Water

    A. Chronic Cardiovascular Conditions

       1. CAD

       2. Hypertension

       3. CHF

       4. PVD

       5. Nursing considerations

         a. physiological principles

         b. psychosocial responses

         c. nursing diagnoses

         d. therapeutic nursing interventions

         e. pharmacological interventions

         f. rehabilitation to maximize function

         g. expected outcomes and outcome measures

         h. prevention and detection strategies

    B. Chronic Respiratory Conditions

       1. COPD

       2. Asthma

       3. Nursing considerations

         a. physiological principles

         b. psychosocial responses

         c. nursing diagnoses

         d. therapeutic nursing interventions

         e. pharmacological interventions

         f. rehabilitation to maximize function

         g. expected outcomes and outcome measures

         h. prevention and detection strategies

    C. Metabolic Conditions

       1. Diabetes

    2. Fluid-electrolyte imbalance
    3. Nursing considerations
      a. physiological principles
      b. psychosocial responses
      c. nursing diagnoses
      d. therapeutic nursing interventions
      e. pharmacological interventions
      f. rehabilitation to maximize function
      g. expected outcomes and outcome measures
      h. prevention and detection strategies

D. Hematologic Conditions
    1. Anemias
    2. Blood dyscrasias
    3. Nursing considerations
      a. physiological principles
      b. psychosocial responses
      c. nursing diagnoses
      d. therapeutic nursing interventions
      e. pharmacological interventions
      f. rehabilitation to maximize function
      g. expected outcomes and outcome measures
      h. prevention and detection strategies

IX. Commonly Occurring Problems Related to the Proper Use and Care of the Body

A. Neurological Conditions
    1. CVA
    2. Parkinsonian syndrome
    3. Alzheimer's disease
    4. Nursing considerations
      a. physiological principles
      b. psychosocial responses
      c. nursing diagnoses
      d. therapeutic nursing interventions
      e. pharmacological interventions
      f. rehabilitation to maximize function
      g. expected outcomes and outcome measures
      h. prevention and detection strategies

B. Musculo-Skeletal Conditions
    1. Osteoarthritis
    2. Fractures
    3. Nursing considerations
      a. physiological principles
      b. psychosocial responses
      c. nursing diagnoses
      d. therapeutic nursing interventions

          e. pharmacological interventions
          f. rehabilitation to maximize function
          g. expected outcomes and outcome measures
          h. prevention and detection strategies
    C. Sensory Alterations
       1. Eye
          a. glaucoma
          b. cataracts
          c. macular degeneration
       2. Ear
       3. Nursing considerations
          a. physiological principles
          b. psychosocial responses
          c. nursing diagnoses
          d. therapeutic nursing interventions
          e. pharmacological interventions
          f. rehabilitation to maximize function
          g. expected outcomes and outcome measures
          h. prevention and detection strategies
X. Meeting Needs for Ego Preservation and Enhancement
    A. Living with stable chronicity
    B. Functional alterations following surgical interventions
    C. Common complications associated with pharmacological treatment
    D. Loss, grief, grieving
    E. Promoting a dignified death

Appendix C

Sample Clinical Evaluation Form

Clinical Laboratory Evaluation Form

NUR 235 Clinical Nursing Practice I

Student Name _____   *Semester* _____ *Year* _____

Clinical Agency _____   *Final Grade*: Pass   Fail

Directions: This evaluation form will be reviewed with students by the course instructor. Students will meet with their clinical instructor at midsemester and at the end of the semester. Prior to each meeting, the student will provide a written self-evaluation of their progress toward meeting the objectives, using the student version of this form, and obtain feedback from the clinical laboratory instructor. Students must meet all objectives according to the rating levels of 2 or 3 to receive a passing grade for the course.

Rating Scale:

1. Performance is not consistently safe, competent, or accomplished within a reasonable time frame, and requires ongoing verbal and physical cues.
2. Performance is safe and competent and is accomplished within a reasonable time frame with minimal guidance required.
3. Performance is safe and competent and is accomplished within a reasonable and efficient time frame and, in most instances, independently. Acts as a resource for fellow students.

Objective	Midterm Evaluation Rate 1, 2, 3	Final Evaluation Rate 1, 2, 3	Date/ Comment
1. Transfer and **apply knowledge from the arts, sciences, and humanities** as it is used with nursing theory in making nursing practice decisions.			
2. Develop **critical thinking skills** in the use of the nursing process to assess, diagnose, plan, implement, and evaluate the care provided to individuals.			
3. Apply the nursing process to design, implement, and evaluate **therapeutic nursing interventions** to provide preventive, curative, supportive, and restorative care for individuals in structured settings, using a variety of technologies.			
4. Demonstrate competence in using a variety of **communication** techniques, including written documentation, in the process of assessment and therapeutic intervention with individuals.			

5. Adapt **teaching-learning** strategies to meet specific needs for health teaching for individuals.			
6. Identify the **scientific support** for assessments and therapeutic nursing interventions.			
7. Identify and begin to **use sources of information, human resources,** and **material resources** to achieve optimum client outcomes in a cost-effective manner.			
8. Apply **group process skills** as a member of a multidisciplinary team within the health care delivery system to develop, implement, and evaluate health care provided to clients.			
9. Articulate principles involved in **advocating** for consumers of health care services, including pertinent **ethical** and **legal** issues.			
10. Demonstrate **accounta-bility** for learning and for nursing actions, based on accepted standards of nursing care and in accord with standards of professional nursing practice.			

Comments: Midsemester   Comments: End of Semester

Appendix D

Sample Anecdotal Notes

Elvira was assigned to care for an elderly patient recovering from a CVA. The patient dropped his dentures, which broke. He was upset, because he couldn't afford to repair or replace them. Elvira contacted social services and asked if something could be done. The social worker met with the patient the same day, and made arrangements to have the dentures replaced through the dental clinic.

Flora was assigned to care for a critically ill 64-year-old woman of Hispanic origin. The patient's large family was crowded into the room, making it difficult to provide nursing care. Flora contacted an interpreter listed in the hospital's volunteer list, and sought his assistance in identifying a family spokesperson, who was asked to arrange a schedule permitting one additional family member to be in attendance with the spokesperson, while others remained in the waiting room. During the postconference, Flora's explanation of her actions reflected sensitivity to sociocultural needs of this patient, which include the presence of a family support system, while addressing the needs of nursing staff to have sufficient space to work with the patient.

Gretchen was assigned to the care of a 55-year-old man who had surgery to fix a compound fracture of the fibula. She charted a temperature of 100.2 as 102 on the unit's vital signs sheet.

Hilda was assisting a nursing technician in making an occupied bed. The patient, an elderly woman, was not draped with a cover sheet or bath blanket, and was clearly uncomfortable in her patient gown. When questioned about the patient's exposure, Hilda replied, "She's not my patient. I was just helping Jessie make the bed." When asked why she didn't teach the technician proper care, or provide such herself, she said, "It's not my responsibility."

Iris was assigned to care for a 6-year-old patient who was admitted to the pediatric unit with a diagnosis of pneumonia and rule-out empyema.

I am grateful to Professor Eileen Geraci and Dr. Patricia Lund for their contributions to this appendix.

Upon arrival on the pediatric unit, Iris was given a copy of the patient's clinical rounds report (the patient—and his chart—were in radiology, where a CT scan was being performed). Iris did not refer to references regarding the patient's diagnosis when questioned about the patient's underlying condition, nor could she report when the child had been admitted, although this was clearly indicated on the clinical rounds report. She told the instructor that the patient had "emphysema." Iris was referred to the numerous references on the unit. After consulting these, she reported to the instructor that the child had "mucous" in his lungs. She was unable to foresee possible plans of care for this patient. When the child returned from radiology, and the report was made available to the physicians, a decision was made to do surgery that evening for decortication of the lung. The instructor informed Iris that this meant that the patient was now "preop," and a preoperative check sheet should be initiated to ensure that all necessary nursing actions were completed prior to the child's scheduled arrival in the OR. Iris appeared unaware of this process, although she had completed a surgical nursing rotation the previous semester.

Appendix E

Sample Agency Affiliation Agreement

AGREEMENT (the "Agreement"), effective as of [date], between [program name] (the "University") and [agency name] (the "Health Care Institution").

WHEREAS, the University desires to establish a clinical program as part of its education of students (the "Students") enrolled in its nurse education program; and

WHEREAS, the Health Care Institution, in the interest of furthering the educational objectives of the University, desires to make its facility available to the Students;

NOW THEREFORE, in consideration of the promises and the mutual covenants, agreements and undertakings hereinafter set forth, it is hereby AGREED:

1. **Planning of Clinical Program.** The University shall be responsible for the planning, implementation, and execution of all educational aspects of the Students' clinical experience.
2. **Philosophy and Objectives of the Nursing Program.** The University will convey to appropriate Health Care Institution personnel information about the philosophy and objectives of the nursing program.
3. **Instruction and Supervision.** The University shall provide faculty (the "Faculty") for teaching and supervision of Students assigned to the Health Care Institution. Faculty shall be responsible for planning and implementing individual Student assignments, and for evaluating and grading Student performance. Faculty may consult with Health Care Institution personnel as appropriate in conducting evaluations of Student performance. The Health Care Institution shall be responsible, with input from the Faculty, for assigning students to clinical areas and patients.
4. **Notice of Program.** The University shall submit to the Health Care Institution at least thirty (30) days prior to commencement of the

Source: Department of Nursing. Western Connecticut State University, Danbury, CT.

clinical program a description of the types of clinical experiences needed, the dates during which such experiences will be needed, the number of Students expected to participate in the clinical program, and the names, professional credentials, and evidence of current licensure of Faculty who will supervise the Students. The University shall inform the Health Care Institution as practicable of any changes in information previously provided to the Health Care Institution regarding the clinical program.

5. **Compliance with Health Care Institution Rules by Faculty.** The University agrees that its Faculty will comply with all rules and regulations of the Health Care Institution.

6. **Compliance with Health Care Institution Rules by Students.** The University will enforce Student compliance with all rules and regulations of the Health Care Institution. The University will enforce Student compliance with any and all instructions of Health Care Institution personnel.

7. **Confidential Information.** The University will assure that Students, Faculty, and University personnel shall not disclose any confidential material or information connected with the Health Care Institution or any of its patients. The University shall enforce compliance by Students and Faculty with Health Care Institution policy on confidentiality.

8. **Withdrawal of Students from the Clinical Program.** The University agrees to withdraw any Student from the clinical area due to health, performance, or other reasons immediately upon the request of the Health Care Institution if such Student's continued participation in the clinical program is detrimental to the Student and/or any patient of the Health Care Institution.

9. **Clinical Experience.** The Health Care Institution will accept, in mutually agreed upon terms, Students from the University for clinical experience. The Health Care Institution shall provide the opportunity for qualified Students to perform clinical work under the supervision of Faculty provided by the University in accordance with the terms of this Agreement. The Health Care Institution shall not be responsible for the supervision, instruction, grading, or education of the Students but shall at all times retain authority and responsibility for the delivery of patient care.

10. **Equipment and Use of Facilities.** The Health Care Institution shall provide: equipment and supplies necessary for the administration of nursing care by the Students; space for conferences connected with the Students' clinical instruction as available; and locker room or equivalent space for use by Students and Faculty as available. Students and Faculty may use the Health Care Institution cafeteria during their clinical experience.

11. **Orientation for Faculty and Students.** The Health Care Institution shall provide orientation for Faculty regarding relevant Health Care Institution information, including policies, procedures, and rules with which Faculty must comply. The University shall provide such orientation to Students.

12. **Emergency Medical Care.** The Health Care Institution will expedite emergency medical care to Students and/or Faculty who become ill or who are injured while on duty at the Health Care Institution. The cost of such care shall be the responsibility of the individual receiving it.

13. **Required Inservices.** The University will provide the Health Care Institution with evidence of mandatory inservices having been provided to Students and Faculty in advance of the first clinical experience as required by the Health Care Institution.

14. **Immunizations and Physical.** The University will provide the Health Care Institution with evidence that Students and Faculty meet the Health Care Institution's requirements for immunization. The University will provide the Health Care Institution with evidence that Students have completed a satisfactory physical exam.

15. **Insurance/Indemnification.** The University and the Health Care Institution agree to be responsible for their own negligent acts. Any claim that the Health Care Institution has against the University based upon the latter's negligence should be presented as a claim as provided by law.

    The University will also carry professional liability insurance coverage in the amount of [amount] for nursing students and clinical instructors.

16. **Evaluations.** Appropriate Health Care Institution personnel will meet at least once each year with the University's nursing program department head for the purpose of evaluating the clinical education program.

17. **Term and Termination of Agreement.** This Agreement shall be effective as of the date first written above, shall be reviewed annually and shall continue in effect for three (3) years, unless either party notifies the other in writing no less than sixty (60) days prior to the annual review date of its intent not to renew. Either party may terminate this Agreement at any time without cause by giving one-hundred-and-twenty (120) days written notice to the other party.

18. **Students and Faculty Not Employees or Agents.** Both the University and the Health Care Institution acknowledge that neither Students nor Faculty are to be considered employees or agents of the Health Care Institution.

19. **Governing Law.** This Agreement shall be construed in accordance with and governed by the laws of the State of Connecticut applying to contracts made and performed in Connecticut.

20. **Entire Agreement and Amendment.** This Agreement is the entire agreement between the parties and supersedes and rescinds all prior agreements relating to the subject matter hereof. This Agreement may be amended only in writing signed by both parties.
21. **Notices.** Any notice required to be given pursuant to the terms of this Agreement shall be in writing and shall be sent, postage prepaid, by certified mail, return receipt requested, to the Health Care Institution or the University at the address set forth below. The notice shall be effective on the date of delivery indicated on the return receipt.

If to the Health Care Institution:

[Name]

Executive Vice President

[Agency]

[Address]

If to the University:

[Name]

Chair, Department of Nursing

[University]

[Address]

22. **Prohibition Against Assignment.** This Agreement may not be assigned by either party without the prior written consent of the other party.
23. **Accommodations for Persons with Disabilities.** In the event that a Student, Faculty, or other University personnel requires accommodation for a disability beyond those accommodations that are currently available at the Health Care Institution, the University shall be responsible for making any arrangements necessary to effectuate the additional accommodation.
24. **Nondiscrimination and Affirmative Action.** The Health Care Institution agrees and warrants that in the performance of this Agreement, it will not discriminate or permit discrimination against any person or group of persons on the grounds of race, color, religious creed, age, marital status, national origin, ancestry, sex, or mental retardation, physical disability, blindness, or other handicap, in any manner prohibited by the laws of the United States or the State of Connecticut.

APPENDIX F

SAMPLE CLINICAL PREPARATION FORMS

SAMPLE CLINICAL PREPARATION FORM FOR A SURGICAL UNIT EXPERIENCE

WEEKLY NURSING CARE PLAN GUIDE

Pt Initials _____ Age _____ Gender _____ Allergies _____

Admitting Dx _____ Secondary Dx _____

Surgical Procedure _____

Diet: Activity:

Treatments:

Medications: Actions: Major Nursing Considerations:

I am grateful to Dr. Laurel Halloran and Dr. Stephanie Golub for their contributions to this appendix.

Admitting Lab Tests: Current Lab Tests: Significance:

Pathophysiology: (Relate to your patient)

Developmental Task: Psychosocial Assessment:

PHYSICAL ASSESSMENT (ROS)

STRENGTHS   WEAKNESSES

General Appearance: _____

Skin: _____

EENT: _____

Mouth/Throat: _____

Neck: _____

Respiratory: _____

Cardiac: _____

Gastrointestinal: _____

Genitourinary: _____

Musculoskeletal: _____

Peripheral Vascular: _____

Neurologic: _____

PROBLEM LIST*

Food, Air, Water	Control of Excessive Forces	Control of Pathogens	Ego Preservation and Enhancement	Proper Use and Care of the Body

My evaluation of this experience:

---

*This follows the conceptual framework of the curriculum within which this clinical experience occurs.

SAMPLE CLINICAL PREPARATION FORM FOR A COMMUNITY HEALTH EXPERIENCE

Student Log for Home Health Nursing
Instructions for Logs:

Purpose: The log is an integral part of your Home Health Nursing clinical experience. Its purposes include the following:

- Collecting and organizing data regarding the client/family to which you are assigned;
- Demonstrating your knowledge of the client/family and your ability to plan for client/family needs; and
- Documenting your development of a long-term therapeutic relationship with the client/family.

Mechanics: Each student purchases a folder which, when opened, contains a pocket on either side. The log is to be submitted at least one day prior to your next clinical day. Logs will be returned to you at the clinical site. Logs may be handwritten, but must be neat and legible. Each client to whom you are assigned is to have a separate folder.

Format for the **left side** of the folder. (This side is completed once for each patient; occasionally, changes in patient situation may be added.)

1. **Data base**—medical diagnoses (include diagnoses from patient history if still valid) and *relevant assessments* you plan to do every visit, unusual physical assessment findings, living arrangement and support systems, services in the home other than nursing
2. **Patient goals**—list all *patient* goals (include those on the 485 and any additional ones you see as relevant)
3. **Medications**—list the medications (with dose and frequency), side effects, and areas for patient teaching
4. **Possible complications**—for which your patient may be at risk
5. **Teaching**—list general areas/topics that you address during this rotation

Format for the *right side* of the folder. (The purpose of entries on this side of the log is to communicate to your instructor your objectives for each weekly home visit and a follow-up description of your results.):

Date: **Patient goals and your related objectives of *each* goal.** Use the following format when describing your objectives:

Description and evaluation of how each objective was met and the patient's response.

I. Patient goal
   e.g., Resume normal pattern of elimination.
   A. Additional Assessments
      (not listed on left side of folder)
      e.g., I plan to do a 48-hour recall to assess the patient's intake of roughage and fluid volume.
   B. Direct Patient Care
      e.g., Administer PRN colace if needed.
   C. Patient Teaching
      e.g., Teach patient about use and side effects of colace. Review other methods of avoiding constipation: increase roughage in diet, increase fluid intake by 8–16 oz per day, increase physical activity by increasing walking 60–100 feet per day.

D. Case Management
   e.g., Inform home health aide
   about patient teaching and add
   monitoring of elimination patterns
   to HHA care plan. Ask HHA to offer
   8 oz of fluid to patient during
   his/her HHA visits.

II. Next Patient Goal
   A. Additional Assessments
   B. Direct Patient Care
   C. Patient Teaching
   D. Case Management

Appendix G

Sample Guidelines for Off-Unit Experiences

General Instructions for Operating Room (OR), Recovery Room (RR), and Same-Day Surgery Experiences

On the Assigned Day:

- Take the patient elevator to the fourth floor.
- Take a right out of the elevator and a left down the hall.
- Stop at Central Supply and pick up a pair of scrubs. You will be asked to sign out for them.
- Go back toward the elevators. About half way down the hall, take a left into a door marked "Staff Locker Rooms."
- Proceed to male or female locker rooms. Change into scrubs.
- Exit from the back door of the locker rooms into the main hall.
- Cross the main hall and put on booties, hat, and get a mask.
- If you are assigned to the OR, go to the control desk on the right.
- If you are assigned to the Same Day Surgery unit, go back down the hall to the Same Day unit.

Notes:

- You must wear uniform or lab coat with name tag and hospital ID to the hospital.
- Do not bring any valuables. Watch, stethoscope, and black ink pen needed.

I am grateful to Dr. Laurel Halloran and to Dr. Patricia Lund for their contributions to this appendix.

- Be on time OR @ 7:00 (late start @ 8:30) [telephone number]
  SD Unit @ 7:00 (late start @ 7:30) [telephone number]
- If you are ill, notify your clinical instructor and your assigned area.
- E*at breakfast!*

To prepare for this experience, read the following:

- [textbook references]

OPERATING ROOM ASSIGNMENT

Directions: Briefly describe your observations regarding the areas listed below. Use a separate sheet of paper and attach this as a cover sheet. Assignment is due within one week following the experience.

1. Describe the steps you took to properly enter the surgical suite.
2. Describe the general purpose and procedure for a surgical scrub.
3. Describe the role and activities of the nurse during the preoperative phase.
4. Describe the roles and activities of the anesthesiologist and the nurse anesthetist in the perioperative period.
5. List the basic principles of surgical asepsis that are followed during surgery.
6. Compare the functions of the circulating nurse and the scrub nurse in the operating room.
7. Describe the safety precautions followed when transferring and positioning a patient on the operating table.
8. Describe the environmental control procedures in the OR aimed at

   - Controlling traffic flow
   - Controlling infection
   - Maintaining open channels of communication
   - Managing stress

9. Describe the types of records the RN must keep during the perioperative period.
10. Describe how the OR is readied for the next surgical case.
11. Give your impressions of this experience.

OR TO RECOVERY ROOM EXPERIENCE

Patient's Age _____ *Type of Surgery* _____

Patient's Developmental Level _____

1. What preoperative instructions were given to this patient? Was any preoperative teaching done in the surgeon's office?
2. What physiologic parameters were assessed prior to surgery?
    A. Laboratory tests? Results?
    B. EKG? Results?
    C. Other testing?
3. Describe the patient's surgical experience.
    A. Preoperative nursing assessment
    B. Preoperative anesthesia assessment
    C. How patient was brought to OR and prepared for anesthesia
    D. Medications used for anesthesia
    E. Preparation of surgical site
    F. The surgery
    G. Medications used to reverse the anesthesia
    H. Transfer to recovery room
4. Describe the parameters assessed on your patient in the recovery room.
    A. Airway: Is an artificial airway present? Is the patient intubated? What is the respiratory rate, depth, and volume? What do you hear when you auscultate the lung fields? Is oxygen in use?
    B. Color: What is the patient's color? Is there any cyanosis or pallor present?
    C. How is cardiac status monitored? What is the apical pulse? Are there any EKG leads present? What is the patient's blood pressure? Assess and record the peripheral pulses.
    D. Operative site: What does the site look like? Note any bleeding or drainage. Are any surgical drains present? What are they and what is their function?
    E. Level of consciousness: Identify the stage of anesthesia the patient is in. What is the patient's LOC?
    F. IV lines: Note flow rate, solution, and site. Why is this solution being used?
    G. Urinary output: Note amount of output. Is a Foley present?
    H. Pain: Evaluate level of pain on a 1 to 10 scale. Evaluate ability to cough, turn, and deep breathe.
    I. Others?
5. Describe how the patient is evaluated for transfer to his/her room. Who makes these assessments/decisions?
6. Describe how the patient is transferred.
    A. Who transports? Why?
    B. Who reports to the floor nurse?
    C. What is reported?
7. Describe the floor nurse's responsibilities upon accepting a patient from the recovery room. Why are these assessments done?
8. Give your impression of this experience.

OBSERVATION OF WELL CHILDREN

Each student is to spend one clinical day visiting a facility appropriate to children, such as a zoo, aquarium, children's museum, or the like. You are to identify the facility and why you chose it, and observe and record the following:

1. Sit or stand quietly and observe at least three (3) different child-adult (could be parent, grandparent, or caretaker) interactions. Briefly describe the individuals involved (age, attire, affect, comfort with the situation), and their interactions within the pair.

2. Assess the interactions observed in relation to theories of growth and development (for example, Erikson, Piaget, Bowen, or Freud). Also assess how the child's needs are being met according to Maslow's hierarchy.

3. Which animals/exhibits did the observed children seem to enjoy? Which ones seemed to make them fearful? Did this vary by age of the child? What did the adult do to help the child overcome fears?

4. Comment on the behaviors observed in terms of your own personal thoughts.

5. Assess the environment in relation to child health and safety:
   A. Are there restrooms with provisions for diaper changes and disposal? Is there soap and paper towels? Can children reach the sinks?
   B. Is food available for lunch and/or snacks? What kinds of food? Is this suitable for the age children you have observed? Why or why not? What does it cost?
   C. What safety measures are there to protect children and parents? Is there a first aid station?
   D. What facilities are there for handicapped adults and children? For very young children/babies? What is needed?
   E. What special provisions are there to enhance the experience for the child (e.g., petting zoo, feeding the baby animals, special tours or story time)?

6. Would you suggest a visit to this facility for a child? Why?

Guidelines for Submission of Report

Your typed report is to be submitted no later than the week following the trip. You should anticipate the time spent on the visit and the writeup to be the equivalent of the time you spend on the pediatric unit, plus the time it takes you to prepare for the clinical experience.

Include either your entry ticket, or a map of the facility, with your report.

Late writeups will not be accepted.

Be sure to cover the questions asked above. Feel free to add extra comments.

Wear casual attire, appropriate to the setting, for this experience. Also, if outdoors, you may want to wear sunglasses, and do your observations of interactions as unobtrusively as possible—observing behavior, and then stepping back from it, sitting down, and writing down your observations. DO NOT trail people, be obtrusive, or follow them around, notebook or clipboard in hand. If anyone does ask what you are doing, show them a copy of this assignment and your student ID.